# Sleep Medicine
# Pearls

# Sleep Medicine Pearls

## RICHARD B. BERRY, MD

Director, Sleep Laboratory
Veterans Affairs Medical Center
Long Beach, California
Associate Professor of Medicine
University of California
Irvine, California

*Series Editors*

### STEVEN A. SAHN, MD

Professor of Medicine and Director
Division of Pulmonary and
  Critical Care Medicine
Medical University of South Carolina
Charleston, South Carolina

### JOHN E. HEFFNER, MD

Professor of Clinical Medicine
University of Arizona Health Sciences Center
Chairman, Academic Internal Medicine
St. Joseph's Hospital and Medical Center
Phoenix, Arizona

HANLEY & BELFUS, INC./Philadelphia

Publisher:     HANLEY & BELFUS, INC.
               Medical Publishers
               210 S. 13th Street
               Philadelphia, PA 19107
               (215) 546-7293, 800-962-1892
               FAX (215) 790-9330
               Website: http://www.hanleyandbelfus.com

**Library of Congress Cataloging-in-Publication Data**

Sleep medicine pearls / Richard B. Berry.
       p.     cm. — (The Pearls Series®)
       Includes bibliographical references and index.
       ISBN 1-56053-273-4 (alk. paper)
       1. Sleep disorders—Case studies.      I. Berry, Richard B., 1947–  .
    II. Series.
       [DNLM:  1.  Sleep Disorders case studies.      WM 188S6324 1998]
       RC547.S55   1999
       616.8′498—dc21
       DNLM/DLC
       for Library of Congress                                   98-29334
                                                                      CIP

SLEEP MEDICINE PEARLS     ISBN 1-56053-273-4

Last digit is the print number: 9 8 7 6 5 4 3 2 1

# CONTENTS

**Patient**                                                                                                    **Page**

**Fundamentals of Sleep Medicine 1**

Sleep Stages and Electroencephalographic Patterns ................................................................... 1

1. A 30-year-old man taking a hypnotic nightly ........................................................................ 3

2. A 30-year-old man with insomnia ......................................................................................... 5

**Fundamentals of Sleep Medicine 2**

Electroencephalographic Lead Placement ................................................................................... 7

3. A 50-year-old man with insomnia ......................................................................................... 9

**Fundamentals of Sleep Medicine 3**

Eye Movement Monitoring ........................................................................................................ 11

**Fundamentals of Sleep Medicine 4**

Eye Movement Patterns ............................................................................................................ 13

4. A 20-year-old man with excessive daytime sleepiness .......................................................... 15

**Fundamentals of Sleep Medicine 5**

Chin (Submental) Electromyography ........................................................................................ 17

5. A 40-year-old man with difficulty falling asleep .................................................................. 19

6. A 30-year-old woman having trouble falling asleep .............................................................. 21

7. A 30-year-old man having difficulty staying awake during the day ....................................... 23

8. A 35-year-old woman with insomnia ..................................................................................... 25

9. A 25-year-old man with a history of sleep walking ............................................................... 27

10. A 20-year-old man with daytime sleepiness .......................................................................... 29

11. A 40-year-old man with a history of snoring and daytime sleepiness ..................................... 31

12. A 34-year-old man with sleep disturbance ............................................................................ 33

**Fundamentals of Sleep Medicine 6**

Additional Sleep Staging Rules ................................................................................................. 35

13. A 30-year-old man with severe snoring and occasional breathing lapses ............................... 38

14. A 35-year-old woman experiencing uncontrollable, brief episodes of sleep ........................... 40

**Fundamentals of Sleep Medicine 7**

Sleep Architecture Definitions ................................................................................................. 43

15. A 23-year-old man with difficulty sleeping .......................................................................... 45

16. A 25-year-old man with daytime sleepiness and fatigue ....................................................... 47

**Fundamentals of Sleep Medicine 8**

Polysomnography ..................................................................................................................... 49

17. A 30-year-old man having difficulty staying awake during the day.................................. 52

18. A 25-year-old man complaining of excessive daytime sleepiness ............................... 54

19. A 40-year-old man with complaints of snoring ......................................................... 56

20. A 40-year-old man with frequent awakenings at night............................................... 58

21. A 50-year-old man with difficulty remaining awake during the day........................... 60

22. A 29-year-old man struggling with daytime sleepiness.............................................. 62

**Fundamentals of Sleep Medicine 9**

Multiple Sleep Latency Test ............................................................................................ 65

23. A 25-year-old man with daytime sleepiness ............................................................. 67

**Fundamentals of Sleep Medicine 10**

Respiratory Definitions ................................................................................................... 69

24. A 45-year-old man with possible sleep apnea ......................................................... 71

25. A 50-year-old man with possible central apnea......................................................... 74

**Fundamentals of Sleep Medicine 11**

Excessive Daytime Sleepiness......................................................................................... 76

26. A 30-year-old man with heavy snoring ................................................................... 78

27. A 33-year-old man complaining of daytime sleepiness............................................ 80

28. A 45-year-old man with a snoring problem.............................................................. 82

29. A 30-year-old woman with severe fatigue................................................................ 84

**Fundamentals of Sleep Medicine 12**

Treatment of Obstructive Sleep Apnea........................................................................... 86

30. A 40-year-old woman with mild sleep apnea ........................................................... 87

31. A 55-year-old man with heavy nighttime snoring and daytime sleepiness ............... 89

32. A 45-year-old man with heavy snoring ................................................................... 92

33. A 30-year-old man with heavy snoring and daytime sleepiness................................ 94

34. A 30-year-old man with weight loss and sleep apnea............................................... 96

35. A 55-year-old man having difficulty with CPAP because of nasal congestion........... 98

36. A 30-year-old man unable to tolerate nasal CPAP ................................................. 100

37. A 55-year-old man unable to use nasal CPAP due to intractable nasal congestion ... 103

38. A 45-year-old man with intolerance to nasal CPAP because of difficulty exhaling ... 105

39. A 55-year-old obese man with desaturation during a nasal CPAP trial .................... 107

40. A 30-year-old woman with fatigue and mild daytime sleepiness............................. 110

41. A 40-year-old man with sleep apnea unable to tolerate nasal CPAP ....................... 113

42. A 45-year-old man still experiencing daytime sleepiness after uvulopalatopharyngoplasty .... 115

43. A 50-year-old man with a return of snoring 6 months after uvulopalatopharyngoplasty.......... 117

44. A 45-year-old man who snores when sleeping on his back....................................... 119

45. A 55-year-old man with severe daytime sleepiness and limited treatment options.................. 121

46. A 50-year-old man needing objective confirmation of his ability to stay awake ....................... 124

47.  A 45-year-old man falling asleep at the wheel while driving ................................... 126

48.  A 30-year-old man with mild daytime sleepiness ........................................... 128

49.  A 30-year-old man with severe snoring ...................................................... 130

50.  A 30-year-old choir singer with heavy snoring .......................................... 133

51.  A 45-year-old man with unexplained daytime sleepiness ......................... 135

52.  A 40-year-old woman with sleep apnea and fatigue .................................. 138

53.  A 50-year-old man with severe hypertension ............................................. 140

54.  A 55-year-old man with premature ventricular contractions during sleep .............................. 143

55.  A 30-year-old pregnant woman with onset of snoring ............................. 146

56.  A 45-year-old man with snoring and hypercapnia ..................................... 148

57.  A 55-year-old man with hypercapnic respiratory failure .......................... 150

58.  A 57-year-old man with severe obstructive sleep apnea treated with oxygen ......................... 153

59.  A 10-year-old boy with large tonsils ........................................................ 155

60.  A 55-year-old man with chronic obstructive pulmonary disease and nocturnal desaturation ... 157

61.  A 60-year-old man with leg swelling ........................................................ 160

62.  A 55-year-old man with chronic obstructive pulmonary disease and severe pedal edema ....... 162

63.  A 60-year-old "pink puffer" with insomnia .............................................. 164

64.  A 55-year-old man with chronic obstructive pulmonary disease and pedal edema ................. 166

65.  A 35-year-old woman with asthma and poor sleep at night ..................... 169

66.  A 55-year-old man with daytime sleepiness .............................................. 172

67.  A 55-year-old man with central sleep apnea ............................................. 175

68.  A 70-year-old man with daytime sleepiness and pedal edema ................. 177

69.  A 60-year-old man with severe congestive heart failure and daytime sleepiness ................... 179

70.  A 60-year-old man with obstructive sleep apnea and numerous central apneas on CPAP ....... 181

71.  A 75-year-old man with a history of polio ................................................. 183

72.  A 40-year-old man who kicks in his sleep ................................................. 185

73.  A 50-year-old man groggy in the morning after treatment for periodic leg movements .......... 187

74.  A 56-year-old man with crawling sensations in his legs at bedtime ......................... 189

75.  A 72-year-old man with worsening symptoms during treatment for restless legs ................... 191

76.  A 58-year-old man with sleep apnea and leg jerks during sleep ............. 193

77.  A 30-year-old man with daytime sleepiness and episodes of weakness ................................. 195

78.  A 23-year-old man with daytime sleepiness but no symptoms of cataplexy .......................... 197

79.  A 25-year-old man with narcolepsy who is still sleepy on medication ................................. 199

80.  A 25-year-old man with frequent episodes of cataplexy .......................... 202

81.  A 35-year-old man with sleep apnea and a short REM latency ................ 204

82.  A 40-year-old man with sleep apnea and persistent daytime sleepiness ................................ 206

83.  A 65-year-old woman with excessive daytime sleepiness and a short REM latency ................ 208

84.  A 35-year-old man requesting stimulant medication ............................... 210

85.  A 64-year-old man with daytime sleepiness since age 21 ....................... 212

86.  A 55-year-old man with violent dreams .................................................... 214

 87. A 25-year-old woman walking in her sleep.................................................. 217

 88. A 20-year-old man with severe "nightmares" ............................................. 220

 89. A 55-year-old man with unusual movements during sleep ........................... 222

**Fundamentals of Sleep Medicine 13**

    Evaluation of Insomnia................................................................................ 225

 90. A 30-year-old woman having difficulty falling asleep ................................ 227

 91. A 30-year-old woman with insomnia ......................................................... 229

 92. A 40-year-old man with difficulty falling asleep after the death of his brother ........ 232

 93. A 40-year-old woman complaining of difficulty falling asleep.................... 235

 94. A 70-year-old man with early morning awakening ...................................... 238

 95. A 44-year-old man with jet lag ................................................................. 240

 96. A 40-year-old woman with fibromyalgia.................................................... 243

 97. A 40-year-old woman with fatigue and disturbed sleep .............................. 245

 98. A 45-year-old man with persistent insomnia while on treatment for depression ........ 247

 99. A 45-year-old man with hyperphagia and hypersomnia............................... 249

100. A 50-year-old veteran of the Vietnam War with upsetting dreams ............... 251

101. A 40-year-old woman with terrifying awakenings ...................................... 254

**Appendix I**   Sleep Disorders Classification ............................................... 257

**Appendix II**   Sleep Stage Characteristics.................................................... 259

**Appendix III** Excessive Daytime Sleepiness/Insomnia................................. 261

**Glossary**.................................................................................................... 263

**Index** ........................................................................................................ 267

# FOREWORD

Sleep—and the lack thereof—has surfaced as a major health issue of the 1990s. Complicated work schedules, regimented lifestyles with early morning wakeups, and the fast pace of even "leisure" time conspire to throw off our delicate rhythms of sleep. As if falling asleep and awakening refreshed are not complicated enough, newly recognized primary sleep disorders and complex effects of underlying medical conditions on sleep quality further challenge many patients each night at "lights out." Not only do difficulties with sleep present risks for diminished functional abilities and altered mood, but emerging data suggest that sleep deprivation can foster or aggravate medical conditions. These negative effects of impaired sleep translate into increased morbidity and mortality.

Considering the central importance of sleep to the well being of every patient, all physicians require a practical working knowledge of the varied disorders associated with impaired sleep. Unfortunately, much of this knowledge base is sequestered within the specialized field of sleep medicine.

We are delighted, therefore, with the efforts of Dr. Richard Berry in writing *Sleep Medicine Pearls*. This 10th book in The Pearls Series® presents the field of sleep medicine with clarity, in a format that allows readers to progress from an understanding of basic sleep physiology to the complexities of sophisticated polysomnographic studies. In so doing, *Sleep Medicine Pearls* provides both a primer for general physicians serving as the first evaluators of patients with sleep-related symptoms and a resource for specialists in training as well as experienced sleep physicians honing their skills. The patient-oriented approach of The Pearls Series® applied to sleep medicine lifts the subject from a didactic discussion to a clinically pertinent review. Clinical Pearls listed at the end of each case emphasize the most important concepts related to the patient's condition.

We anticipate that *Sleep Medicine Pearls* will further the skills of practicing physicians in the field of sleep medicine and provide valuable assistance in helping their patients get a good night's rest, so that they may awaken to a healthy and productive day.

STEVEN A. SAHN, MD
JOHN E. HEFFNER, MD

# *Acknowledgments*

I wish to acknowledge the help of the staff of the Sleep Disorders Laboratory at the Long Beach Veterans Affairs Medical Center, including Clinical Director Michael J. Dickel, PhD, and Sleep Technicians Jerome Bower and Kerry Kouchi. Walter Thill of the medical media department provided invaluable assistance with many of the graphics. The encouragement and guidance of David P. White, MD, of the Brigham and Women's Hospital in Boston during the planning stage of this book also are greatly appreciated. Finally, the patience and hard work of Hanley & Belfus editor Jacqueline M. Mahon were essential to completion of the book.

RICHARD B. BERRY, MD

# PREFACE

*Sleep Medicine Pearls,* an exploration of the diagnostic tools and physiologic principles of sleep medicine, offers 101 cases covering a wide spectrum of disorders that affect sleep. The patient presentations and the questions and discussions challenge readers at all levels with varying degrees of complexity.

This book differs from others in The Pearl Series® in that 13 sections of basic didactic material, called Fundamentals of Sleep Medicine, are included for the many physicians who have received little or no formal training in sleep medicine. The cases following each Fundamental illustrate the concepts outlined in that tutorial section. There also is a convenient Glossary of sleep medicine terms at the back of the book.

Some of the discussions center on problems in diagnosis or sleep monitoring; others evaluate complex treatment choices. The goal was to present information relevant to the everyday interpretation of sleep studies and to the treatment of a wide variety of sleep problems. I hope that *Sleep Medicine Pearls* is useful not only to physicians who are new to sleep medicine, but also to more experienced doctors caring for patients with sleep disorders.

RICHARD B. BERRY, MD

## *Dedication*

I dedicate this book to my mother, Sarah Ramseur Berry, and to the memory of my father, Louie Berry, DDS.

## Sleep Stages and Electroencephalographic Patterns

Sleep is divided into **nonrapid eye movement** (NREM) and **rapid eye movement** (REM) sleep. NREM sleep is further subdivided into stages 1–4. Stages 1 and 2 are light sleep; stages 3 and 4 are deep sleep, also called slow wave or delta sleep. Time is divided into **epochs** (commonly 30 seconds each). The sleep stage assigned to each epoch is the stage occupying the majority of time within that epoch. Sleep staging criteria depend on electroencephalographic (EEG), eye movement or electro-oculographic (EOG), and chin (submental) electromyographic (EMG) recordings.

| Sleep Stages | Recorded For Staging |
|---|---|
| Wake — stage W | EEG — central, occipital |
| NREM sleep | EOG — eye movement |
| Stage 1 | EMG — chin/submental |
| Stage 2 | |
| Stage 3 | |
| Stage 4 | |
| REM sleep — stage REM | |

Recognition of certain characteristic EEG patterns is essential for sleep staging (see figure next page). EEG terminology defines waves by their frequency in cycles per second, or hertz (Hz). The classically described frequency ranges are: delta ($<4$ Hz), theta ($4$–$7$ Hz), alpha ($8$–$13$ Hz), beta ($>13$ Hz). Alpha waves are commonly noted when the patient is in an awake but relaxed state with the eyes closed. They are best recorded over the occiput and are attenuated when the eyes are open. Bursts of alpha waves also are seen during brief awakenings from sleep called **arousals.**

Stage 1 is scored when alpha activity occupies less than 50% of an epoch. The EEG of stage 1 shows a low-voltage, mixed-frequency pattern with theta wave activity. Near the transition from stage 1 to stage 2 sleep, vertex sharp waves — high in amplitude but short in duration — occur. Stage 2 is defined by the presence of either sleep spindles or K complexes. **Sleep spindles** are oscillations of 12–14 Hz with a duration of 0–1.5 seconds. They may persist into stages 3 and 4, but usually do not occur in stage REM. The **K complex** is a high-amplitude, biphasic wave of at least 0.5-second duration. As classically defined, a K complex consists of an initial sharp, negative voltage (by convention an upward deflection) followed by a positive deflection (down) slow wave. Spindles frequently are superimposed on K complexes.

As sleep deepens, slow (delta) waves appear. These are high-amplitude, broad waves. In human sleep scoring, by convention, slow waves are defined as EEG activity slower than 2 Hz (longer than 0.5-second duration) that has an amplitude (peak to peak) of $\geq75$ microvolts. Stage 3 is scored when 20–50% of an epoch has slow wave activity meeting this criteria. Stage 4 is scored when more than 50% of an epoch contains slow wave activity.

As a K complex resembles slow wave activity, differentiating the two is sometimes difficult. However, by definition a K complex should stand out (be distinct) from the lower-amplitude, background EEG activity. Therefore, a continuous series of high-voltage slow waves would not be considered to be a series of K complexes.

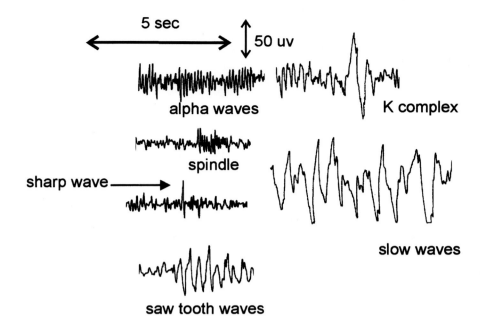

alpha waves

K complex

spindle

sharp wave

slow waves

saw tooth waves

Stage REM is not defined by a characteristic EEG wave pattern, although saw-tooth waves may be present. **Saw-tooth waves** are in the theta frequency range and may be notched. The EEG of stage REM looks much like that of stage 1 sleep—a low-voltage, mixed-frequency pattern.

## REFERENCES

1. Rechtschaffen A, Kales A (eds): A Manual of Standardized Terminology Techniques and Scoring System for Sleep Stages of Human Sleep. Los Angeles, Brain Information Service/Brain Research Institute, UCLA, 1968.
2. Williams RL, Karacan I, Hursch CJ: Electroencephalography of Human Sleep: Clinical Applications. New York, John Wiley & Sons, 1974.
3. West P, Kryger MH: Sleep and respiration: Terminology and methodology. Clin Chest Med (Symposium on Sleep Disorders) 1985; 6:691–718.

# PATIENT 1

### A 30-year-old man taking a hypnotic nightly

A 30-year-old man was studied for complaints of frequent awakenings during the night. He had been using triazolam, a benzodiazepine hypnotic, for 5 years to maintain sleep. Several physicians had encouraged him to discontinue this medication but he had been unable to do so. The patient gave a history of snoring, and a sleep study was ordered to eliminate the possibility that the frequent awakenings were secondary to obstructive sleep apnea. He was asked to reduce the dose of triazolam from .25 mg to .125 mg for 1 week and then discontinue the medication for at least 2 weeks before the upcoming sleep study.

*Figure:* A sample tracing of the central electroencephalogram (EEG) taken during the sleep study is shown below.

*Question:* Do you think the patient complied with the request to discontinue triazolam?

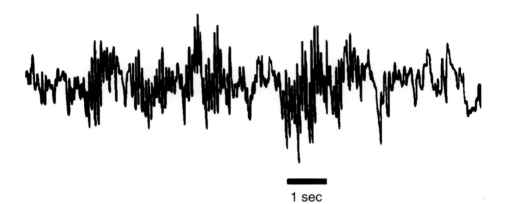

1 sec

***Diagnosis:*** Frequent sleep spindles suggest continued benzodiazepine use.

***Discussion:*** Benzodiazepine use often is associated with a large increase both in spindle activity (12–14 Hz) and the amount of stage 2 sleep. This medication also slightly curtails sleep stages 3 and 4 and reduces REM sleep. Sleep spindles are secondary to thalamocortical oscillations and are characteristic of stage 2 sleep. When the healthcare provider first is learning sleep staging, some difficulty distinguishing sleep spindles from alpha activity may be encountered. Alpha activity (8–13 Hz) is somewhat slower. Additionally, spindles usually occur in short bursts, unlike the almost continuous spindle activity noted in the present study. A typical EEG tracing (see below) shows a sleep spindle during stage 2 sleep (*A*) followed by lengthy alpha activity (*B*).

In the present case, the tremendous amount of spindle activity (see figure on page 3) suggests that the patient had continued to take triazolam. A urine drug screen at the time of the sleep study revealed the presence of a benzodiazepine. When confronted with this evidence, the patient admitted that he was dependent on the medication.

A                     B

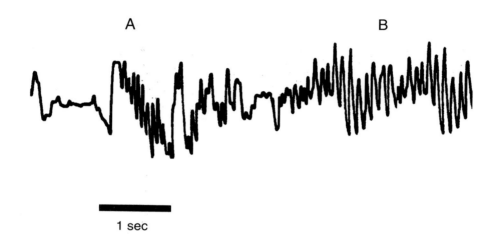

1 sec

## Clinical Pearls

1. Ubiquitous sleep spindle activity suggests that the patient is on a benzodiazepine.
2. Urine drug screens are useful in patients possibly dependent on medication who are undergoing a sleep study "off" medication.
3. Knowledge of medications the patient is taking (or is refraining from taking) at the time of the sleep study often is important in interpreting the results.

## REFERENCES
1. Johnson LC, Hanson K, Bickford RG: Effect of flurazepam on sleep spindles and K complexes. Electroencephalogr Clin Neurophysiol 1976; 40:67–77.
2. Johnson LC, Spinweber CL, Seidel WF, et al: Sleep spindle and delta changes during chronic use of a short acting and a long acting benzodiazepine hypnotic. Electroencephalogr Clin Neurophysiol 1983; 55:662-667.
3. Obermeyer WH, Beneca RM: Effects of drugs on sleep. Neurol Clin (Sleep Disorders II) 1996; 14:827–840.

# PATIENT 2

## A 30-year-old man with insomnia

A 30-year-old man with insomnia of 5-year duration underwent a sleep study. The 15-second sleep tracing shown below (central and occipital EEG) illustrates a transition from wakefulness to sleep. The tracing was preceded by an epoch of sleep with prominent alpha activity for the entire 30 seconds (stage Wake). Alpha activity stopped during the 15-second tracing and was absent for the remainder of the epoch (stage 1).

*Question:* Where does alpha activity stop—at point *A* or *B*?

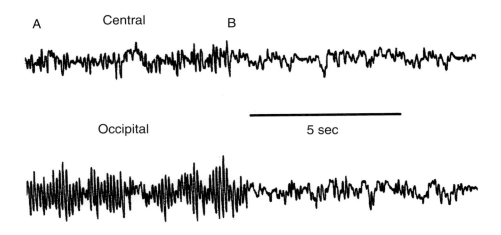

***Answer:***   Prominent alpha activity ends at point *B*.

***Discussion:*** While recording occipital EEG leads is optional, failure to do so may underestimate the degree of wakefulness. Occipital leads allow more precise monitoring of the timing of sleep onset. The transition from drowsy stage Wake to stage 1 sleep is characterized by a reduction in alpha wave activity to less than 50% of the epoch. Unfortunately, this reduction does not always mean sleep is present. Alpha activity also is suppressed when the eyes are open. Such a state usually is accompanied by rapid eye movements (see Fundamentals 4) or blinks.

The EEG of eyes-open wakefulness typically has considerable high-frequency activity. In contrast, the EEG of stage 1 has low-voltage, slower activity in the theta range. During biocalibrations at the start of the sleep study, patients are asked to close and then open their eyes. This allows the sleep scorer to note the EEG and eye lead patterns of eyes-open and eyes-closed wakefulness for the patient.

In the tracing below, alpha activity is prominent in the central leads until the command "eyes open" (*EO*) is given. Note the eye blinks (*EB*) in the right (ROC-A₁) and left (LOC-A₂) eye leads. In this tracing, alpha activity is more prominent in the central leads than in the occipital leads and also is quite prominent in the eye leads. The presence of rapid eye movements or blinks in the second part of the tracing is typical of eyes-open wakefulness.

In the present patient, alpha activity is not prominent from point *A* to point *B* in the central EEG lead (see figure on page 5). However, in the occipital lead clear-cut, high-amplitude alpha activity persists until point *B*, demonstrating the utility of occipital leads in detecting alpha activity and sleep onset. After point *B*, waves in the theta range (lower frequency) become more prominent. The transition from alpha activity to theta activity at point *B* is consistent with transition from stage Wake to stage 1 sleep.

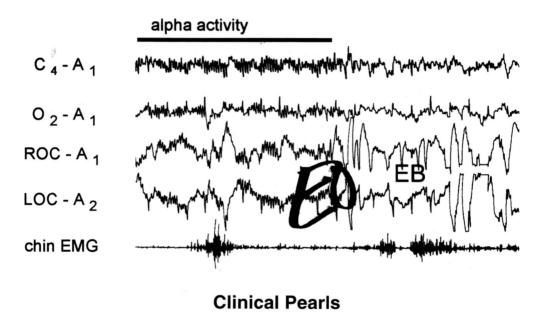

**alpha activity**

$C_4$-$A_1$

$O_2$-$A_1$

ROC - $A_1$

LOC - $A_2$

chin EMG

## Clinical Pearls

1. Alpha activity is usually more prominent in occipital than central EEG tracings.
2. Prominent alpha activity in the EEG is common during drowsy (eyes-closed) wakefulness.
3. Alpha activity is suppressed during wakefulness when the eyes are open.

## REFERENCES

1. Rechtschaffen A, Kales A (eds): A Manual of Standardized Terminology Techniques and Scoring System for Sleep Stages of Human Sleep. Los Angeles, Brain Information Service/Brain Research Institute, UCLA, 1968.
2. West P, Kryger MH: Sleep and respiration: Terminology and methodology. Clin Chest Med (Symposium on Sleep Disorders) 1985; 6:691–718.

## Electroencephalographic Lead Placement

Standard monitoring to detect the presence and stage of sleep requires only a few of the traditional EEG leads. The international 10–20 nomenclature for EEG electrode placement is used. The 10–20 terminology refers to the fact that the electrodes are positioned at either 10% or 20% of the distance between landmarks (see figure). Standard landmarks include the nasion (bridge of the nose) and inion (prominence at the base of the occiput). The distance between the two preauricular points also is an important standard. In the 10–20 system *even*-numbered subscripts refer to the *right* side of the head and *odd*-numbered subscripts to the *left*. For example $C_3$ and $C_4$ are the left and right **central leads,** respectively. These are placed along a line running between the two preauricular points and down 20% of this distance from the vertex.

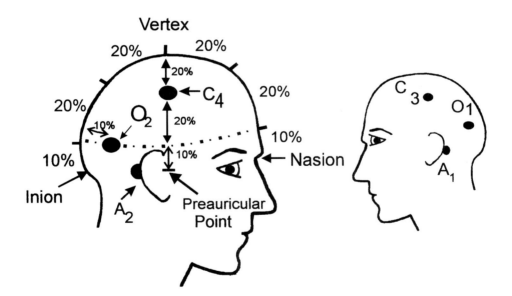

Central leads are the minimum required for staging sleep. Sleep spindles, K complexes, and slow waves can all be seen in these leads. The other important sleep EEG leads are the right and left **occipital leads ($O_2$ and $O_1$).** These are placed slightly off midline and above the level of the inion and preauricular points (as shown in the figure). The occipital leads are important for detecting alpha waves. Sometimes alpha waves will be detected in the occipital leads and not the central leads. Recognition of alpha activity is important for detecting transitions between wake and sleep.

Standard EEG monitoring for sleep studies is referential—the voltage difference between an exploring electrode and a reference electrode is recorded. The electrode pair (exploring electrode–reference electrode) is called a derivation. The standard reference electrodes are the left and right **mastoid leads ($A_1$ and $A_2$).** The mastoid electrode on the opposite side of the head from the exploring electrode usually is chosen as the reference ($C_3$–$A_2$ or $C_4$–$A_1$, $O_2$–$A_1$ or $O_1$–$A_2$) to produce the greatest voltage difference. Typically, the $C_3$, $C_4$, $O_2$, $O_1$, $A_2$, and $A_1$ leads all are placed. However, only one set of central and occipital leads are recorded at one time (for example, $C_3$–$A_2$ and $O_1$–$A_2$). The other leads are available if one of the monitored leads becomes defective during the night, allowing continued recording without awakening the patient to place new leads.

### EEG Monitoring

| Electrodes | Right | Left |
|---|---|---|
| Central | $C_4$ | $C_3$ |
| Occipital | $O_2$ | $O_1$ |
| Mastoid | $A_2$ | $A_1$ |

The visual appearance of the EEG tracings depends not only on lead placement but also on the paper speed, amplifier gain, and filter settings. The standard paper speed for sleep studies is 10 millimeters per second. At this speed, 30 seconds (the usual epoch length) is 30 centimeters or one page of standard paper. Other time scales are better for respiratory events. The paper speed for clinical EEG studies usually is 15–30 mm/sec. This faster speed is useful for recognition of seizure activity. The standard EEG amplifier gain adjustment for sleep studies is 50 microvolts equals 1 centimeter of pen deflection. Calibration of the EEG amplitude is important for detecting stages 3 and 4 sleep because they have an EEG voltage criteria.

### REFERENCES

1. Rechtschaffen A, Kales A (eds): A Manual of Standardized Terminology Techniques and Scoring System for Sleep Stages of Human Sleep. Los Angeles, Brain Information Service/Brain Research Institute, UCLA, 1968.
2. Williams RL, Karacan I, Hursch CJ: Electroencephalography of Human Sleep: Clinical Applications. New York, John Wiley & Sons, 1974.

# PATIENT 3

## A 50-year-old man with insomnia

A 30-second epoch of the central EEG ($C_3$–$A_1$) was recorded during the sleep study of this patient and is shown below as two 15-second segments. The dotted lines show 75 microvolts (µv) of deflection. The dark bars above the segments mark slow wave activity meeting voltage criteria ($\geq$75 µv peak to peak). The numbers above the bars are the approximate durations in seconds.

*Question:* What stage is this epoch?

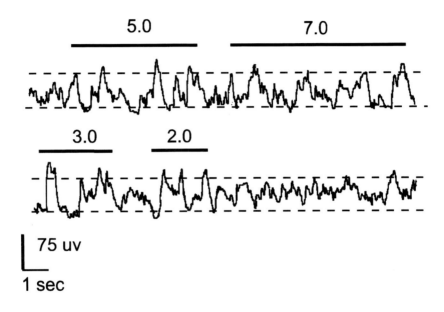

***Answer:*** This epoch is in stage 4.

***Discussion:*** Identification of sleep stages 3 and 4 depends on determining the amount of slow wave activity meeting voltage criteria. Slow wave activity for the purpose of sleep staging is slower than 2 Hz (longer than 0.5-second duration) and the amplitude is $\geq 75$ $\mu$v peak to peak. In recording calibration, a typical standard is 50 $\mu$v equals 1 cm pen deflection. Thus, 75 $\mu$v is equivalent to a pen deflection of 1.5 cm. Stage 3 is scored when 20–50% of the epoch has slow wave activity meeting voltage criteria (6–15 seconds of a 30-second epoch). Stage 4 is scored when more than 50% of an epoch contains such slow wave activity. Stage 2 has less than 20% (6 seconds in a 30-second epoch) of slow wave activity. Of course, to be scored as stage 2 the epoch also must meet other criteria for stage 2 (sleep spindles or K complexes).

As humans age, the amplitude of the EEG during sleep diminishes. Therefore, slow wave activity may be present in older patients but may not meet voltage criteria. In young subjects, stage 3 is relatively brief, and most slow wave sleep is stage 4. In older subjects, most of slow wave sleep is stage 3. Some authorities are against using a voltage criteria for scoring sleep, but this is the standard practice. Note that the amplitude of the slow wave activity recorded can be diminished if the low-frequency filter is set too high (½ amp equals 1 or higher, meaning that a signal of 1 Hz is reduced to 50% of its original amplitude by the filter). Thus, it is important to know the filter settings and to be informed if they are changed (e.g., to diminish artifact) during the night.

In the present case, approximately 17 seconds of the 30-second epoch contained slow wave activity meeting voltage criteria. Therefore, the epoch is scored as stage 4. Note that most of the high-voltage, slow wave activity was present in the first portion of the epoch. In actual practice, detailed measurement of the duration of slow wave activity is unnecessary. An "eyeball estimate" usually suffices. Epochs that are on the borderline between stages 2 and 3 or stages 3 and 4 may necessitate more careful examination, but for most clinical studies such precision is not warranted. Even authorities on sleep staging can disagree on whether a given segment of the record meets criteria. Faster EEG activity often is superimposed on underlying slow activity, making visual interpretation somewhat arbitrary. Many sleep laboratories report the sum of stages 3 and 4.

## Clinical Pearls

1. Scoring of stages 3 and 4 depends on identification of the percentage of the epoch occupied by slow wave activity meeting voltage (amplitude) criteria.

2. The appearance of a record and the amount of slow wave sleep scored depends on the voltage calibration of the EEG leads and the filter settings (especially the low-frequency filter).

REFERENCES
1. Rechtschaffen A, Kales A (eds): A Manual of Standardized Terminology Techniques and Scoring System for Sleep Stages of Human Sleep. Los Angeles, Brain Information Service/Brain Research Institute, UCLA, 1968.
2. Tyner FS, Knot JR, Mayer WB: Fundamentals of EEG technology. New York, Raven Press, 1983.

## Eye Movement Monitoring

Electro-oculographic (eye movement) leads typically are placed at the outer corners of the eyes—at the right outer canthus (ROC) and the left outer canthus (LOC). In a common approach, two eye channels are recorded and the eye electrodes are referenced to the opposite mastoid (ROC-A$_1$ and LOC-A$_2$). However, some sleep centers use the same mastoid electrode as a reference (ROC-A$_1$ and LOC-A$_1$). To detect vertical as well as horizontal eye movements, one electrode is placed slightly above and one slightly below the eyes (see figure).

Recording of eye movements is possible because a **potential difference** exists across the eyeball: front positive (+), back negative (−). Eye movements are detected by electro-oculographic recording of voltage changes. When the eyes move toward an electrode, a positive voltage is recorded (see figure below). By standard convention, polygraphs are calibrated so that a negative voltage causes an upward pen deflection (negative polarity up). Thus, eye movement toward an electrode results in a downward deflection.

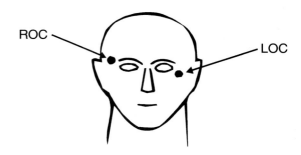

Note that movement of both of the eyes is always toward one electrode and away from the other because eye movements are conjugate. If the eye channels are calibrated with the same polarity settings, eye movements produce out-of-phase deflections in the two eye tracings (e.g., one up, one down). The schematic below shows the recorded results of eye movements to the right and left, assuming both amplifier channels have negative polarity up. Remember, this means an upward deflection occurs when the eyes move away from an electrode. The same approach can be used to understand the tracings resulting from vertical eye movements. Because ROC is positioned above the eyes (and LOC below), upward eye movements are toward ROC and away from LOC. Thus, upward eye movement results in a downward deflection in the ROC tracing and an upward deflection in the LOC tracing.

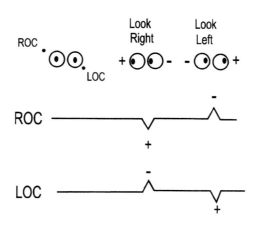

## Key Points

1. Conjugate eye movements produce out-of-phase deflections when the usual two-channel method properly calibrated for monitoring eye movements is applied.

2. Eye movements can be recorded because a voltage difference exists between the front (+) and the back (−) of each eye.

## REFERENCES

1. Rechtschaffen A, Kales A (eds): A Manual of Standardized Terminology Techniques and Scoring System for Sleep Stages of Human Sleep. Los Angeles, Brain Information Service/Brain Research Institute, UCLA, 1968.
2. West P, Kryger MH: Sleep and respiration: Terminology and methodology. Clin Chest Med (Symposium on Sleep Disorders) 1985; 6:691–718.

## Eye Movement Patterns

The tracings below show two important patterns of eye movements recorded during sleep. ROC and LOC are right and left outer canthus electrodes; $A_1$ and $A_2$ are the left and right mastoid electrodes, respectively. Slow rolling eye movements are characterized by a smooth undulation of the tracings (*A*). This pattern frequently is seen during drowsy wakefulness and stage 1 sleep. Slow rolling eye movements also may be seen following arousals (brief awakenings) or after a shift to a lighter stage of sleep. Rapid eye movements (REMs) are sharper, and the baseline between the movements usually is flat (*B*). Even sharper movements are seen with eye blinks.

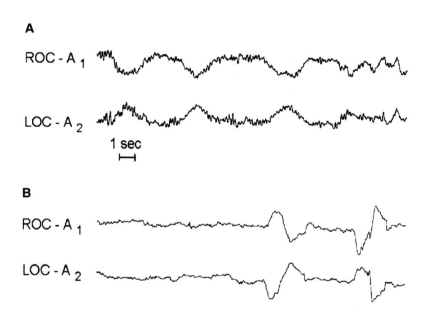

During wakefulness with eyes open, eye blinks or rapid eye movements are common. In an eyes-closed drowsy state, slow rolling eye movements and EEG alpha activity are noted. Slow rolling eye movements continue to be present after the transition from stage Wake to stage 1 sleep (alpha activity in less than 50% of the epoch). As sleep progresses to stage 2, these movements disappear. During slow wave sleep, eye movements are not seen. However, slow wave activity usually is noted in the eye movement channels. With the onset of stage REM, REMs appear episodically.

REMs are characteristic of stage REM sleep, and they are critical to the detection of this stage. The REM density (number of REMs per minute of REM sleep) increases during the night. Early episodes of REM sleep sometimes are difficult to recognize because REMs are relatively infrequent. At times it also may be difficult to differentiate between a brief episode of slow rolling eye movements and REMs. A useful approach is to find a period of unequivocal REM sleep (usually in the last part of the recording) and note the appearance of the patient's stage REM sleep. Remember that REMs can be seen during wakefulness (eyes open). However, in contrast to stage REM, during wakefulness the chin EMG amplitude is not reduced and the EEG may have more prominent, high-frequency activity.

# Key Points

1. Slow rolling eye movements may be seen during drowsy wakefulness and stage 1 sleep.
2. The presence of REMs is a defining characteristic of REM sleep.
3. REMs in early episodes of REM sleep are infrequent (lower REM density) and identification of REM sleep may be more difficult.
4. Identification of early periods of REM sleep may be aided by observing the patterns during unequivocal stage REM sleep later in the night.

## REFERENCES

1. Rechtschaffen A, Kales A (eds): A Manual of Standardized Terminology Techniques and Scoring System for Sleep Stages of Human Sleep. Los Angeles, Brain Information Service/Brain Research Institute, UCLA, 1968.
2. West P, Kryger MH: Sleep and respiration: Terminology and methodology. Clin Chest Med (Symposium on Sleep Disorders) 1985; 6:691–718.

# PATIENT 4

## A 20-year-old man with excessive daytime sleepiness

A 20-year-old patient was evaluated in the sleep laboratory for excessive daytime sleepiness. Sleep was recorded in 30-second epochs.

*Figure:* Below is the last half of an epoch (15 seconds). The electrode $C_4$ (right central) and $O_2$ (right occipital) are referenced to the left mastoid ($A_1$). The right outer canthus (ROC) and left outer canthus (LOC) electrodes are referenced to the opposite mastoid electrodes ($A_1$ and $A_2$, respectively). The chin electromyogram (EMG) also is shown.

*Question:* Are rapid eye movements present at point *A*, point *B*, or both?

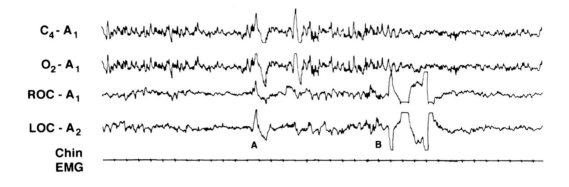

*Answer:*    Rapid eye movements are present at point *B*.

*Discussion:*    High-voltage EEG activity also may be picked up by electro-oculography (EOG). In the standard two-channel scheme for monitoring eye movements, with both channels having the same polarity, large-amplitude EEG activity (K complexes, slow waves) produces deflections that are in-phase (both up or down) in the two eye channels. In contrast, conjugate eye movements produce out-of-phase deflections (one up, one down) in the two eye channels. During stages 3 and 4, it also is common to detect considerable amounts of slow wave activity in the eye lead tracings.

Sleep is staged by epochs (usually 30 seconds). When there is a transition of sleep stages within an epoch, the convention is to score the epoch according to which stage occupied the majority of the epoch. However, epochs are not scored in isolation. For example, eye movements are not present in every epoch of REM sleep: epochs with eye movements sometimes are referred to as **phasic REM** and epochs without eye movements as **tonic REM.** Tonic REM epochs must otherwise meet criteria for stage REM (same EEG and EMG) and are contiguous with epochs of phasic REM. Rules for identifying epochs of tonic REM are discussed in Fundamentals 6.

In the present patient, the tracing shows a K complex at point *A* and two rapid eye movements at point *B*. At point *A* the deflections in both eye channels are in-phase, but at point *B* they are out-of-phase. In the first part of the tracing, the K complex without slow waves is consistent with stage 2 sleep. In the second part, the appearance of REMs with a low-amplitude chin EMG is consistent with REM sleep. However, as point *B* occurs near the end of the epoch, the epoch was scored as stage 2 sleep, and the subsequent epoch was scored as stage REM.

## Clinical Pearls

1.  In the standard two-channel EOG method, high-amplitude EEG activity picked up by the eye leads produces deflections that are in-phase (assuming both channels have the same polarity setting).

2.  When a sleep stage transition occurs within an epoch, the epoch is scored according to which stage occupies the majority of the epoch.

## REFERENCES

1. Rechtschaffen A, Kales A (eds): A Manual of Standardized Terminology Techniques and Scoring System for Sleep Stages of Human Sleep. Los Angeles, Brain Information Service/Brain Research Institute, UCLA, 1968.
2. Williams RL, Karacan I, Hursch CJ: Electroencephalography (EEG) of Human Sleep: Clinical Applications. New York, John Wiley & Sons, 1974.
3. West P, Kryger MH: Sleep and respiration: Terminology and methodology. Clin Chest Med (Symposium on Sleep Disorders) 1985; 6:691–718.

## Chin (Submental) Electromyography

Staging sleep depends on electroencephalographic (EEG), eye movement, and chin electromyographic (EMG) criteria. Usually, three EMG leads are placed in the mental and submental areas (see figure). The voltage between two of these three is monitored (for example, EMG1-EMG3). If either of these leads fail, the third lead can be substituted.

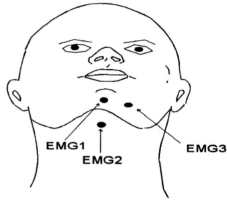

The chin EMG is an essential element only for identifying stage REM sleep. In stage REM, the chin EMG is **relatively reduced**: the amplitude is equal to or lower than the lowest EMG amplitude in NREM sleep. If the EMG gain is adjusted high enough to show some activity in NREM sleep, a drop in activity often is seen on transition to REM sleep. Depending on the gain, a reduction in the EMG amplitude from wakefulness to sleep and often a further reduction on transition from stage 1 to stage 4 may be seen. The reduction in the chin EMG amplitude during REM sleep is a reflection of the generalized skeletal-muscle hypotonia present in this sleep stage.

In the tracings below, there is a fall in chin EMG amplitude just before the REMs (*arrows*) occur. The combination of REMs, a relatively reduced chin EMG, and a low-voltage mixed-frequency EEG is consistent with stage REM. Note that a reduction in airflow follows the onset of REMs. Even in normal persons, a reduction in airflow often occurs during **phasic REM** (stage REM with eye movements present).

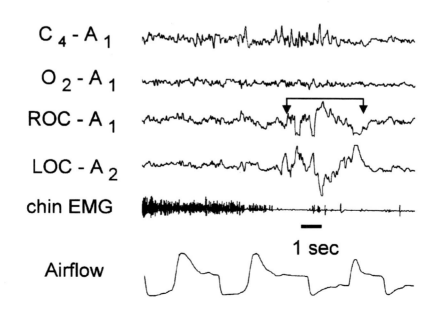

$C_4 - A_1$

$O_2 - A_1$

ROC - $A_1$

LOC - $A_2$

chin EMG

1 sec

Airflow

While the chin EMG amplitude may progressively decrease with the transition from wakefulness to stage 4 NREM sleep, this change is not a requirement for the staging of sleep. In the 15-second tracings below, the chin EMG actually was higher in stage 3 than in stage 2 sleep.

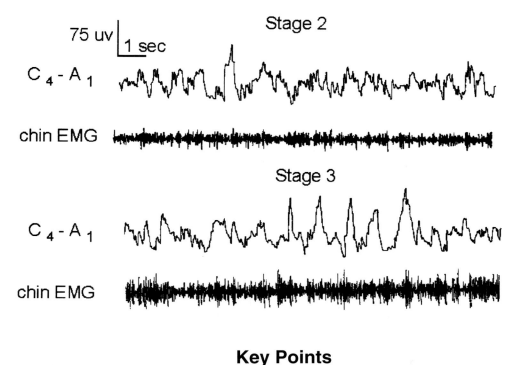

## Key Points

1. Recording of EMG activity in the chin area helps identify stage REM.
2. The amplitude of chin EMG activity is relatively reduced in stage REM compared to NREM sleep. That is, the amplitude of the chin EMG in REM sleep is equal to or lower than the lowest level recorded in NREM sleep.

REFERENCES
1. Rechtschaffen A, Kales A (eds): A Manual of Standardized Terminology Techniques and Scoring System for Sleep Stages of Human Sleep. Los Angeles, Brain Information Service/Brain Research Institute, UCLA, 1968.
2. Williams RL, Karacan I, Hursch CJ: Electroencephalography (EEG) of Human Sleep: Clinical Applications. New York, John Wiley & Sons, 1974.

# PATIENT 5

## A 40-year-old man with difficulty falling asleep

A 40-year-old man was evaluated for difficulty falling asleep. The tracing below was recorded soon after lights out. $C_4$-$A_1$ and $O_2$-$A_1$ are the central and occipital EEG channels; ROC-$A_1$ and LOC-$A_2$ are the right and left eye movement (EOG) channels. The chin EMG also is presented.

*Question:* What sleep stage is shown?

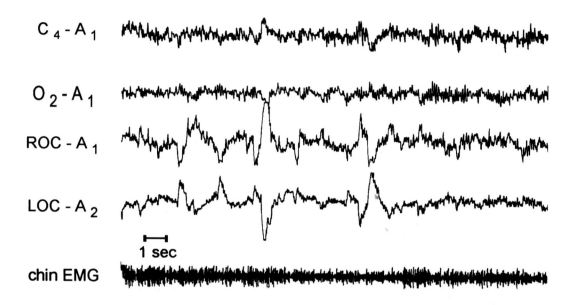

*Answer:* The sleep stage shown is Wake (eyes open).

*Discussion:* The appearance of stage W (wakefulness) depends on whether the eyes are open or closed and if the subject being monitored is alert or drowsy. When the patient is alert, the EEG shows a low-voltage, high-frequency pattern. When the patient is tense, **muscle artifact** consisting of a mixed high-frequency pattern can be seen in the tracings—the EEG electrodes are recording the EMG activity of the underlying scalp muscles. Note the change in the EEG below when the patient is asked to grit his teeth.

With relaxation, lower frequency activity appears in the waking EEG. However, alpha activity (8–13 Hz) usually is not prominent until the eyes are closed (having the eyes open attenuates the alpha activity). REMs or eye blinks are commonly seen during eyes-open wakefulness. The level of the chin EMG amplitude tends to be relatively high unless the amplifier gain is very low.

With eye closure and the onset of a drowsy, relaxed state, prominent alpha activity usually appears, the background EEG frequency slows, and slow rolling eye movements are present. The chin EMG amplitude may fluctuate as the patient drifts in and out of a drowsy state

In the present case, REMs are seen in the eye leads (sharp, out-of-phase deflections), and the EEG tracings show a low-voltage, fast-frequency pattern (see figure on page 19). The chin EMG amplitude is relatively high. Toward the end of the tracing, more prominent alpha activity is seen as REMs vanish (probable eye closure). This pattern is different from stage REM, which also contains REMs. In that stage, the EEG exhibits a lower frequency and the chin EMG amplitude is relatively reduced. Stage REM for this patient was associated with a flat-line EMG tracing.

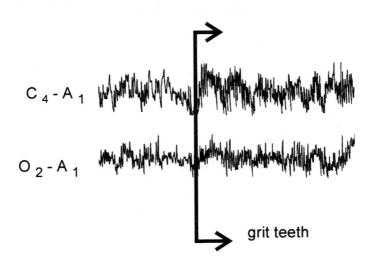

## Clinical Pearls

1. Stage Wake (eyes open) may feature REMs but differs from stage REM in the amplitude of the chin EMG and the pattern of the EEG.

2. Muscle artifact may be present in the EEG and EOG channels if the subject being monitored is tense. The artifact usually diminishes as the patient becomes drowsy and falls asleep.

## REFERENCES
1. Rechtschaffen A, Kales A (eds): A Manual of Standardized Terminology Techniques and Scoring System for Sleep Stages of Human Sleep. Los Angeles, Brain Information Service/ Brain Research Institute, UCLA, 1968.
2. Carskadon MA, Rechtschaffen A: Monitoring and staging human sleep. *In* Kryger MH, Roth T, Dement WC (eds): Principles and Practice of Sleep Medicine. Philadelphia, WB Saunders Co., 1994, pp 943–960.

# PATIENT 6

## A 30-year-old woman having trouble falling asleep

A 30-year-old woman who complained of difficulty falling asleep was monitored in the sleep laboratory. Sixty-six epochs (each 30 seconds long) of stage Wake were recorded before the first epoch of sleep (stage 1 in this case).

*Figure:* A 15-second tracing was obtained soon after lights out. The central and occipital EEG tracings are $C_4$–$A_1$ and $O_2$–$A_1$, respectively. ROC-$A_1$ and LOC-$A_2$ are the eye movement (EOG) tracings.

*Question:* What is the sleep stage and sleep latency?

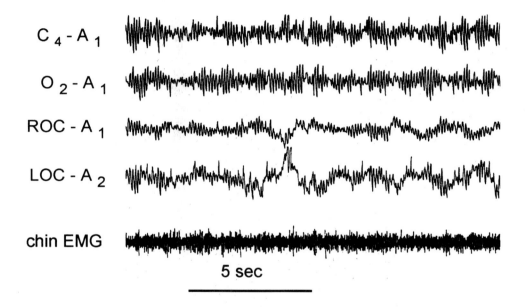

*Answer:*    The sleep stage is Wake. The sleep latency is 33 minutes.

*Discussion:*    Sleep latency is defined as the time from lights out until the first epoch of any stage of sleep. In most age groups this occurs within 30 minutes. Several factors must be considered when evaluating sleep latency. The bedtime in the laboratory should mimic the patient's normal bedtime. Time before lights out (and after electrode placement) should be allowed for adaptation to the surroundings. Many normal people experience some difficulty falling asleep in a new environment. Changes in sleep latency and sleep architecture that result from sleeping in a novel environment are termed the **first-night effect.** Most research studies of the effects of medication or interventions on sleep architecture include an adaptation night to attempt to control for this effect. In contrast, some patients with psychophysiologic insomnia may fall asleep more easily in a new environment.

Determining **sleep onset** is an important part of sleep staging. The usual progression at sleep onset is from stage Wake (eyes open) to drowsy wakefulness (eyes closed) and finally to stage 1 sleep. In general, the EEG in stage Wake with the eyes open is composed of low-amplitude, high-frequency activity. REMs and eye blinks may be present. The amplitude of the chin EMG is relatively high. As the person becomes drowsy, the eyes close and slow rolling eye movements and alpha activity (8–13 Hz) are prominent. Stage 1 is scored when alpha activity is present in less than 50% of the epoch. Slow rolling eye movements commonly persist into stage 1 sleep. The EMG amplitude may or may not decrease (depends on amplifier gain).

In patients who do not produce prominent alpha activity, this progression to sleep is more difficult to detect, and the exact timing of transition from wakefulness to stage 1 sleep may be indeterminate. The typical characteristics of the transition—attenuation of higher frequencies and increased theta activity (4–7 Hz)—can be subtle in these patients. However, the onset of stage 2 sleep is more easily determined, and for this reason many sleep centers also compute a latency to stage 2 sleep or a latency to **sustained sleep** (defined as three consecutive epochs of sleep).

Recognition of alpha activity can be enhanced by monitoring occipital leads and by carefully observing the EEG during **biocalibrations** to note the patterns of eyes-open and eyes-closed periods. (For a detailed discussion of biocalibrations, see Fundamental 8.) Briefly, the patient is recorded opening and closing the eyes and looking right, left, up, and down. The resultant displays provide the EEG patterns for eyes-open and eyes-closed wakefulness and for deflections in the eye movement channels during REMs. Comparisons can assist in recognition of stage W and stage 1 in difficult cases.

In the present case, the sleep tracing shows almost continuous alpha activity (8–13 Hz), which is consistent with stage Wake (drowsy, eyes closed). The eye leads show some slow rolling eye movements. The EMG activity is relatively high. We are told that 66 epochs (33 minutes) of stage W were recorded after lights out and before the first epoch of sleep. Thus, the sleep latency is 33 minutes. This is a long sleep latency and is consistent with the patient's complaints of difficulty initiating sleep.

## Clinical Pearls

1. The sleep latency is prolonged past 30 minutes in patients with sleep-onset insomnia.
2. The timing of sleep onset can be difficult to determine in patients who do not produce significant alpha activity. Monitoring occipital leads can help detect alpha activity.
3. The timing of lights out in the laboratory should mimic the patient's normal bedtime.
4. The first-night effect can increase the sleep latency.

## REFERENCES

1. Agnew HW, Webb WB, Williams RL: The first-night effect: An EEG study of sleep. Psychophysiology 1966; 2:263–266.
2. Carskadon MA, Rechtschaffen A: Monitoring and staging human sleep. *In* Kryger MH, Roth T, Dement WC (eds): Principles and Practice of Sleep Medicine. Philadelphia, WB Saunders Co., 1994, pp 943–960.

# PATIENT 7

## A 30-year-old man having difficulty staying awake during the day

A 30-year-old man was monitored for complaints of excessive daytime sleepiness. In the 15-second tracing below, $C_4$–$A_1$ and $O_2$–$A_1$ are the central and occipital EEG tracings and ROC-$A_1$ and LOC-$A_2$ are the right and left eye movement (EOG) tracings. The chin EMG tracing also is shown.

*Question:*   What is this sleep stage?

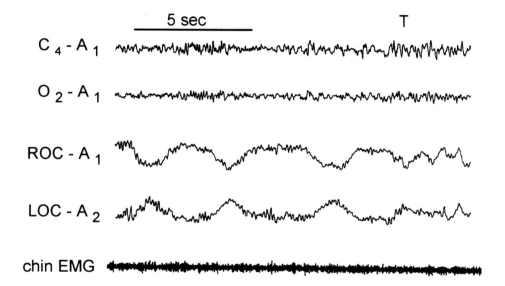

*Answer:* The tracings indicate stage 1 sleep.

*Discussion:* The stage 1 EEG is characterized by low-voltage, mixed-frequency activity (4–7 Hz). Stage 1 is scored when less than 50% of an epoch contains alpha waves and criteria for deeper stages of sleep are not met. Slow rolling eye movements often are present in the eye movement tracings, and the level of muscle tone (EMG) is equal or diminished compared to that in the awake state.

Some patients do not exhibit much alpha activity, making detection of sleep onset difficult. The ability of a patient to produce alpha waves can be determined from biocalibrations at the start of the study. The patient is asked to lie quietly with eyes open and then with the eyes closed. Alpha activity usually appears with eye closure. When patients do not produce significant alpha activity or when differentiating eyes-open wakefulness (attenuates alpha) from stage 1 sleep, several points are helpful. First, with the eyes open, eye movements usually are much sharper than slow rolling eye movements (blinks or REMs). Second, the EEG of wakefulness (when no alpha is present) tends to have more high-frequency components. Note the slower (wider) EEG activity at point *T* in the figure. This activity is in the theta range. Third, often the easiest method to determine sleep onset in difficult cases is to find the first epoch of unequivocal sleep (usually stage 2) and work backward. The examiner can be confident of the point of sleep onset within one or two epochs.

In the present case, alpha activity for less than 50% of the epoch; the presence of low-amplitude, mixed-frequency EEG activity and slow rolling eye movements; and the absence of spindles or K complexes (stage 2) classify this tracing as stage 1 sleep.

## Clinical Pearls

1. The stage 1 EEG is characterized by low-amplitude and mixed-frequency activity with alpha activity present less than 50% of the time.

2. In cases were determination of sleep onset is difficult, find the first epoch of unequivocal stage 2 sleep and work backward toward the beginning of the night.

## REFERENCES

1. Rechtschaffen A, Kales A (eds): A Manual of Standardized Terminology Techniques and Scoring System for Sleep Stages of Human Sleep. Los Angeles, Brain Information Service/Brain Research Institute, UCLA, 1968.
2. Carskadon MA, Rechtschaffen A: Monitoring and staging human sleep. *In* Kryger MH, Roth T, Dement WC (eds): Principles and Practice of Sleep Medicine. Philadelphia, WB Saunders Co., 1994, pp 943–960.

# PATIENT 8

## A 35-year-old woman with insomnia

A 35-year-old woman was monitored for complaints of insomnia. The 15-second tracing below was recorded soon after sleep onset.

*Question:* What stage of sleep is illustrated? What is the large-amplitude EEG deflection?

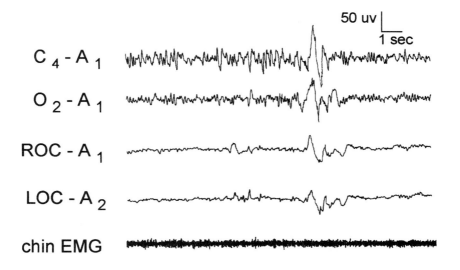

*Answer:*   The patient is in stage 2 sleep. The large-amplitude deflection is a K complex.

*Discussion:*   Stage 2 sleep is characterized by the presence of one or more sleep spindles (bursts of 12–14 Hz activity) or K complexes (large-amplitude, biphasic EEG deflections). To qualify as stage 2, an epoch also must contain less than 20% of slow (delta) wave EEG activity. Slow wave activity is defined as waves with a frequency < 2 Hz and a minimum peak-to-peak amplitude of 75 microvolts. Stage 2 occupies the greatest proportion of the total sleep time and accounts for roughly 40–50% of sleep.

In the present case, the tracing shows the presence of a K complex and no slow wave activity. Therefore, the sleep is stage 2. Note that the K complex is transmitted to the eye leads, resulting in deflections in the EEG and eye leads that are in-phase. This occurs when all channels are calibrated with the same polarity (by convention, negative polarity up).

## Clinical Pearls

1. Stage 2 is scored when one or more sleep spindles or K complexes are noted but the epoch does not have enough slow wave activity to meet criteria for stage 3 sleep.
2. Stage 2 sleep accounts for the largest proportion of the total sleep time.
3. When the EEG and eye channels are properly calibrated, a K complex produces in-phase (same direction) deflections in the two eye lead channels.

## REFERENCES

1. Rechtschaffen A, Kales A (eds): A Manual of Standardized Terminology Techniques and Scoring System for Sleep Stages of Human Sleep. Los Angeles, Brain Information Service/Brain Research Institute, UCLA, 1968.
2. Carskadon MA, Rechtschaffen A: Monitoring and staging human sleep. *In* Kryger MH, Roth T, Dement WC (eds): Principles and Practice of Sleep Medicine. Philadelphia, WB Saunders CO., 1994, pp 943–960.

# PATIENT 9

## A 25-year-old man with a history of sleep walking

A 25-year-old man was monitored for complaints of sleep walking. These episodes had been present since childhood. The 15-second tracing below occurred just before body movements were noted during sleep.

*Question:* In which half of the night is this event likely to have occurred?

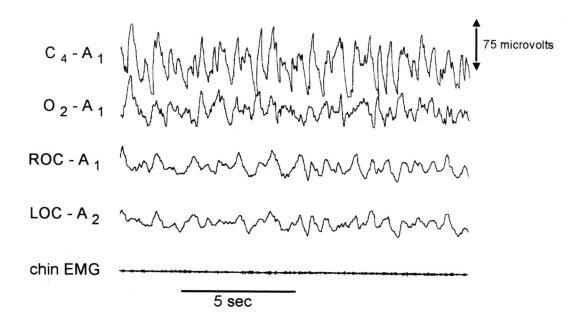

*Answer:* This event occurred during stage 4 NREM sleep in the first half of the night.

*Discussion:* Stages 3 and 4 NREM sleep are called slow wave, delta, or deep sleep. Stage 3 is scored when slow wave activity (frequency < 2 Hz and amplitude 75 microvolts) is present for 20–50% of the epoch. Stage 4 is scored when more than 50% of the epoch is occupied by slow wave activity meeting the above criteria. Spindles may be present in the EEG. Frequently, the high-voltage EEG activity is transmitted to the eye leads. The EMG often is lower than during stages 1 and 2 sleep, but this is variable. Stage 3 sleep in younger patients often is brief and represents a transition from stage 2 to stage 4 sleep. In older patients, the EEG amplitude is lower, and the total amount of slow wave sleep is reduced. In these patients, the amount of stage 3 sleep may exceed the amount of stage 4 sleep.

During the night there are three to five cycles of NREM sleep with episodes of REM sleep between the cycles. The amplitude of the slow waves (and amount of slow wave sleep) is highest in the first sleep cycles. Typically, stages 3 and 4 occur mostly in the early portions of the night. The episodes of REM sleep occur about every 90–120 minutes, and they are of longer duration as the night progresses. An overview of the cyclic nature of sleep can be shown using a **hypnogram** (see figure below). Note the periods of slow wave sleep (*A, B,* and *C*) in the early part of the night and longer REM episodes (*dark bars*) during the second half of the night.

Several **parasomnias** (disorders associated with sleep) occur in stages 3 and 4 sleep and therefore can be predicted to occur in the early part of the night. These include **somnambulism** (sleep walking) and night terrors. In contrast, parasomnias occurring in REM sleep (for example, nightmares) are more common in the early morning hours.

In the present case, the epoch of sleep displayed on page 27 occurred about 1 hour after sleep monitoring had begun. High-amplitude, slow wave activity occupies essentially all of the tracing. Note that slow wave activity also is present in the eye leads. The chin EMG activity is relatively low. After this epoch the patient was noted to sit up and "pick at the bed sheets." The presence of body movements occurring out of slow wave sleep is consistent with a mild form of somnambulism.

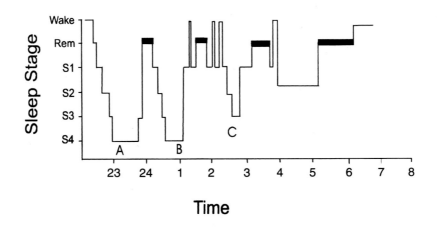

## Clinical Pearls

1. Sleep occurs in cycles of NREM sleep separated by periods of REM sleep.
2. Stages 3 and 4 sleep occur mostly in the first few cycles of NREM sleep.
3. Parasomnias originating in slow wave sleep tend to occur in the early part of the night.

## REFERENCES
1. Williams RL, Karacan I, Hursch CJ: Electroencephalography (EEG) of Human Sleep: Clinical Applications. New York, John Wiley & Sons. 1974.
2. Carskadon MA, Rechtschaffen A: Monitoring and staging human sleep. *In* Kryger MH, Roth T, Dement WC (eds): Principles and Practice of Sleep Medicine. Philadelphia, WB Saunders Co., 1994, pp 943–960.

# PATIENT 10

## A 20-year-old man with daytime sleepiness

A 20-year-old man was monitored for complaints of increased daytime sleepiness. The recording below was obtained about 100 minutes after lights out.

*Question:* What stage of sleep is shown?

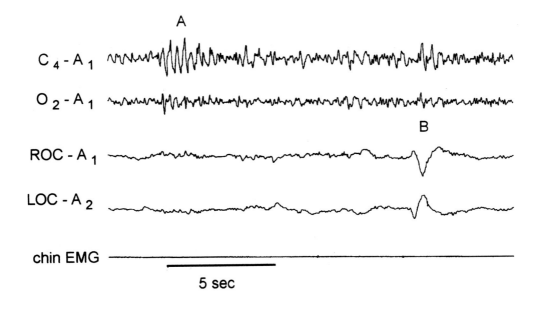

*Answer*:    The tracing displays stage REM sleep.

*Discussion:*    Stage REM sleep is characterized by a low-voltage, mixed-frequency EEG, the presence of episodic REMs, and a relatively low-amplitude chin EMG. Saw-tooth waves (see figure, point *A*) also may occur in the EEG. There usually are three to five episodes of REM sleep during the night, which tend to increase in length as the night progresses. The number of eye movements per unit time (REM density) also increases during the night. Not all epochs of REM sleep contain REMs. Epochs of sleep otherwise meeting criteria for stage REM and contiguous with epochs of unequivocal stage REM (REMs present) are scored as stage REM. (See Fundamental 6 for a detailed discussion of this concept.)

Stage REM is associated with many unique, physiologic changes, such as widespread **skeletal muscle hypotonia.** Skeletal muscle hypotonia is a protective mechanism to prevent the acting out of dreams. In a pathologic state known as the REM behavior disorder, muscle tone *is* present, and body movements and even violent behavior can occur during REM sleep.

Important respiratory changes occur during REM sleep. The pattern of breathing becomes more irregular. REM sleep is not homogeneous, and periods of **phasic activity** (eye movements present) are associated with the most significant changes. Even in normal subjects, a reduction in tidal volume may be seen during bursts of eye movement. As more eye movements occur in the early-morning REM episodes, this is the time of the most profound changes in ventilation. The diaphragm becomes the only active inspiratory muscle during REM sleep, and the ventilatory responses to hypoxia and hypercapnia are reduced. Hence, patients with lung disease typically experience the most severe arterial oxygen desaturation episodes during early-morning REM. Upper-airway muscle activity also is reduced during periods of phasic REM, possibly explaining why some patients have obstructive apnea only during REM sleep.

Many nonrespiratory physiologic changes, such as nocturnal penile tumescence, occur during REM sleep as well. Dreaming is more common and more complex in stage REM. Nightmares also occur during this sleep stage.

In the present case, REMs (see figure, point *B*); a low-voltage, mixed-frequency EEG; and a low-amplitude EMG are consistent with REM sleep. The saw-tooth waves (at point *A*) are not an essential part of the definition of stage REM, but are a clue that REM sleep is present.

## Clinical Pearls

1. Saw-tooth waves are a clue that REM sleep is present.

2. Alterations in ventilation are common during phasic REM sleep (eye movements present). Episodes of reduction in tidal volume and upper airway muscle activity are associated with bursts of eye movements.

3. As eye movements are more common (higher REM density) during early-morning episodes of REM sleep, this is the time of the greatest changes in ventilation.

4. Patients with lung disease typically have the most severe arterial oxygen desaturations during the early-morning periods of REM sleep.

## REFERENCES

1. Gould GA, Gugger M, Molloy J, et al: Breathing pattern and eye movement density during REM sleep in humans. Am Rev Respir Dis 1988; 138:874–877.
2. Wiegand L, Zwillich CW, Wiegand D, et al: Changes in upper airway muscle activation and ventilation during phasic REM sleep in normal men. J Appl Physiol 1991; 71:488–497.

# PATIENT 11

## A 40-year-old man with a history of snoring and daytime sleepiness

A 40-year-old man was monitored in the sleep laboratory because of a history of snoring and daytime sleepiness. The following tracings (*A* and *B*) show different chin EMG patterns.

*Question:*   Rapid eye movements are present in both *A* and *B*. Which tracing is stage REM?

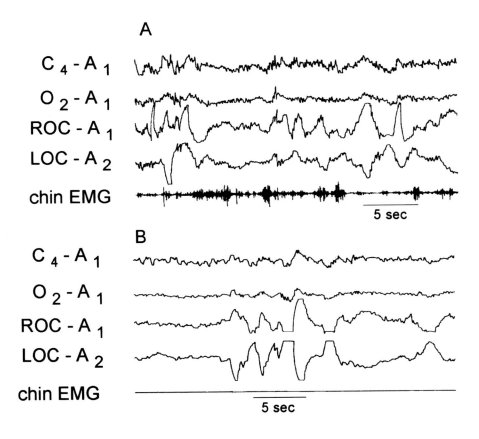

***Answer:*** Tracing *B* is stage REM; tracing *A* is stage Wake.

***Discussion:*** Staging sleep depends on EEG, eye movement, and chin (submental) EMG criteria. However, the **chin EMG** is an essential element only for identifying stage REM sleep. The chin EMG must be **relatively reduced** in stage REM: the amplitude must be equal to or lower than the lowest EMG amplitude in NREM sleep. If the EMG gain is adjusted high enough to show some activity in NREM sleep, a drop in activity on transition to REM sleep may be evident. Depending on the gain, there usually is a reduction in the EMG amplitude from wakefulness to sleep and often a further reduction on transition from stage 1 to stage 4. It is essential that the EMG gain is high enough to see some activity during wakefulness. Obviously, if the EMG trace shows a flat line during wakefulness, no further decreases in EMG activity will be detected.

In the present case, the tracings demonstrate the utility of the chin EMG in identifying REM sleep. In both *A* and *B* the EEG is low voltage, and REMs are present. However, in *B* the EMG is reduced compared to *A*. This reduced level of EMG activity was seen throughout the night in REM sleep. A more subtle finding is that more high-frequency activity is present in the central EEG of *A* compared to *B*. The lack of more prominent alpha activity in *A* (stage Wake) is due to the fact that the eyes were probably open (REMs). The eye movements in eyes-closed wakefulness are usually of the slow rolling type. The EMG of REM sleep can show phasic bursts of activity; however, the tonic activity is reduced. Nevertheless, these tracings illustrate the difficulty in distinguishing REM sleep from wakefulness with REMs. The appearance of REM sleep varies between patients. There are patients in whom REM sleep may look like tracing A! Thus, it is essential to find a period of unequivocal REM in each patient and note that patient's characteristic pattern of eye movements and chin EMG amplitude.

## Clinical Pearls

1. The chin EMG is reduced in stage REM compared to wakefulness. This fact is useful in differentiating eyes-open wakefulness (with REMs) from stage REM sleep.

2. The chin EMG amplitude in a given stage depends on the amplifier gain. The gain should be high enough so that a reduction in amplitude is evident as sleep progresses from wakefulness to slow wave sleep/REM.

3. Identification of early periods of REM sleep can be aided by observing the pattern of unequivocal periods of REM later in the recording period.

REFERENCES

1. Rechtschaffen A, Kales A (eds): A Manual of Standardized Terminology Techniques and Scoring System for Sleep Stages of Human Sleep. Los Angeles, Brain Information Service/Brain Research Institute, UCLA, 1968.
2. Williams RL, Karacan I, Hursch CJ: Electroencephalography (EEG) of Human Sleep: Clinical Applications. New York, John Wiley & Sons, 1974.

# PATIENT 12

## A 34-year-old man with sleep disturbance

A 34-year-old man complained of excessive daytime sleepiness despite sleeping at least 9 hours per night. On awakening, he never felt refreshed. He had no bed partners and lived by himself.

*Physical Examination:*   Normal.

*Sleep Study:*   A total sleep time (minutes of stages 1–4 and REM sleep) of 420 minutes was noted.

*Figure:*   Three hundred events such as the one illustrated below were recorded.

*Question:*   How can these events explain why the patient is sleepy despite the normal total sleep time?

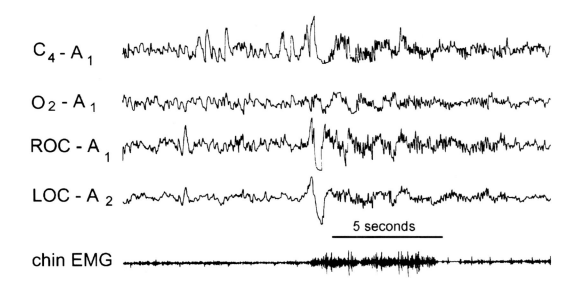

*Answer:* Frequent arousals result in sleep fragmentation and daytime sleepiness.

*Discussion:* Arousal from sleep denotes a transition from a state of sleep to wakefulness. Frequent arousals can cause daytime sleepiness by shortening the total amount of sleep. The EEG will show brief changes (1–5 seconds) consistent with wakefulness and then a rapid return to a pattern consistent with sleep. A given epoch (30-second period) may be classified as sleep despite the brief "micro-awakening." Considerable experimental evidence suggests that frequent, brief arousals prevent sleep from being restorative even if the total amount of sleep is normal. Thus, the restorative function of sleep depends on **continuity** as well as **duration.**

Many disorders that are associated with excessive daytime sleepiness also are associated with frequent, brief arousals. For example, patients with obstructive sleep apnea frequently have arousals coincident with apnea/hypopnea termination. Periodic limb movements in sleep may trigger brief arousals and cause daytime sleepiness. Therefore, determination of the frequency of arousals has become a standard part of the analysis of sleep architecture during sleep testing.

The criteria used to define arousal have been somewhat variable. A preliminary report from the Atlas Task Force of the American Sleep Disorders Association (ASDA) recommended that an arousal be scored in nonrapid eye movement (NREM) sleep when there is "an abrupt shift in EEG frequency, which may include theta, alpha, and/or frequencies > 16 Hz, but not spindles," of 3-second or longer duration. The 3-second duration was chosen for methodological reasons; shorter arousals may also have physiologic importance. To be scored as an arousal, the shift in EEG frequency must follow at least 10 continuous seconds of any stage of sleep.

Arousals in NREM sleep may occur without a concurrent increase in the submental EMG amplitude. In REM sleep, however, the required EEG changes must be accompanied by a concurrent increase in EMG amplitude for an arousal to be scored. This extra requirement was added because spontaneous bursts of alpha rhythm are a fairly common occurrence in REM (but not NREM) sleep.

Finally, according to these preliminary recommendations, increases in the chin EMG in the absence of EEG changes are not considered evidence of arousal in either NREM or REM sleep. Similarly, sudden bursts of delta (slow wave) activity in the absence of other changes do not qualify as evidence of arousal. Because cortical EEG changes must be present to meet the above definition, such events also are termed **electrocortical arousals.** Note that the preliminary ASDA guidelines represent a consensus on events likely to be of physiologic significance. The committee recognized that other EEG phenomena, such as delta bursts, also can represent evidence of arousal in certain contexts.

The frequency of arousals usually is computed as the **arousal index** (number of arousals per hour of sleep). Relatively little data is available to define a normal range for the arousal index. Normal young adults studied after adaptation nights frequently have an arousal index of five per hour or less. In one study, however, normal subjects of variable ages had a mean arousal index of 20 per hour, and the arousal index was found to increase with age.

In the present patient, a delta wave followed by speeding of the EEG for more than 3 seconds and an increase in the chin EMG amplitude are present (see figure). The arousal index (number of arousals/hour of sleep) for this case is

$$[300/(420/60)] = 42.8/hr.$$

Excessive daytime sleepiness generally is associated with an arousal index of > 25/hour.

## Clinical Pearls

1. Frequent, brief electrocortical arousals can result in excessive daytime sleepiness even if the total sleep time is normal.

2. The scoring of arousals is based on changes in the EEG in NREM sleep or the EEG and chin EMG in REM sleep.

3. The arousal index (arousals per hour of sleep) is an important index of sleep fragmentation and the restorative quality of sleep.

## REFERENCES

1. Bonnet MH: Performance and sleepiness as a function of frequency and placement of sleep disruption. Psychophysiology 1986; 23:263–71.
2. American Sleep Disorders Association—The Atlas Task Force: EEG arousals: Scoring rules and examples. Sleep 1992; 15:174–184.
3. Roehrs T, Merlotti L, Petrucelli N, et al: Experimental sleep fragmentation. Sleep 1994; 17:438–443.
4. Mathur R, Douglas NJ: Frequency of EEG arousals from nocturnal sleep in normal subjects. Sleep 1995; 18:330–333.

## Additional Sleep Staging Rules

The EEG, EOG and chin EMG characteristics of the different stages of sleep are discussed in Patients 1–12 and summarized in Appendix 2. There are additional scoring rules to handle special situations. These rules are necessary because K complexes, sleep spindles, and REMs are episodic.

The **three-minute rule** concerns stage 2 sleep. This rule, as outlined by the classic sleep staging manual of Rechtschaffen and Kales, states that if the period of time **between spindles or K complexes** is shorter than 3 minutes *and* if the intervening sleep would otherwise meet criteria for stage 1 (less than 50% alpha activity) with no evidence of intervening arousal, then this period of sleep is scored as stage 2. If the period of time is 3 minutes or longer, then the intervening sleep is scored as stage 1.

**Figure 1** (below) shows five epochs (30 seconds each) of sleep, with K complexes (*K*) in epochs 69 and 73. The central and occipital EEG tracings in epochs 70–72 are assumed not to contain sleep spindles, K complexes, or evidence of arousal. The time between the K complexes is less than 3 minutes; therefore, this intervening sleep is scored as stage 2.

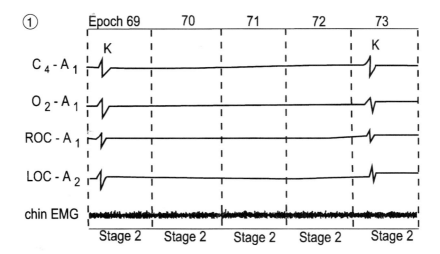

Staging of REM sleep also requires special rules (**REM rules**) to define the beginning and end, because REMs are episodic, and the three indicators of stage REM (EEG, EOG, EMG) may not change to (or from) the REM-like pattern simultaneously. Rechtschaffen and Kales recommend that any section of the record that is *contiguous* with stage REM and displays a relatively low-voltage, mixed-frequency EEG be scored as stage REM *regardless* of whether REMs are present, providing the EMG is at the stage REM level. To be **REM-like**, the EEG must not contain spindles, K complexes, or slow waves.

**Figure 2** (next page) shows four epochs, with a K complex in epoch 69 and REMs in epoch 72. After epoch 69 there are no K complexes or sleep spindles, and the EMG falls to the REM level during the last part of epoch 70. Hence, epoch 71 meets criteria for REM sleep except that there are no eye movements. Epoch 71 is scored as stage REM because it is contiguous with an epoch of unequivocal REM sleep (epoch 72). Epoch 70 also does not contain K complexes or sleep spindles, but is scored as stage 2 by the three-minute rule.

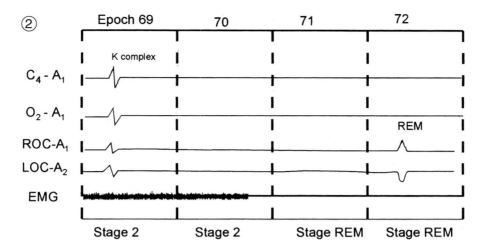

These rules are more difficult to apply if arousals break the continuity of sleep. With respect to the three-minute rule, sleep following an arousal is scored according to its nature. In **Figure 3** (below), a brief arousal occurs at the end of epoch 71 (alpha waves in EEG, increased EMG). The sleep before the arousal is scored by the three-minute rule as stage 2. Epoch 71 is scored as stage 2 because most of the epoch is

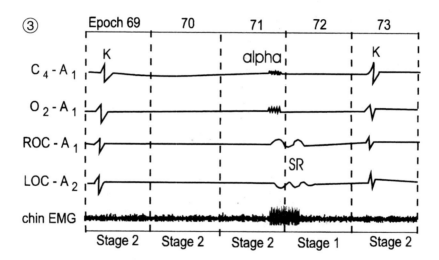

stage 2. Epoch 72 is scored as stage 1 because there are no K complexes or spindles, and the slow rolling eye movements (*SR*) following the arousal are more characteristic of stage 1 than stage 2.

In REM sleep, bursts of alpha waves are common and do not signify an arousal *unless the chin EMG amplitude also increases*. Deciding how to score an epoch of sleep with a REM-like EEG/EMG but no REMs that is separated from contiguous unequivocal REM sleep by an intervening arousal is sometimes difficult. The decision in this case is between stage REM and stage 1 sleep (with an EMG at the REM level). The EEGs of stage 1 and REM sleep are similar but subtle differences are present:

| REM sleep EEG | Stage 1 EEG |
| --- | --- |
| Saw-tooth waves may occur | No saw-tooth waves |
| Alpha waves 1–2 Hz slower than wakefulness | Vertex sharp waves may occur |

A very brief arousal and/or the presence of saw-tooth waves in the sleep following the arousal is evidence that the sleep after the arousal is still stage REM (until definite evidence for another sleep stage is noted). Conversely, a prolonged arousal (with persistent alpha waves) followed by slow rolling eye movements is evidence that the arousal induced a change from stage REM to stage 1 sleep. Sharp waves or **incipient spindles** (shorter than 0.5-second duration) on the EEG also are evidence for stage 1. If stage 1 is scored following the arousal, all subsequent epochs are scored as stage 1 until evidence of another sleep stage is noted (spindles or K complexes—stage 2).

In **Figure 4** (below), a brief arousal signified by EEG alpha waves and an EMG increase occurs at the end of epoch 70. Epoch 70 is scored as REM because the majority of the epoch is REM-like, and it is contiguous with an epoch of unequivocal REM sleep. Epoch 72 contains a K complex and is scored as stage 2.

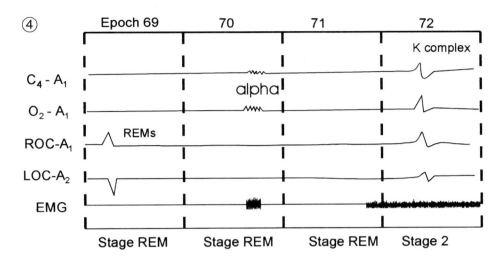

Epoch 71 is scored as stage REM because the arousal was brief and the EEG and EMG are REM-like for most of the epoch.

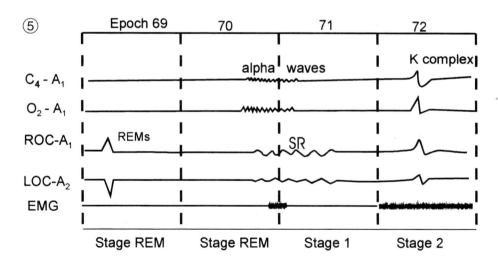

An epoch containing slow rolling eye movements and following a prolonged arousal is illustrated in **Figure 5**. This epoch is labeled stage 1.

The reader is referred to reference 1 for special rules governing the unusual case in which spindles occur during REM sleep

## REFERENCES

1. Rechtschaffen A, Kales A (eds): A Manual of Standardized Terminology Techniques and Scoring System for Sleep Stages of Human Sleep. Los Angeles, Brain Information Service/Brain Research Institute, UCLA, 1968.
2. Carskadon MA, Rechtschaffen A: Monitoring and staging human sleep. *In* Kryger MH, Roth T, Dement WC (eds): Principles and Practice of Sleep Medicine. Philadelphia, WB Saunders Co., 1994, pp 943–960.

# PATIENT 13

**A 30-year-old man with severe snoring and occasional breathing lapses**

A 35-year-old man was evaluated for a history of loud snoring and possible sleep apnea. Below is a schematic representation of five epochs of the patient's sleep. Assume that epoch 69 is stage 2 sleep (a K complex is shown). No K complexes, sleep spindles, or arousals are noted in epochs 70–75. The EEG in these epochs otherwise meets criteria for stage 2.

*Question:* What sleep stage is scored in epochs 70–75?

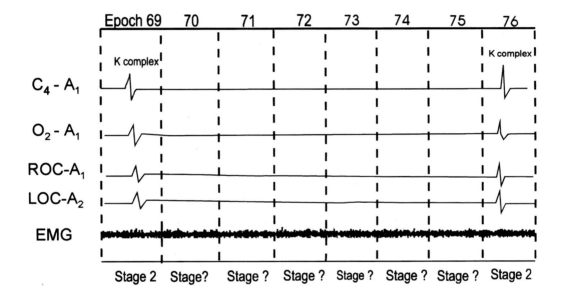

*Answer:* Epochs 70–75 are scored as stage 1 because the interval between K complexes is longer than 3 minutes.

*Discussion:* Stage 2 is characterized by the presence of either sleep spindles, which are bursts of 12–14 Hz activity, or K complexes, which are large-amplitude, biphasic EEG deflections. To qualify as stage 2, an epoch also must contain less than 20% of slow (delta) wave EEG activity. Slow waves are large-amplitude ($>$ 75 microvolts) deflections with a frequency of $<$ 2 Hz. K complexes and sleep spindles are episodic and may not occur in each epoch.

According to the three-minute rule, if the period of time **between spindles or K complexes** is shorter than 3 minutes *and* if the intervening sleep would otherwise meet criteria for stage 1 (less than 50% alpha activity) with no evidence of intervening arousal, then this period of sleep is scored as stage 2. If the period of time is 3 minutes or longer, then the intervening sleep is scored as stage 1.

In the current patient, the time between intervening K complexes in epochs 69 and 76 is longer than 3 minutes; therefore, the intervening sleep is scored as stage 1. The 3-minute time frame is somewhat arbitrary. It was selected based on the spindle-to-spindle and K complex-to-K complex intervals typically observed.

## Clinical Pearl

Use the three-minute rule to stage sleep occurring *between* K complexes or spindles which would otherwise meet criteria for stage 2 sleep except that K complexes or sleep spindles are absent.

## REFERENCES

1. Rechtschaffen A, Kales A (eds): A Manual of Standardized Terminology Techniques and Scoring System for Sleep Stages of Human Sleep. Los Angeles, Brain Information Service/Brain Research Institute, UCLA, 1968.
2. Carskadon MA, Rechtschaffen A: Monitoring and staging human sleep. *In* Kryger MH, Roth T. Dement WC (eds): Principles and Practice of Sleep Medicine. Philadelphia, WB Saunders Co., 1994, pp 943–960.

# PATIENT 14

## A 35-year-old woman experiencing uncontrollable, brief episodes of sleep

A 35-year-old woman was evaluated for possible narcolepsy. A schematic representation of eight epochs of the patient's sleep is shown. A K complex occurs in epoch 69 (stage 2 sleep). The chin EMG amplitude decreases at the start of epoch 70 and briefly increases at the end of epoch 75. A REM occurs in epoch 76.

*Question:* What sleep stage is scored in epochs 70–75?

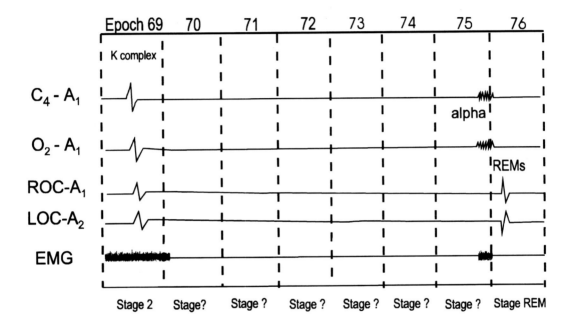

*Answer:* Epochs 70–75 are scored as stage REM.

*Discussion:* Stage REM is characterized by a low-amplitude, mixed-frequency EEG and an absence of sleep spindles and K complexes. The eye movement channels show REMs and the chin EMG is relatively reduced (equal to or lower than the lowest level of NREM sleep). These EEG, EOG, and EMG characteristics may not all start or end at the same time. REMs are episodic and may not occur in all epochs of REM sleep. Therefore, the **REM rule** is useful for scoring epochs that do not contain REMs: Any section of record contiguous with stage REM in which the EEG is relatively low-voltage and mixed-frequency (no spindles, K complexes) is scored stage REM *regardless* of whether or not REMs are present, providing the EMG is at the stage REM level. The rule holds for both the beginning and end of a segment of REM sleep. During sleep scoring, once unequivocal REM sleep is noted, the examiner should work backward to determine if preceding epochs meet the above criteria for REM sleep (see Fundamentals 6).

At the transition from NREM to REM sleep, the above REM rule takes precedence over the three-minute rule. However, when an arousal separates the end of unequivocal stages 2–4 NREM sleep and the beginning of unequivocal REM sleep, the scoring of the intervening sleep prior to the arousal is more problematic. The arousal may or may not signify a change in sleep stage. The EEGs of stage 1 and REM sleep can look similar. If the EMG of the period in question is at the REM level, the decision is between stage 1, stage 2 (based on the three-minute rule), or stage REM. The scoring manual recommends scoring sleep **between the last spindle or K complex and an arousal** as stage 2 if the time duration is less than 3 minutes. If the segment is *longer than 3 minutes,* the sleep is scored as *stage REM* (rather than stage 1—an exception to the three-minute rule).

In the example below, note the arousal at the end of epoch 72. Sleep after the arousal is scored on the basis of the REM rule. Sleep before the arousal is scored according to a combination of the three-minute rule and the REM rule.

On the other hand, if an arousal is prolonged or followed by an obvious change to stage 1 sleep (slow rolling eye movements), then the sleep following the arousal is scored as stage 1 until unequivocal evidence for another sleep stage is present. The presence of saw-tooth waves favors stage REM.

In the present case, epoch 76 is unequivocal REM sleep (see figure on page 40). Epochs 70–75 have a REM-like EEG and EMG except for a brief arousal at the end of epoch 75. The choices for epochs 70–75 include stages 1, 2, or REM sleep. As the interval after the last K complex (epoch 69) exceeds 3 minutes, it is not stage 2 sleep. Thus, the choices are stage 1 or REM sleep. Epochs 70–75 look like REM sleep, except for the absence of REMs, and are contiguous with unequivocal REM sleep. Therefore, they are scored as stage REM.

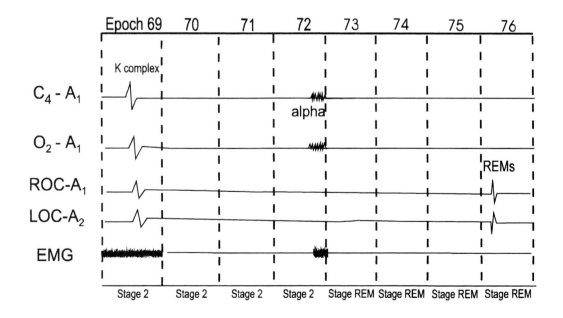

# Clinical Pearls

1. Sleep that is contiguous with an epoch of unequivocal REM sleep and meets criteria for stage REM, except that no REMs are present, is scored as stage REM (REM rule).

2. To identify the start of an episode of REM sleep, first identify an epoch of unequivocal REM (REM-like EEG, REMs present, EMG at REM level) and then work backward using the REM rule. To determine the end of an episode of REM, work forward from an epoch of unequivocal REM sleep.

3. When a brief arousal separates unequivocal stages 2–4 NREM sleep and the start of REM sleep, epochs with a REM-like EEG and EMG prior to the arousal are scored as stage 2 if the arousal occurred less than 3 minutes after the last sleep spindle or K complex. Otherwise, the segment is considered stage REM sleep (combination of three-minute rule and REM rule).

## REFERENCES

1. Rechtschaffen A, Kales A (eds): A Manual of Standardized Terminology Techniques and Scoring System for Sleep Stages of Human Sleep. Los Angeles, Brain Information Service/Brain Research Institute, UCLA, 1968.
2. Carskadon MA, Rechtschaffen A: Monitoring and staging human sleep. *In* Kryger MH, Roth T, Dement WC (eds): Principles and Practice of Sleep Medicine. Philadelphia, WB Saunders Co., 1994, pp 943–960.

## Sleep Architecture Definitions

A number of variables have been defined to help characterize the quantity, composition, and quality of sleep.

Standard Sleep Variables

| | |
|---|---|
| Time in bed (TIB) | Monitoring period—lights out to lights on |
| Movement time | Epochs in which stage is indeterminant due to artifact |
| Total sleep time (TST) | Total minutes of sleep (stages 1–4 and REM) |
| Wake after sleep onset (WASO) | Minutes of wake after initial sleep onset and before the final awakening |
| Sleep period time (SPT) | TST + WASO |
| Sleep efficiency (%) | (TST * 100) / TIB |
| Sleep latency (min) | Time from *lights out* to the first epoch of sleep |
| REM latency (min) | Time from *sleep onset* to the first epoch of REM sleep |

Any condition that results in frequent or prolonged awakenings (sleep-maintenance insomnia) results in an increased WASO. Even if the WASO is small, it is possible to have a low sleep efficiency if the final awakening occurs early in the monitoring period (early-morning awakening).

The sleep latency reflects how rapidly the patient fell asleep. Patients with sleep-onset insomnia (difficulty in initiating sleep) typically have a long sleep latency (more than 30 minutes). Some sleep laboratories also compute the latency to stage 2 sleep. The REM latency is the time from the first sleep (not lights out) to the first epoch of REM sleep. The normal REM latency, usually 70–120 minutes, can be reduced in narcolepsy, sleep apnea, depression, and after withdrawal of REM-suppressing medications. REM latency is discussed in Patient 16 and Fundamentals 9.

The division of total sleep time among the sleep stages often is called the **sleep architecture.** A common approach is to express the minutes spent in each stage of sleep as a percentage of either TST or SPT. There are few widely accepted normative values for sleep architecture. In this book, the normal ranges are the mean ± standard deviations as presented by Williams, et al., and the values are age- and sex-dependent. The fraction of slow wave sleep (stages 3 and 4) decreases considerably with age, while the amount of sleep stages 1 and 2 and WASO increase. The fraction of REM sleep changes little after young adulthood. The table on the following page shows typical values for normal sleep at two different ages and in a patient with severe obstructive sleep apnea.

## Key Point

---

The normal ranges for many parameters of sleep architecture, particularly the amount of slow wave sleep, are age-dependent.

---

| | Normal Sleep (% SPT) | | Obstructive Sleep Apnea (% SPT) |
|---|---|---|---|
| | Age 20 | Age 60 | |
| Wake | 1 | 8 | 10 |
| Stage 1 | 5 | 10 | 25 |
| Stage 2 | 45 | 57 | 55 |
| Stages 3 and 4 | 21 | 2 | 0 |
| Stage REM | 28 | 23 | 10 |

## REFERENCES

1. Williams RL, Karacan I, Hursch CJ: Electroencephalography (EEG) of Human Sleep: Clinical Applications. New York, John Wiley & Sons, 1974, pages 49–60.
2. Bonnet MH: Sleep deprivation. *In* Kryger MH, Roth T, Dement W (eds): Principles and Practice of Sleep Medicine. Philadelphia, WB Saunders, 1994, pp 50–67.

# PATIENT 15

## A 23-year-old man with difficulty sleeping

A 23-year-old man was monitored because he complained of poor sleep. He admitted to the sleep technician that he had taken his usual benzodiazepine sleeping pill before arriving in the sleep laboratory because he feared that otherwise he would be unable to sleep.

***Physical Examination:*** Normal.

***Sleep Study***

| | | | |
|---|---|---|---|
| Time in bed (monitoring time) | 450 min (430–454) | Sleep Stages | % SPT |
| Total sleep time (TST) | 428.5 min (405–434) | Stage Wake | 1 (0–1) |
| Sleep period time (SPT) | 432.5 min (410–439) | Stage 1 | 6 (3–6) |
| WASO | 4 min | Stage 2 | 71 (40–51) |
| Sleep efficiency | .95 (.91–.99) | Stages 3 and 4 | 7.8 (16–26) |
| Sleep latency | 5 min (3–26) | Stage REM | 15.2 (22–34) |
| REM latency | 120 min (78–99) | | |

( ) = normal values for age; sleep efficiency = (TST * 100) / TIB

***Question:*** What is abnormal about the sleep architecture?

*Answer:* The percentages of stages 3, 4, and REM sleep are reduced, and the amount of stage 2 sleep is increased. The REM latency also is mildly increased.

*Discussion:* Sleep architecture can be altered by several factors, including sleep disorders, coexistent medical disorders, prior sleep for the last week (sleep deprivation), medications (or withdrawal), beverages, and exposure to a novel sleep environment (the first-night effect). It is essential to know the patient's normal sleep patterns and recent sleep history (sleep diary). An earlier-than-normal bedtime during the sleep study can increase the sleep latency. A later-than-normal bedtime can decrease the REM latency. Prior sleep deprivation can cause a rebound in the amount of slow wave and REM sleep.

While it is important to know the patient's medication intake, it is equally important to know if usual medications (or beverages) were not taken (see table). Abrupt withdrawal of certain medications can profoundly affect sleep architecture. Withdrawal of stimulants or tricyclic antidepressants (REM suppressors) can cause a rebound in the amount of REM sleep and/or shorten the REM latency. Abrupt withdrawal of medications decreasing a given sleep stage can cause a rebound in the amount of that sleep stage.

### Common Medications Affecting Sleep Architecture

| Decrease REM sleep | Increase REM sleep |
|---|---|
| Ethanol | Nefazadone |
| Tricyclic antidepressants | Reserpine |
| Trazadone | Withdrawal of REM-suppressing medications |
| Selective serotonin reuptake inhibitors | |
| MAO inhibitors | |
| Lithium | |
| Amphetamines | Decrease SWS |
| Methylphenidate | Benzodiazepines |
| Clonidine | |

SWS = slow wave sleep

In the current case, the total amount of sleep and sleep efficiency were normal. However, the amounts of stages 3, 4, and REM sleep were reduced. This change is not unusual with benzodiazepines, which tend to decrease slow wave sleep and, to a lesser degree, REM sleep. The amounts of stage 2 sleep and sleep spindle activity were increased tremendously.

## Clinical Pearls

1. Analysis of sleep architecture can provide important insight into the causes of sleep disturbance.

2. A medication history (including over-the-counter medications) and a history of the pattern of sleep for several days prior to the sleep study are essential when analyzing sleep architecture.

3. The lights-out time should always mimic the patient's usual bedtime, if possible.

## REFERENCES

1. Williams RL, Karacan I, Hursch CJ: Electroencephalography (EEG) of Human Sleep: Clinical Applications. New York, John Wiley & Sons, 1974, pages 49–60.
2. Bonnet MH: Sleep deprivation. *In* Kryger MH, Roth T, Dement W (eds): Principles and Practice of Sleep Medicine. Philadelphia, WB Saunders, 1994, pp 50–67.
3. Obermeyer WH, Benca RM: Effects of drugs on sleep. Neurol Clin (Sleep Disorders II) 1996; 14:827–840.

# PATIENT 16

## A 25-year-old man with daytime sleepiness and fatigue

A 25-year-old man developed daytime sleepiness and fatigue during the last year. He had broken up with his girlfriend and was quite depressed. He had trouble waking up and getting out of bed in the morning. Recently, his primary care physician began him on 20 mg of fluoxetine every morning. There was no history of cataplexy (muscle weakness triggered by emotion) or sleep paralysis. The patient had never been told that he snored.

***Physical Examination:*** Normal.

***Sleep Study***

| | | Sleep Stages | % SPT |
|---|---|---|---|
| Time in bed (monitoring time) | 457.5 min (430–454) | | |
| Total sleep time (TST) | 406.5 min (405–434) | | |
| Sleep period time (SPT) | 432.5 min (410–439) | Stage Wake | 6 (0–1) |
| WASO | 26 min | Stage 1 | 8 (3–6) |
| Sleep efficiency | .89 (.91–.99) | Stage 2 | 49 (40–51) |
| Sleep latency | 15 min (3–26) | Stages 3 and 4 | 25 (16–26) |
| REM latency | 140 min (78–99) | Stage REM | 12 (22–34) |

( ) = normal values for age; sleep efficiency = (TST * 100) / TIB

***Questions:*** What is abnormal about the sleep architecture? What is the most likely cause?

**Diagnosis:** Prolonged REM latency and decreased REM sleep probably secondary to medication.

**Discussion:** The **REM latency** is the time from the first epoch of sleep until the first epoch of stage REM—usually about 70–120 minutes, depending on the age of the patient. Alterations in REM latency can be due to the presence of disease processes, but many other factors increase or decrease this time period as well (see table below).

Narcolepsy, a disorder causing excessive daytime sleepiness, often is associated with a very short REM latency (10–15 minutes) referred to as **sleep-onset REM.** However, this finding is neither specific for nor always present in narcolepsy. Obstructive sleep apnea or any other cause of REM deprivation also may be associated with a short REM latency. Depression typically causes only modest shortening (40–50 minutes); however, depression can have an effect as extreme as narcolepsy.

The propensity for REM sleep is associated with the daily (circadian) change in body temperature. By delaying bedtime, the time of sleep onset may move closer to the time of initial REM sleep. Usually this is not a problem, unless the lights-out time is much later than the patient's normal bedtime. Abrupt withdrawal of REM-suppressing medications also can reduce REM latency.

A medication history is essential for proper interpretation of the sleep study results. If a diagnosis of narcolepsy is suspected, patients usually are asked to stop medications altering REM latency for at least 2 weeks prior to the sleep study, because changes in REM latency are an essential part of diagnostic criteria. In other cases, prolonged withdrawal of such medications may not be possible. A common mistake is to withhold REM-suppressing medications just before the sleep study. This may cause a rebound in the amount of REM sleep and possibly shorten the REM latency.

In the present case, the sleep architecture is fairly normal except for the prolonged REM latency, decreased amount of REM sleep, and slightly decreased sleep efficiency (increased stage W as % of SPT). The changes in REM sleep are most likely secondary to the use of fluoxetine (Prozac), a selective serotonin reuptake inhibitor (SSRI) antidepressant. Sleep efficiency often is decreased in patients with depression. In some of these patients, treatment with SSRIs improves sleep quality. In others, the medications themselves disturb sleep. However, when this patient was seen for discussion of the sleep study results, he claimed to be feeling better and denied any symptoms of daytime sleepiness.

### Common Factors Altering REM Latency

| Short REM latency | Long REM latency |
|---|---|
| Narcolepsy | First-night effect |
| Prior REM deprivation (e.g., sleep apnea) | Medical disease (COPD, chronic pain syndromes) |
| Depression, schizophrenia | Ethanol |
| Withdrawal of REM suppressants | REM-suppressant medications (tricyclic antidepressants, trazadone, SSRIs [fluoxetine, sertaline], lithium, stimulants [amphetamine, methylphenidate], clonidine) |
| Later-than-normal bedtime | |

COPD = chronic obstructive pulmonary disease, SSRI = selective serotonin reuptake inhibitor

## Clinical Pearls

1. The REM latency is the time from the first epoch of sleep until the first epoch of stage REM.

2. A short REM latency is associated with withdrawal of REM-suppressant medications as well as several sleep disorders, including narcolepsy, sleep apnea, and depression.

### REFERENCES
1. Standards of Practice Committee, American Sleep Disorders Association: The clinical use of the multiple sleep latency test. Sleep 1992; 15:268–276.
2. Obermeyer WH, Benca RM: Effects of drugs on sleep. Neurol Clin (Sleep Disorders II) 1996; 14:827–840.

## Polysomnography

Polysomnography is the term used to denote the continuous and simultaneous recording of multiple variables during sleep.

### Routinely Monitored Variables

| Variables | Purpose | Methods |
|---|---|---|
| EEG (central, occipital), right and left EOG, chin EMG | Detect the presence and stage of sleep | Scalp/face surface electrodes |
| EKG | Measures cardiac rate and rhythm | |
| Airflow (nasal and oral) | Detects apnea and hypopnea | Thermistors, thermocouples Pneumotachograph in mask, nasal pressure |
| Respiratory effort | Detects respiratory effort | Respiratory movement— chest and abdominal bands (piezoelectric, impedance) Intercostal EMG Esophageal pressure |
| Anterior tibialis EMG | Detects periodic leg movements | Separate channel for each leg or one common channel Alternate: leg movement transducers |
| Arterial oxygen saturation | Measures $SaO_2$ Detects desaturation | Pulse oximetry |

EEG = electroencephalogram, EOG = electro-oculogram, EMG = electromyogram, EKG = electrocardiogram

A typical twelve-channel recording montage (the set of variables being recorded):

| Channel | Variable | Channel | Variable |
|---|---|---|---|
| 1 | Central EEG | 7 | Right leg EMG |
| 2 | Occipital EEG | 8 | Left leg EMG |
| 3 | Right EOG | 9 | Airflow |
| 4 | Left EOG | 10 | Chest movement |
| 5 | Chin EMG | 11 | Abdominal movement |
| 6 | EKG 12 | | $SaO_2$ |

These variables usually are recorded on a polygraph, using a standard paper speed of 10 mm/sec, and/or digitally acquired on a computer system.

Sleep monitoring also requires continuous **visual and auditory monitoring** of the patient. This is especially important to detect changes in the sleeping posture (supine—lateral decubitus) and allows the patient to signal the technician if assistance is needed. Visual monitoring generally is accomplished via a low-light camera system with video monitors in the recording room. Video recording is needed for evaluation of parasomnias. Systems are available to allow synchronization of the polysomnographic recording and the video record. Where evaluation for possible nocturnal seizures is a consideration, a full EEG montage also should be recorded.

The signal from each variable recorded enters the system via an amplifier that must be correctly adjusted (sensitivity, low filter, high filter, polarity). EEG, EOG, and EMG channel AC amplifiers are calibrated with a standard voltage signal (usually 50 micovolts) that is available by pushing a button on the polygraph. The sensitivity is adjusted so that the desired output signal (pen deflection) for a given voltage input is obtained (see table below). Low- and high-frequency filters attenuate signals with frequencies outside (below and above, respectively) the desired range of recorded frequency. While filters reduce artifact from unwanted signals, they also can impair recording of desired variables. For example, the low filter must be set high enough so that slow waves and eye-movement signals are not attenuated.

### Polysomnograph Calibration

|  | Sensitivity | Low Filter (Hz) | High Filter (Hz) |
|---|---|---|---|
| EEG (central, occipital) | 5 μv/mm | 0.3 | 30 |
| EOG | 5 μv/mm | 0.3 | 30 |
| EMG (chin, legs) | 5–10 μv/mm | 10.0 | 30 |
| EKG | 50 μv/mm | 0.3 | 30 |

Filter settings are given as ½ amplitude frequency (the amplitude of a signal at this frequency is attenuated by 50%).

Deflections from a calibration signal of 50 microvolts are shown in the sample tracing at right. The smaller signal in the chin EMG channel is secondary to the higher low-frequency (LF) setting.

A **biocalibration procedure** is performed while signals are acquired with the patient connected to the monitoring equipment. This procedure permits checking of amplifier settings, integrity of monitoring leads/transducers, and recording abilities of airflow and respiratory effort transducers as well as leg EMG. It also provides a record of the patient's EEG and eye movements during wakefulness with eyes closed and open.

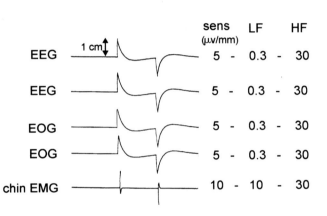

| Biocalibration | What To Check (Technician and Scorer) |
|---|---|
| Eyes closed | Alpha EEG activity, slow rolling eye movements |
| Eyes open | Attenuation of alpha EEG activity, pattern of eyes-open wakefulness |
| Look right, look left; look up, look down; blink eyes | Integrity, amplitude, polarity of eye channels, pattern of REMs |
| Grit teeth | Chin EMG<br>Adjust chin EMG gain so that some activity is present during relaxed wakefulness |
| Breathe in, breathe out | Airflow channel working<br>Airflow, chest, abdomen tracings should have same polarity and be of reasonable amplitude<br>Direction of inspiration (upward deflection) |
| Hold breath | Apnea occurrence |
| Wiggle right toe, left toe | Leg movements |

The next figure is a sample tracing during eye movement biocalibration. The patient has been asked to hold the head still and look in different directions (*Left, Right, Down, Up*) and then blink (*B*) the eyes.

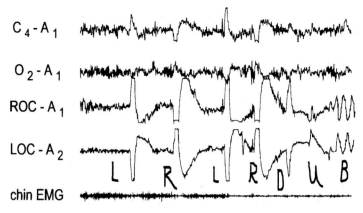

Next, respiratory channels (recording airflow and chest/abdominal movement) are adjusted so that tidal breathing induces a reasonable deflection in all three channels (see figure below) with the same polarity (inspiration up, *arrows*). Amplifier gain (sensitivity) and chest/abdominal band positions may need adjustment. The patient is asked to breathe in and hold the breath to simulate apnea, then resume normal breathing.

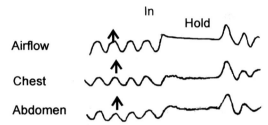

The patient is then asked to wiggle the right and left toes to check the ability of the anterior tibialis EMG to detect leg movements (see tracing below).

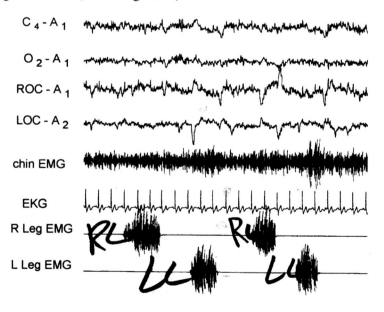

## REFERENCES

1. Harris CD: Recording montage. *In* Shepard JW (ed): Atlas of Sleep Medicine. Mount Kisco, NY, Futura Publishing Co., 1991, pp 1–5.
2. Introduction to the Polysomnograph (video/manual). Available from: Synapse Media, 4702 Cloudcrest Drive, Medford, Oregon; Tel. 800/949-8195.

# PATIENT 17

## A 30-year-old man having difficulty staying awake during the day

A 30-year-old man was studied to evaluate complaints of excessive daytime sleepiness. An artifact was noted in his recording. The EEG leads $C_4$–$A_1$ and $O_2A_1$, both eye leads (ROC-$A_1$ and LOC-$A_2$), a chin EMG, and an EKG lead were monitored. After the initial artifact was noted, the EEG leads were "double referenced" ($C_4$-$A_{12}$ and $O_2$-$A_{12}$), meaning the combined leads $A_1$ and $A_2$ were used as the reference for the central and occipital EEG derivations (see figure).

***Question:*** What is the artifact?

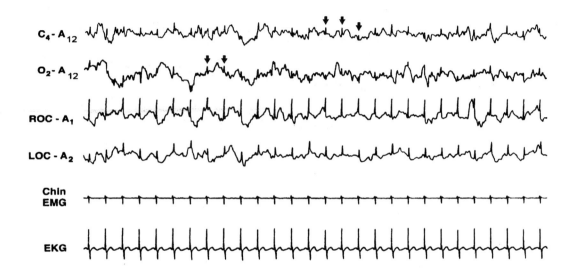

*Answer:*   It is an EKG artifact, minimized by double referencing.

*Discussion:*   The **EKG artifact** is one of the most common and easily recognizable recording artifacts. It can be identified by sharp deflections in the signals of affected channels corresponding exactly in time to the QRS of the EKG. Fortunately, this artifact does not interfere a great deal with visual sleep staging, as the artifact does not mimic usual EEG patterns. The artifact can be minimized by placing the mastoid electrodes sufficiently high (behind the ear) so that they are over bone instead of neck tissue (fat). **Double refer-**
**encing** to both mastoid electrodes also can minimize EKG artifact. This works because if the EKG voltage vector is toward one mastoid, it is away from the other. Hence, the EKG component of the two signals ($C_4$-$A_1$ and $C_4$-$A_2$) tend to cancel each other out.

In the present case, EKG artifact is prominent in the eye leads and chin EMG (see figure). It is less prominent in the EEG leads (*arrows*) because of double referencing. The artifact is larger than desirable, but the record still can be scored.

## Clinical Pearls

1. EKG artifact can be easily recognized as sharp deflections in the affected leads corresponding to the QRS complex in the EKG lead.

2. Proper application of the mastoid electrodes and double referencing can prevent or minimize this artifact.

## REFERENCE

1. Harris CD, Dexter D: Recording artifacts. *In* Shepard JW (ed): Atlas of Sleep Medicine. Mount Kisco, New York, Futura Publishing, 1991, pp 50–51.

# PATIENT 18

## A 25-year-old man complaining of excessive daytime sleepiness

A 25-year-old man was being monitored for complaints of excessive daytime sleepiness. After several minutes of recording, the patient was noted to scratch his chin, and a humming noise was heard from the polygraph pens. A portion of the tracing is shown below.

*Question:* What artifact is responsible for the humming?

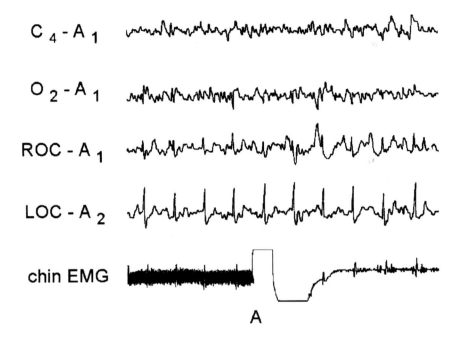

**Answer:** There is a sixty-cycle artifact in the chin EMG channel.

**Discussion:** Sixty-cycle artifact is a common problem in sleep-study recording. It is caused by 60-Hz electrical activity from power lines and can be minimized by correct application of electrodes and proper design of the sleep laboratory. When prominent, the artifact causes a characteristic humming of the pens as they oscillate at 60 cycles per second. The artifact usually is easy to spot in the EEG and EOG leads, but may be more subtle in the EMG leads. Most EEG amplifiers have a 60-cycle notch amplifier to minimize the recording of this signal. If a 60-cycle filter is out (disengaged), the amplitude of the artifact increases tremendously (see figure below). If the paper speed is increased to 60 millimeters per second, then there will be 10 cycles in 1 centimeter (1/6 sec).

EEG amplifiers are alternating current (AC)–coupled, which allows them to record low-voltage EEG activity (50 microvolts) while rejecting high-voltage direct current (DC) activity. Differential amplifiers can record low-voltage physiologic signals by amplifying the difference in voltage between two elec-

trodes while rejecting the common-mode signal consisting of higher-voltage, 60-Hz, background activity. When recording the voltage difference between two electrodes, the background AC activity is rejected only if the electrode impedances are low and fairly equal. If one electrode is faulty (disconnected or high impedance), then the 60-Hz AC activity will be more prominent. Although most AC amplifiers have notch filters to minimize AC activity, these filters may not prevent 60-Hz activity from being prominent when electrode impedances are very different. The ideal impedance of electrodes is below 5 kilohms. Electrode impedance should be checked by the sleep technician after electrode application.

In the present case, when the patient scratched his chin he moved one of the EMG electrodes, altering its impedance (see figure on page 54, point A). The problem was fixed (see tracing subsequent to A) by switching to a spare chin EMG electrode that had been placed in the submental area. Note the considerable EKG artifact in the left eye channel in this tracing.

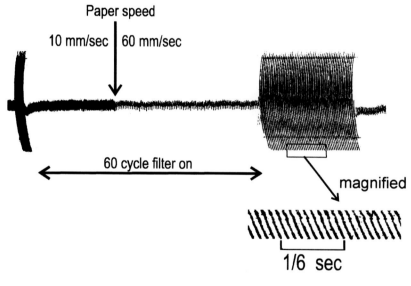

Paper speed

10 mm/sec | 60 mm/sec

60 cycle filter on

magnified

1/6 sec

## Clinical Pearls

1. Sixty-cycle artifact causes a humming in the recording pens.
2. Causes of sixty-cycle artifact include high and unequal electrode impedances (faulty attachment), lead failure, and interference from nearby power lines.
3. Sixty-cycle filters can minimize 60-cycle interference, but the problem often requires switching to a different electrode.

### REFERENCE
1. Harris CD, Dexter DD: Recording artifacts. *In* Shepard JW (ed): Atlas of Sleep Medicine. Mount Kisco NY, Futura Publishing Co, 1991, pp 19–23.

# PATIENT 19

## A 40-year-old man with complaints of snoring

An obese 40-year-old man was monitored in the sleep laboratory. The EEG, EOG, and EMG tracings showed a definite artifact. Below is a sample 15-second tracing.

*Questions:*  What is this type of artifact? How can it be minimized?

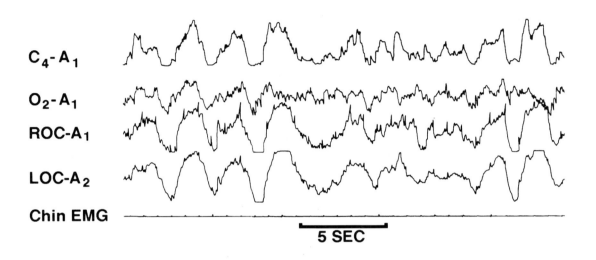

**Answers:** This is sweat or respiratory artifact. It can be minimized by cooling the patient.

**Discussion:** Sweat artifact is characterized by a slowly undulating movement of the baseline of affected channels. The movement may or may not be synchronous with the patient's respiration. When in-phase with the patient's respiration, the artifact also is called respiratory artifact.

Sweat artifact is believed to be secondary to the effects of perspiration. Sweat alters the electrode potential, thereby producing an artifact that mimics delta waves and results in overscoring of stages 3 and 4 NREM sleep. When the artifact is not present in all channels, sweat artifact probably is altering the signal of one or more electrodes on the side the patient is lying on. For example, if the patient is sleeping with the left side down and $C_4$-$A_1$, $O_2$-$A_1$, and ROC-$A_1$ are affected, but LOC-$A_2$ shows no artifact, then lead $A_1$ requires attention. Switching to $C_3$-$A_2$ or $C_4$-$A_2$ may be tried, but if switching electrodes does not solve the problem, then other actions are necessary. Options include reducing the room temperature, uncovering the patient, and/or using a fan. As a last-ditch alternative, the setting of the low-frequency filter may be increased (e.g., from 0.3 to 1). Unfortunately, this maneuver decreases the amount of delta activity recorded, but still may be preferable to a totally unscorable record. Sweat artifact can be prevented by maintaining a low room temperature, especially when very obese or heavily perspiring patients are studied.

In the present case, the sweat artifact is present in leads referenced to both $A_1$ and $A_2$. The room temperature was lowered, and the patient was uncovered. Over the next 15 minutes, the artifact resolved.

## Clinical Pearls

1. Sweat or respiratory artifact is characterized by a slowly undulating baseline.
2. Maintaining a sufficiently cool room temperature is essential when studying obese patients.
3. Changing the electrodes to those opposite the side the patient is lying on can eliminate the artifact in some cases.
4. If all electrodes are involved, use a fan or lower the room temperature.

## REFERENCE

1. Harris CD, Dexter D: Recording artifacts. *In* Shepard JW (ed): Atlas of Sleep Medicine. Mount Kisco, New York, Futura Publishing, 1991, pp 50–51.

# PATIENT 20

## A 40-year-old man with frequent awakenings at night

A 40-year-old man was monitored in the sleep laboratory. The EEG, EOG, and EMG tracings showed a definite artifact. Below is a sample 15-second tracing.

*Questions:*   What is the artifact? Which lead is responsible for the problem?

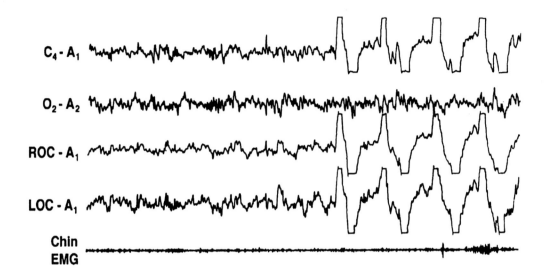

*Answer:* This artifact is due to electrode popping in lead $A_1$.

*Discussion:* Electrode popping is a common and severe artifact that makes the staging of sleep very difficult. It is characterized by sudden, high-amplitude deflection (channel blocking) secondary to an electrode pulling away from the skin (sudden loss of signal). The popping tends to be regular and corresponds to body movement during breathing. Electrode popping often is caused by the patient lying on one mastoid electrode or pulling on an electrode during respiration. Popping also can occur if the electrode gel dries out during the night.

This artifact frequently can be handled by switching to an alternate lead. For example, if $O_2$ is the problem, the exploring occipital electrode is switched to $O_1$. This is one reason that redundant electrodes are routinely placed. Alternatively, the offending electrode is repaired by adding electrode gel, or replaced.

In the present case, the regular high-voltage deflections are noted in all EEG and EOG channels except $O_2$-$A_2$. The common electrode to all the affected channels is $A_1$; therefore, the problem is most likely in electrode $A_1$. The patient was sleeping on his left side. After changing the reference electrode to $A_2$ ($C_3$-$A_2$, ROC-$A_2$, LOC-$A_2$) the problem was eliminated. The change could have been to $C_4$-$A_2$, but using an exploring electrode opposite the reference is preferable (if possible) as this produces a larger voltage signal.

## Clinical Pearls

1. Electrode popping artifact is a sudden, high-voltage deflection occurring at regular intervals usually coincident with respiration.
2. Electrode popping artifact is due to an electrode pulling away from the skin.
3. The offending electrode sometimes can be identified by noting if the affected channels have a common electrode.
4. Recording from alternative electrodes may eliminate the problem.

## REFERENCE

1. Harris CD, Dexter D: Recording artifacts. *In* Shepard JW (ed): Atlas of Sleep Medicine. Mount Kisco, New York, Futura Publishing, 1991, pp 30–31.

# PATIENT 21

## A 50-year-old man with difficulty remaining awake during the day

A 50-year-old man was undergoing sleep monitoring as an evaluation for excessive daytime sleepiness. He snored heavily and underwent polysomnography to rule out obstructive sleep apnea.

*Sleep Study:*    The tracing (see figure) looked much like REM sleep except for an unusual pattern in the eye leads showing deflections only in the right eye lead (points *A*).

*Questions:*    What sleep stage is shown? How do you know that the eye leads were working?

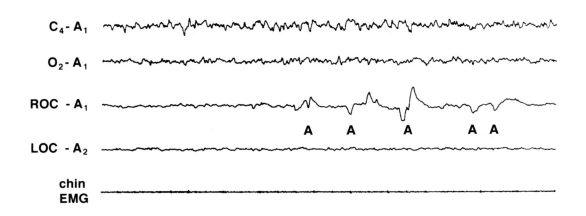

***Answers:*** Stage REM in a patient with an artificial left eye. Check the biocalibrations.

***Discussion:*** Biocalibrations are an important initial part of all sleep studies (see Fundamentals 8). Patients are asked to look left, right, up, and down to test the effectiveness of both the eye electrodes and the amplifier settings at detecting eye movements.

In this study, no movement was seen in LOC-A$_2$, during biocalibration. The technician questioned the patient, who reported that he had an artificial (glass) left eye. At the usual amplifier settings, movements of the right eye (relatively far away) did not result in deflections in LOC-A$_2$. The absence of any deflection in the EEG leads coincident with the deflections in ROC-A$_1$ indicated that these deflections were due to eye movements and not to transmitted EEG activity. The eye movements, low-voltage EEG, and low-amplitude EMG are consistent with stage REM sleep.

## Clinical Pearls

1. Always check biocalibrations prior to sleep study interpretation.
2. Pay special attention to the deflections resulting from voluntary eye movements. In the usual two-channel setup for detecting eye movements, proper calibration should result in reasonably sized, out-of-phase deflections.

### REFERENCES

1. Rechtschaffen A, Kales A (eds): A Manual of Standardized Terminology Techniques and Scoring System for Sleep Stages of Human Sleep. Los Angeles, Brain Information Service/Brain Research Institute, UCLA, 1968.
2. Carskadon MA, Rechtschaffen A: Monitoring and staging human sleep. *In* Kryger MH, Roth T, Dement WC (eds): Principles and Practice of Sleep Medicine. Philadelphia, WB Saunders Co., 1994, pp 943–960.

# PATIENT 22

## A 29-year-old man struggling with daytime sleepiness

A 29-year-old, generally healthy man was studied to evaluate complaints of daytime sleepiness. He was taking no medications, and his wife reported only occasional snoring. During the initial part of the test, the technician noted considerable sweat artifact (the air conditioner thermostat was malfunctioning). The low-frequency filter (½ amp) setting on the EEG channels was increased from 0.3 to 1 to control the artifact after only 30 minutes of recording.

***Physical Examination:*** Unremarkable.

***Sleep Study***

| | | Sleep Stages | % SPT |
|---|---|---|---|
| Time in bed (monitoring time) | 435 min (430–454) | | |
| Total sleep time (TST) | 406.5 min (405–434) | Stage Wake | 1 (0–1) |
| Sleep period time (SPT) | 432.5 min (410–439) | Stage 1 | 6 (3–6) |
| WASO | 26 min | Stage 2 | 60 (40–51) |
| Sleep efficiency | .93 (.91–.99) | Stages 3 and 4 | 8 (16–26) |
| Sleep latency | 2.5 min (3–26) | Stage REM | 25 (22–34) |

( ) = normal values for age, sleep efficiency = (TST * 100) / TIB

***Question:*** Can you explain the abnormality in sleep architecture?

***Answer:*** Reduced recording of slow wave activity secondary to the low-frequency filter setting.

***Discussion:*** The high- and low-frequency filter settings can significantly alter the EEG amplifier response to a signal. The low filter settings can dramatically reduce the amplitude of slow wave activity if set too high. A ½ amp low-filter setting of 0.3 Hz means that a sine wave input of 0.3 Hz is attenuated by 50%. On some amplifiers, a low filter setting of 0.3 means that a signal of 0.3 Hz is attenuated by 70.7 or 80% of the original signal. Regardless of the exact meaning for a given amplifier, a low filter setting of 0.3 does not significantly attenuate the majority of slow wave activity (< 2 Hz). However, a low filter setting of 1 Hz does produce considerable attenuation of slow wave activity. Thus, less activity meets the minimum voltage criterion of 75 microvolts.

At the bottom of the page is a tracing showing the effect of changing the low filter from a ½ amp setting of 0.3 Hz (usual setting) to 1 Hz. Note the abrupt reduction in the slow wave activity.

Setting the low-frequency filter of the eye movement channels too high also markedly reduces eye movement amplitude. The low filter settings usually recommended for EEG and EOG leads is 0.3 Hz. For EMG and EKG channels, a low filter setting (½ amp) of 10 is used, as the relevant activity is of a much higher frequency. Filter settings are sometimes given as time constants. Most alternating-current amplifiers employ resistance-capacitance (RC) circuits as input filters. In a simple, low filter RC circuit, the frequency (fc) at which the output voltage across the resistor is attenuated to 70.7% of the input voltage is related to the time constant (Tc) by the formula

$$fc = 1 / (2\pi \ Tc).$$

The $Tc = RC$ where R is the resistance and C the capacitance. Since amplifiers are routinely calibrated by step (square wave) voltage changes rather than sine wave signals, the time constant can be noted from the time it takes for the deflection to return to baseline. In RC circuits, an increase in step voltage produces an abrupt increase in voltage across the resistor, then an exponential fall in voltage to 1/e (0.37) of the maximum voltage in one time constant. When the ½ amp frequency is higher, the time constant is smaller (more rapid fall).

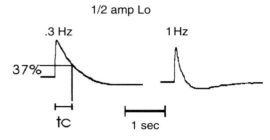

In the present case, the change in low filter settings was the most likely cause for the small amount of slow wave sleep recorded. When the study was scored without using voltage criteria, a higher but still subnormal amount of slow wave sleep was scored. The low filter setting should be increased only as a last resort (see treatment of sweat artifact, Patient 19).

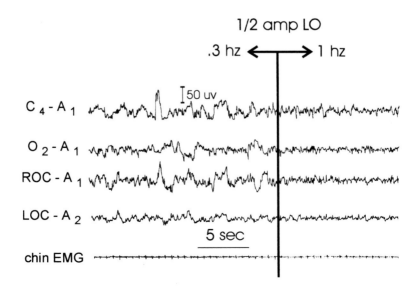

# Clinical Pearls

1. The filter settings should be recorded during calibration and any changes during sleep monitoring noted. The sleep scorer should be informed of any changes.

2. A higher-than-recommended low filter setting in the EEG leads (especially the central EEG) decreases the amplitude of slow wave activity and hence the amount of slow wave sleep that is scored.

## REFERENCES

1. Tyner FA, Knott JR, Mayer WB, Jr: Fundamentals of EEG technology. New York, Raven Press, 1983, pp 89–119.
2. Fisch BJ: Spehlman's EEG Primer. New York, Elsevier, 1991, pp 51–60.

## Multiple Sleep Latency Test

The multiple sleep latency test (MSLT) consists of sleep monitoring during four or five naps spread over the day, usually at two-hour intervals (8 AM, 10 AM, 12 noon, 2 PM, 4 PM). Generally, the test is preceded by nocturnal polysomnography. In the morning, the patient changes into comfortable street clothes, and **nap monitoring** begins 1.5 to 3 hours after nocturnal recording has ceased. The patient is instructed to fall asleep at lights out and is given 20 minutes to do so. Once sleep is attained, the patient is given another 15 minutes to reach stage REM sleep. The nap test is stopped if the patient fails to fall asleep within 20 minutes, fails to reach REM sleep within 15 minutes of sleep onset, or after the first epoch of unequivocal REM sleep. After nap termination, the patient is instructed to get out of bed until the next nap opportunity. The **sleep latency** (time from lights out until the *beginning* of the first epoch of any stage of sleep) and the **REM latency** (time from the first sleep until the beginning of the first epoch of REM sleep) are determined for each nap.

Results of the MSLT in normal subjects show a mean sleep latency longer than 15 minutes and zero to one REM periods in five naps. However, some otherwise normal subjects have a mean sleep latency in the 10–15 minute range. This range represents mild sleepiness, and a mean sleep latency ≤ 10 minutes is considered abnormal. A mean sleep latency of 5–10 minutes represents moderate sleepiness; shorter than 5 minutes is severe (pathological) sleepiness. It is important not to confuse mean MSLT sleep latency with *nocturnal* sleep latency. A short sleep latency at the regular bedtime is not abnormal. However, a majority of patients with narcolepsy have a *nap* sleep latency shorter than 5 minutes, and patients with moderate-to-severe sleep apnea usually have a mean nap sleep latency shorter than 10 minutes.

The presence of two or more REM periods in five naps is characteristic of **narcolepsy**. However, this finding is not specific to this syndrome and can occur with any cause of REM sleep deprivation or disturbance. Sleep apnea and, occasionally, psychiatric disorders can be associated with a short REM latency. Acute withdrawal of REM-suppressing medications (tricyclic antidepressants, lithium, serotonin reuptake inhibitors, stimulants) can be associated with REM sleep during naps. Ideally, any medication affecting either the sleep latency or the REM latency should be withdrawn for 2 weeks before the sleep study and MSLT. (When this is not practical, the medications should *not* be abruptly discontinued just prior to testing.) Most sleep centers have the patient keep a sleep log (diary) of the amount and pattern of sleep during the 2 weeks preceding the MSLT, because sleep loss or disturbance during this period can affect the sleep latency.

Proper interpretation of the MSLT requires analysis of the **nocturnal polysomnogram**. Note if the amount and quality of sleep was adequate and if sleep disorders were present that could affect the sleep latency. Specific conditions such as sleep apnea or periodic leg movements in sleep should be documented. Decreased amounts of REM sleep (or REM-sleep fragmentation) during the night from any cause can increase the number of REM periods recorded on the MSLT. For example, sleep apnea is a common cause of two or more REM periods on the MSLT.

The standard MSLT criteria for narcolepsy are: mean sleep latency shorter than 5 minutes and two or more REM episodes in five naps. Narcoleptic patients with a longer sleep latency (5–10 minutes) and two more REM onsets often show a shorter sleep latency on retesting. When sleep apnea is present, interpretation of the MSLT is problematic. The sleep apnea should be treated first. If narcolepsy is suspected, a repeat sleep study showing adequate sleep (sufficient treatment of sleep apnea) should be performed, followed by an MSLT. When treatment is with nasal continuous positive airway pressure (CPAP), both the repeat sleep study and the MSLT are performed on the prescribed level of CPAP.

# Key Points

1. Proper interpretation of an MSLT requires analysis of: the preceding nocturnal sleep study, a careful medication history, and sleep habits (diary) for at least 1 week preceding the MSLT.
2. The mean nap sleep latency is a measure of the tendency to fall asleep during normal waking hours.
3. The number of naps with REM sleep can provide evidence for narcolepsy.

## REFERENCES

1. Richardson GS, Carskadon MA, Flagg W: Excessive daytime sleepiness in man: Multiple sleep latency measurements in narcoleptic and control subjects. Electroencephalogr Clin Neurophysiol 1978; 45:621–627.
2. Carskadon MA: Guidelines for the multiple sleep latency test. Sleep 1986; 9:519–524.
3. Standards of Practice Committee, American Sleep Disorders Association: The clinical use of the multiple sleep latency test. Sleep 1992; 15:268–276.

# PATIENT 23

## A 25-year-old man with daytime sleepiness

A 25-year-old man complained that for 2 years he'd had problems with sleepiness during the day. A nocturnal sleep study failed to show any abnormality. A multiple sleep latency test (MSLT) was performed the next day.

*Figure:* The results of the five naps are shown below in tabular format. The sleep stage of each 30-second epoch is listed below the epoch number.

*Questions:* What is the sleep latency and REM latency of each nap? What is the mean sleep latency for the MSLT?

**Nap 1**     R = REM, LO = lights out, W = stage Wake

| epoch | 70 | 71 | 72 | 73 | 74 | 75 | 76 | 77 | 78 | 79 | 80 |
|-------|----|----|----|----|----|----|----|----|----|----|----|
| stage | LO | W | W | W | 1 | 1 | 1 | 1 | 2 | 2 | R |

**Nap 2**

| epoch | 90 | 91 | 92 | 93 | 94 | 95 | 96 | 97 | 98 | 99 | 100 |
|-------|----|----|----|----|----|----|----|----|----|----|-----|
| stage | LO | W | W | 1 | 1 | 1 | 1 | 1 | 2 | 2 | 2 |
| epoch | 101 | 102 | 103 | 104 | 105 | 106 | 107 | 108 | 109 | 110 | 111 |
| stage | 2 | 3 | 3 | 3 | 4 | 4 | 4 | 4 | 4 | 4 | 4 |
| epoch | 112 | 113 | 114 | 115 | 116 | 117 | 118 | 119 | 120 | 121 | 122 |
| stage | 2 | 3 | 3 | 3 | 4 | 4 | 4 | 4 | 4 | 4 | 4 |

**Nap 3**

| epoch | 130 | 131 | 132 | 133 | 134 | 135 | 136 | 137 | 138 | 139 | 140 |
|-------|-----|-----|-----|-----|-----|-----|-----|-----|-----|-----|-----|
| stage | LO | W | W | W | 1 | 1 | 1 | 1 | 1 | 1 | 1 |
| epoch | 141 | 142 | 143 | 144 | 145 | 146 | 147 | 148 | 149 | 150 | 151 |
| stage | 2 | 2 | 2 | 2 | 3 | 3 | 3 | 3 | R | R | |

**Nap 4**

| epoch | 160 | 161 | 162 | 163 | 164 | 165 | 166 | 167 | 168 | 169 | 170 |
|-------|-----|-----|-----|-----|-----|-----|-----|-----|-----|-----|-----|
| stage | LO | W | W | W | W | W | 1 | 1 | W | W | 1 |
| epoch | 171 | 172 | 173 | 174 | 175 | 176 | 177 | 178 | 179 | 180 | 181 |
| stage | 2 | 3 | 3 | 3 | 4 | 4 | 4 | R | R | | |

**Nap 5**

| epoch | 190 | 191 | 192 | 193 | 194 | 195 | 196 | 197 | 198 | 199 | 200 |
|-------|-----|-----|-----|-----|-----|-----|-----|-----|-----|-----|-----|
| stage | LO | W | W | W | W | W | W | W | W | W | W |
| epoch | 201 | 202 | 203 | 204 | 205 | 206 | 207 | 208 | 209 | 210 | 211 |
| stage | W | W | W | W | W | W | W | W | W | W | W |
| epoch | 112 | 113 | 114 | 115 | 116 | 117 | 118 | 119 | 120 | 121 | 122 |
| stage | W | W | W | W | W | W | W | W | W | W | W |
| epoch | 123 | 124 | 125 | 126 | 127 | 128 | 129 | 130 | 131 | 132 | 133 |
| stage | W | W | W | W | W | W | W | W | | | |

| *Answers:* | Sleep Latency | REM Latency |
|---|---|---|
| Nap 1 | 1.5 min (3 epochs) | 3 min (6 epochs) |
| Nap 2 | 1.0 min (2 epochs) | none |
| Nap 3 | 1.5 min (3 epochs) | 7.5 min (15 epochs) |
| Nap 4 | 2.5 min (5 epochs) | 6 min (12 epochs) |
| Nap 5 | 20 min | none |
| Mean | 5.3 min | |

*Discussion:* The patient is given 20 minutes after lights out to fall asleep for each MSLT nap. If sleep does not occur, then the sleep latency is set at 20 minutes by convention. Once sleep is attained, the patient is given another 15 minutes to attain REM sleep. The **sleep latency** is the time from lights out until the first epoch of any stage of sleep. The **REM latency** is the time from the first epoch of sleep until the first epoch of REM sleep. There is a normal variation in sleep latency over the day in most subjects, with the minimum usually occurring near noon or early afternoon (naps 3 or 4) and the maximum in the late afternoon. The propensity of REM also varies, with REM periods most likely to occur in the morning naps.

In the present patient, the mean sleep latency was consistent with moderate-to-severe sleepiness. Note that in nap 5 no sleep was attained, and the sleep latency was set at 20 minutes. The patient had difficulty falling asleep in this nap because he was "nervous and ready to go home." If nap 5 were excluded, the mean sleep latency would be much lower. REM sleep was present in three of five naps. In nap 4, epochs of wakefulness were noted between sleep onset and the first epoch of REM. The intervening wakefulness was included in the computation of the REM latency. The findings of this study were interpreted in light of the nocturnal polysomnographic findings and clinical history, and a diagnosis of narcolepsy was supported. Narcolepsy is discussed in detail in later cases (e.g., Patients 77 and 78.

# Clinical Pearls

1. If no sleep is attained after 20 minutes of monitoring during an MSLT, then the nap is terminated, and the sleep latency is considered to be 20 minutes.

2. Sleep latency can vary considerably between naps in the MSLT. This is the reason for five naps spread out over the normal waking period.

## REFERENCES

1. Richardson GS, Carskadon MA, Flagg W: Excessive daytime sleepiness in man: Multiple sleep latency measurements in narcoleptic and control subjects. Electroencephalogr Clin Neurophysiol 1978; 45:621–627.
2. Carskadon MA: Guidelines for the multiple sleep latency test. Sleep 1986; 9:519–524.
3. Standards of Practice Committee, American Sleep Disorders Association: The clinical use of the multiple sleep latency test. Sleep 1992; 15:268–276.

## Respiratory Definitions

**Apnea** is defined as an absence of airflow at the nose and mouth for 10 seconds or longer. This time duration is arbitrary, but widely applied. The presence or absence of respiratory (inspiratory effort) determines the type of apnea: **central apnea** is defined by an absence of inspiratory effort; **obstructive apnea** occurs despite persistent respiratory effort; and **mixed apnea** has an initial central part (no inspiratory effort) and a terminal obstructive portion. In the figure below, respiratory effort (signaled by movement) is detected by bands around the chest and abdomen. In central apnea, no movement of the chest and abdomen are detected during the apnea. In obstructive apnea, respiratory effort persists during the apnea. Note that during obstructive apnea, the chest and abdomen move in a paradoxical manner (one inward and the other outward; see *diamonds*). In mixed apnea, an initial central portion of the apnea (point *C*) is followed by an obstructive portion.

**Hypopnea** is defined as a reduction in airflow for 10 seconds or longer. The required amount of reduction varies among sleep laboratories, but generally airflow must be reduced by 33–50% of the baseline. Sometimes a drop in arterial oxygen saturation (desaturation) also is required. Hypopneas can be central (a reduction in inspiratory effort) or obstructive (increased upper airway resistance). Unless the pressure difference across the upper airway is measured, hypopneas cannot always be definitively classified. Obstructive hypopneas often are associated with paradoxical movement of the chest and abdomen.

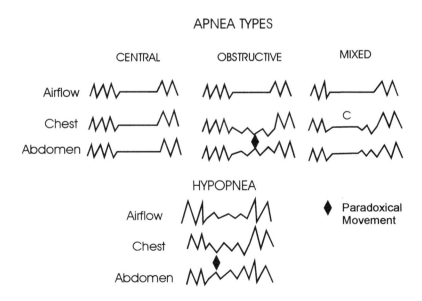

The apnea index (AI), hypopnea index (HI), and the apnea + hypopnea index (AHI) are all defined as the total number of events divided by the total sleep time in hours. The AHI, also called the respiratory disturbance index, commonly is used to quantify the average severity of respiratory disturbances during the night. An AHI < 5/hr is considered normal in adults. Rough guidelines for severity are: AHI < 20 mild, 20–40 moderate, and > 40 severe.

Arterial oxygen saturation ($SaO_2$) is measured during sleep studies using pulse oximetry (finger or ear probes). A desaturation is defined as a decrease in $SaO_2$ of 4% or more from baseline. Note that the nadir in $SaO_2$ commonly *follows* apnea (hypopnea) termination by approximately 6–8 seconds (longer in severe desaturations). This delay is secondary to circulation time and instrumental delay (the oximeter averages over several cycles before producing a reading). In the figure below, the apneas and the corresponding nadirs in saturation are identified. Various measures have been applied to assess the severity of desaturation, including computing the number of desaturations below 85% as well as the mean and minimum saturations.

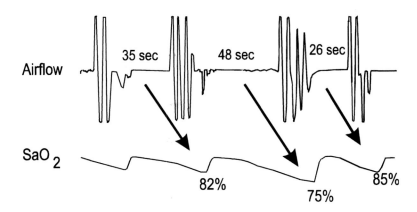

## REFERENCES

1. Block AJ, Boysen PG, Wynne JW, et al: Sleep apnea, hypopnea, and oxygen desaturation in normal subjects: A strong male predominance. N Engl J Med 1979; 330:513–517.
2. West P, Kryger MH: Sleep and respiration: Terminology and methodology. Clin Chest Med (Symposium on Sleep Disorders) 1985; 6:691–718.

# PATIENT 24

## A 45-year-old man with possible sleep apnea

A 45-year-old man underwent polysomnography for evaluation of suspected sleep apnea. Apnea detection was performed by monitoring airflow with a thermocouple and measuring exhaled $CO_2$.

*Figure:*   Although the thermocouple revealed apnea (no deflections), the $CO_2$ tracing revealed persistent deflections that differed from those observed during the pre-apnea period.

*Questions:*   Is apnea present? If so, why is the exhaled $CO_2$ tracing fluctuating?

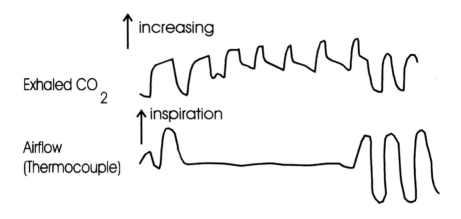

*Answers:* Apnea is present. The $CO_2$ tracing fluctuates due to persistent exhalation during obstructive (inspiratory) apnea.

*Discussion:* Monitoring of airflow during sleep studies may be performed by several methods, the most common of which features temperature-sensitive devices placed near the nose and mouth. Airflow causes a change in the temperature of the devices which results in a change in voltage (**thermocouple**) or resistance (**thermistor**) of the transducer. The alteration in the signal originating from these transducers when appropriately amplified causes a deflection in the airflow tracing. Although convenient, temperature-sensitive devices do not always accurately reflect the *magnitude* of change in airflow and sometimes can be misleading. During apnea, the tracing may continue to fluctuate secondary to changes in temperature from contact with the patient's body or room air.

**Pneumotachographs** accurately measure flow and can provide information about the shape of the airflow profile. However, they require masks covering the nose and mouth and therefore are less comfortable. Measurement of the pressure difference across a known resistance (the pneumotachograph wire screen) when calibrated reflects the flow rate (flow = pressure / resistance). Pneumotachographs also can reveal detail not seen in thermocouple monitoring, such as vibration in the flow (snoring), a flat profile (airflow limitation), or expiratory puffs of air during inspiratory apnea.

Another method for monitoring airflow is to measure **exhaled $CO_2$**. As expired air is rich in $CO_2$ while ambient air has essentially none, respiration is detected by fluctuations in measured $CO_2$. Air is sampled via a small nasal or nasal-oral cannula by continuous suction and is measured downstream at an analyzer. The increases in $CO_2$ values (reflecting exhalation) are slightly time-delayed because there is a finite time for the sampled air to reach the analyzer. The plateau value of measured $CO_2$ (end tidal $PCO_2$) can provide an estimate of arterial $PCO_2$ and is increased during periods of hypoventilation. Apnea is detected by an absence of deflection in the $CO_2$ tracing. This method of monitoring airflow is widely used in pediatric sleep monitoring because children with "sleep apnea" frequently have long periods of hypoventilation (increased end tidal $PCO_2$) rather than discrete apneas or hypopneas.

However, the method can be misleading in adults. During apnea (absence of inspiratory airflow), small expiratory puffs may continue. These small exhalations are rich in $CO_2$ and can cause significant deflections in the $CO_2$ signal, giving a false impression about the nature of airflow ($CO_2$, not airflow, is measured).

Recently measurement of nasal pressure has been used to detect airflow. Pressure just inside the nasal inlet is measured by connecting nasal cannulas (oxygen- or $CO_2$-monitoring) directly to sensitive **pressure transducers**. The pressure deflections are reasonable, semiquantitative estimates of the magnitude and shape of airflow. This method works similarly to a pneumotachograph by measuring the pressure drop across the resistance of the nasal inlet. The major difficulty with this method is that oral airflow is not detected. Simultaneous use of an oral thermocouple can solve this problem.

The Vsum signal of respiratory inductance **plethysmography** can provide a semiquantitative estimate of tidal volume (see figure below). In this method, changes in the inductance of coils in bands around the rib cage (RC) and abdomen (AB) during respiratory movement are translated into voltage signals. The sum of the two signals (Vsum = [a * RC] + [b * AB]) can be calibrated by choosing appropriate constants: a and b. During apnea, the two signals cancel (a * RC = –b * AB) and Vsum is close to zero.

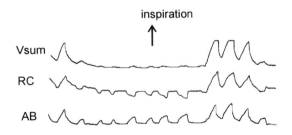

In the present case, simultaneous monitoring with a pneumotachograph (see figure next page) showed that the fluctuations in $CO_2$ during apnea were secondary to small expiratory puffs (rich in $CO_2$) during inspiratory apnea.

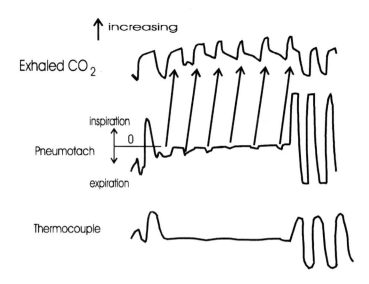

## Clinical Pearls

1. Temperature-sensitive devices for monitoring air flow can be inaccurate because they sometimes do not reflect the *magnitude* of airflow.

2. Pneumotachography accurately measures flow and provides a detailed airflow profile that may include information not seen in thermocouple monitoring.

3. Other options for apnea detection include nasal cannulas connected to pressure transducers and respiratory inductance plethysmography.

REFERENCES

1. Tobin M, Cohn MA, Sackner MA: Breathing abnormalities during sleep. Arch Intern Med 1983; 143:1221–8.
2. Kryger MH: Monitoring respiratory and cardiac function. *In* Kryger MH, Roth T, Dement WC (eds): Principles and Practice of Sleep Medicine. Philadelphia, WB Saunders, 1994, pp 984–993.
3. Monserrat JP, Farré R, Ballester E, et al: Evaluation of nasal prongs for estimating nasal flow. Am J Respir Crit Care Med 1997; 155:211–215.
4. Norman RG, Ahmed MM, Walsleben JA, et al: Detection of respiratory events during NPSG: Nasal cannula/pressure sensor versus thermistor. Sleep 1997; 20:1175–1184.

# PATIENT 25

## A 50-year-old man with possible central apnea

A 50-year-old, obese man was evaluated at another hospital for complaints of excessive daytime sleepiness. He underwent a sleep study in which many apneas were noted. Because of minimal movement in the chest and abdominal bands, the apnea was labeled as central by the technician scoring the study.

A second sleep study was performed on presentation to this sleep laboratory because the patient's history suggested obstructive apnea.

*Figure:* A sample tracing of one of the recorded events is shown below.

*Question:* What type of apnea is present?

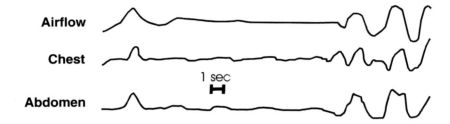

*Diagnosis:* Obstructive apnea. There is minimal chest and abdominal movement due to obesity.

*Discussion:* The diagnosis of obstructive apnea depends on demonstration of apnea despite continued inspiratory effort. This usually is accomplished by detecting chest and abdominal movement. During obstructive apnea/hypopnea, the chest and abdominal tracings may show paradoxical motion (one in, the other out). Sometimes changes in phase between chest and abdomen are more subtle. In the following tracings from a patient with obstructive apnea, paradox is not present in the initial part (*a*) but is obvious in the last part of the tracing (*b*). Paradoxical movement tends to be most pronounced in REM sleep, when there is hypotonia of the chest wall muscles.

Some of the many different methods of detecting movement include piezo-electric transducers in

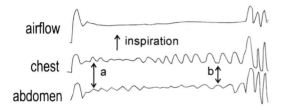

bands, mercury strain gauges, and respiratory impedance plethysmography (RIP). RIP converts changes in the impedance of a coil in a band around the body secondary to changes in the enclosed area during chest/abdominal excursions into a voltage signal. The rib cage (RC) and abdominal (AB) signals are then added (Vsum = [a * RC] + [b * AB]). If the coefficients a and b are selected by calibration, Vsum is a reasonable estimate of tidal volume (see Patient 24). During obstructive apnea, the rib cage and abdominal contributions to Vsum cancel (a * RC = −b * AB), and Vsum is close to zero (apnea). In all the above methods, a change in body position may alter the ability to detect chest/abdominal move-

ment. This may require adjusting band placement or amplifier sensitivity. In addition, very obese patients may show little chest/abdominal wall movement despite considerable inspiratory effort. Thus, one must be cautious about making the diagnosis of central apnea solely on the basis of surface detection of inspiration effort.

The most sensitive method of detecting respiratory effort is to measure the **esophageal pressure.** Changes in esophageal pressure are estimates of pleural pressure changes. In the past, this method required esophageal balloons, which were uncomfortable and difficult to use. Recently, esophageal pressure has been measured using small, soft, fluid-filled catheters (pediatric feeding tubes) connected to pressure transducers, such as the disposable transducers commonly used in intensive care units. In one study using both RIP and esophageal pressure monitoring, apneas were found to have been correctly classified by RIP alone in 91% of patients. Thus, monitoring chest and abdominal movement is satisfactory for most patients. In a few patients, obstructive apneas may be incorrectly labeled as central if esophageal pressure monitoring is not performed.

In the present case, definite chest and abdominal movements are evident, although of a small magnitude. The simultaneous esophageal pressure trace (see figure below) reveals that inspiratory effort clearly is present and increasing during the event. Therefore, the event is an obstructive apnea.

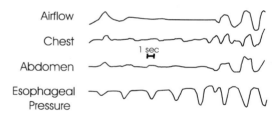

## Clinical Pearls

1. Chest and abdominal movements during obstructive apnea may be small in magnitude and difficult to detect in some obese individuals.

2. The most sensitive method of detecting respiratory effort is to monitor the esophageal pressure.

3. During obstructive apnea and hypopnea, the chest and abdomen movements may be out-of-phase, demonstrating a subtle difference rather than an obvious paradox.

## REFERENCES

1. Staats BA, Bonekat HW, Harris CD, et al: Chest wall motion in sleep apnea. Am Rev Respir Dis 1984; 130:59–63.
2. Flemale A, Gillard C, Dierckx JP: Comparison of central venous, esophageal and mouth occlusion pressure with water-filled catheters for estimating pleural pressure changes in healthy adults. Eur Resp J 1988; 1:51–57.
3. Kryger MH: Monitoring respiratory and cardiac function. *In* Kryger MH, Roth T, Dement WC (eds): Principles and Practice of Sleep Medicine. Philadelphia, WB Saunders, 1994, pp 984–993.

# Excessive Daytime Sleepiness

Excessive daytime sleepiness (EDS) is the most common complaint evaluated by sleep disorder specialists. Sleep apnea is the usual cause. However, do not automatically assume that every patient with EDS and snoring has sleep apnea. All of the causes of daytime sleepiness listed below must be carefully considered. Note that it is common for more than one of these disorders to be present in a given individual. Also, become acquainted with the patient's medical history, and explore a relevant review of symptoms. For example, congestive heart failure is commonly associated with a type of central sleep apnea (Patient 69), and patients with renal failure often have periodic leg movement (PLM) in sleep. Hypothyroidism and acromegaly are predisposing conditions for sleep apnea. In addition, some medications can cause daytime sleepiness or fatigue.

Patients with some of the disorders listed below may present with complaints of insomnia (difficulty initiating and maintaining sleep) rather than EDS. In fact, patients with PLM more commonly present with nocturnal awakenings than EDS. Problems with insomnia also may predominate in those with depression. Even patients with sleep apnea (for which EDS is a cardinal manifestation) may seek medical evaluation primarily because of frequent nocturnal awakenings rather than daytime sleepiness.

**Causes of Excessive Daytime Sleepiness**

| Disorders | Evaluation |
|---|---|
| Sleep apnea syndromes | All cases |
| Upper airway resistance syndrome | History |
| Narcolepsy | Self-rating scales of sleepiness |
| Depression | Sleep-wake diary |
| Periodic leg (limb) movements in sleep | Polysomnography |
| Idiopathic hypersomnia | |
| Withdrawal from stimulants | Selected cases |
| Inadequate sleep | MSLT (narcolepsy) |
| Drug dependence/abuse | Drug screen |

A good **history** is essential in evaluating patients with EDS. Differentiating complaints of fatigue and daytime sleepiness can be difficult. Quantifying the degree of daytime sleepiness is challenging because patients tend to underestimate. Questionnaires such as the Epworth Sleepiness Scale are attempts to standardize the evaluation of self-rated symptoms of sleepiness. However, the results may not always correlate with objective measures of sleepiness. Certainly the patient should be questioned about which activities are compromised by decreased alertness (e.g., driving, work, social situations). The normal bedtime, waketime, and average hours of sleep also should be recorded. Surprisingly, the simple answer for some patients is that they are trying to exist on an inadequate amount of sleep. Many sleep disorders centers have patients fill out a sleep-wake diary for 2 weeks before being evaluated. This diary documents patterns of sleep and daytime sleepiness.

Questioning bed partners is absolutely essential in evaluating patients with EDS. A history of loud **snoring** and observed **gasping** or **apnea** is suggestive of obstructive sleep apnea syndrome, whereas a history of **leg jerks** or kicking suggests periodic limb movements in sleep. The **age at onset** of symptoms provides a clue to the disorder. While sleep apnea can start at any age, it typically presents in middle-aged or older individuals. In contrast, narcolepsy usually starts in late adolescence or the 20s. The patient should be questioned about **cataplexy** (loss of muscle tone during moments of increased emotion such as laughter), which is characteristic of narcolepsy. **Sleep paralysis** (inability to move while still awake, at sleep onset, or after awakening) and **hypnagogic hallucinations** (vivid sensory imagery, usually visual, occurring at sleep onset while still awake) also are common in narcolepsy, but can occur in normal individuals as well. Symptoms of **depression** suggest that this common disorder is the cause of daytime sleepiness.

Physical examination should pay special attention to the blood pressure, upper airway (nose, mouth, and throat), neck circumference, and signs of right or left heart failure or hypothyroidism.

<table>
<tr><td colspan="2" align="center">History in EDS</td></tr>
<tr>
<td>Age of onset, duration of symptoms<br>Daily activities impaired (driving, work, social situations)<br>Medications, ethanol, sleeping pill use<br>Recent weight gain/loss<br>Sleep habits: bedtime, duration of sleep</td>
<td>Bed partner observations: snoring, gasping, apnea, leg kicks<br>Symptoms of narcolepsy: cataplexy, sleep paralysis, hypnogogic hallucinations<br>Symptoms of depression</td>
</tr>
</table>

In addition to the history and physical examination, a nocturnal sleep study (polysomnography) is required for most patients presenting with EDS. The severity of the disorder frequently is underestimated by the patient. Moreover, several disorders may be present in the same individual (narcolepsy, obstructive sleep apnea, and periodic limb movements in sleep). If a diagnosis of narcolepsy is suspected, an MSLT following the nocturnal sleep study can be useful. The MSLT provides objective evidence of the tendency to fall asleep during the day.

## REFERENCES

1. Moldofsky H: Evaluation of daytime sleepiness. *In* Phillipson EA, Bradley TA (eds): Breathing Disorders. Clin Chest Med Philadelphia, WB Saunders, 1991, pp 417–425.
2. Johns MW: Sleepiness in different situations measured by the Epworth Sleepiness Scale. Sleep 1994; 17:703–710.
3. American Sleep Disorders Association: International Classification of Sleep Disorders: Diagnostic and Coding Manual. Rochester, Minnesota, ASDA, 1997.

# PATIENT 26

## A 30-year-old man with heavy snoring

A 30-year-old man was referred for evaluation of heavy snoring. He denied excessive daytime sleepiness. The patient's wife reported that he stopped breathing during the night.

*Physical Examination:*　Blood pressure 150/85, pulse 88/min. HEENT: edematous palate. Neck: 18-inch circumference. Chest: clear. Cardiac: normal. Extremities: no edema.

*Sleep Study:*　Total sleep time: 350 minutes (normal 400–443). Total apneas: 200 (5% central, 30% mixed, 65% obstructive). Total hypopneas: 50.

*Figure:*　A typical apnea is illustrated below. Chest and abdomen tracings show movements of these areas (respiratory effort).

*Questions:*　Which type of apnea is illustrated? What is the diagnosis?

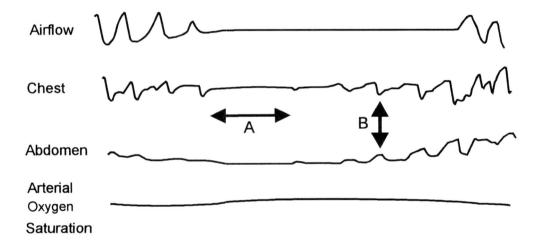

*Answers:*   The illustrated event is a mixed apnea. The diagnosis is obstructive sleep apnea.

*Discussion:*   An obstructive apnea is one in which ventilatory effort is present. A mixed apnea is composed of an initial central apnea (no inspiratory effort) followed by an obstructive portion. Most patients with obstructive sleep apnea have predominantly mixed or obstructive apneas. However, a small fraction of central events is not unusual. Both mixed and obstructive apneas have the same clinical significance and usually the same etiology (upper airway obstruction).

The initial, central portion of a mixed apnea is believed to be due to the hyperventilation following the preceding apnea. As the patient returns to sleep, the $PCO_2$ is below the apneic threshold (the level of $CO_2$ that triggers ventilation). The result is an absence of inspiratory effort (central apnea). During the apnea, the $PCO_2$ rises until inspiratory effort returns. However, apnea persists despite the return of inspiratory effort secondary to an obstructed upper airway. Adequate treatment of upper airway obstruction prevents apnea and post-apnea hyperventilation. Thus, both the central and obstructive components of mixed apneas are eliminated by effective treatments such as tracheostomy or nasal continuous positive airway pressure (CPAP). Some central apneas may persist, but usually resolve with time.

In the current case, the illustrated event is a mixed event with an initial central portion (*A*) followed by an obstructive portion. Paradoxical motion is seen in the chest and abdomen tracings during the obstructive portion (*B*). The patient was treated with nasal CPAP which virtually eliminated mixed and obstructive apnea (AHI = 5/hr). A few central apneas and hypopneas persisted in REM sleep.

## Clinical Pearls

1. Many patients with the obstructive sleep apnea syndrome have both mixed and obstructive apneas. The underlying pathogenesis of both is upper airway obstruction.

2. In most cases of obstructive sleep apnea, adequate treatment of upper airway obstruction eliminates both obstructive and mixed apnea.

## REFERENCES

1. Sanders MH: Nasal CPAP effect on patterns of sleep apnea. Chest 1984; 86:839–844.
2. Dempsey JA, Skatrud JB: A sleep-induced apneic threshold and its consequences. Am Rev Respir Dis 1986; 133:1163–1170.
3. Iber C, Davies SF, Champan RC, Mahowald MM: A possible mechanism for mixed apnea in obstructive sleep apnea. Chest 1986; 89:800–805.

# PATIENT 27

## A 33-year-old man complaining of daytime sleepiness

A 33-year-old man was evaluated for daytime sleepiness of 3-year duration. His wife reported that he snored heavily and stopped breathing when sleeping on his back.

**Physical Examination:**   Normal except for mild obesity (140% of ideal body weight) and a long, edematous palate and uvula.

**Sleep Study:**   No apneas were noted; however, 400 events such as the one illustrated below were recorded. Airflow was monitored with a thermocouple and a pneumotachograph. Respiratory effort was detected by recording esophageal pressure with a thin, fluid-filled catheter.

**Questions:**   What is the diagnosis? What is the illustrated event?

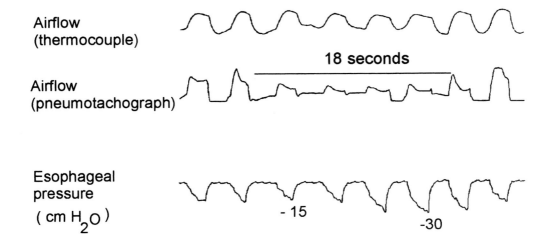

***Diagnosis:*** Obstructive sleep apnea (hypopnea) syndrome. The event is an obstructive hypopnea.

***Discussion:*** While the definition of apnea is well standardized, the definition of hypopnea varies among clinicians. All agree that hypopnea is a reduction in airflow (or tidal volume) by 33–50% of the preceding baseline for 10 seconds or longer. Some also require an associated arterial oxygen desaturation of 2–4%. As most airflow monitoring is done with thermocouples or thermistors, the airflow signal is *qualitative* and may not accurately reflect the decrease in airflow during hypopnea. The classification of an event as an apnea or hypopnea may depend on the sensitivity of the airflow recording device or the amount of amplifier gain. With these diagnostic limitations in mind, most clinicians adjust the hypopnea criteria for each sleep study to identify events likely to be of physiologic significance.

Hypopneas are central (due to a reduction in ventilatory effort), obstructive (due to partial upper airway obstruction/increased resistance), or a combination (mixed type). However, unless airflow and the pressure drop across the upper airway are measured *quantitatively,* precise classification is impossible. Although esophageal (or supraglottic) pressure monitoring is not routinely performed, the obstructive nature of a hypopnea be inferred by noting rib cage or abdominal paradox (inward movement during inspiration) during the event. This is a manifestation of the resistive load (upper airway narrowing) placed on the respiratory muscles. One study found that a 50% reduction in thoracoabdominal motion (Vsum), as measured with respiratory inductance plethysmography (RIP), correlated with the frequency of arterial oxygen desaturation and arousal from sleep. In RIP, changes in the inductance of bands around the chest and abdomen during breathing are converted to voltage signals, and the sum of the voltages from thoracic and abdominal movement are calibrated to provide an estimate of tidal volume. This method is not as widely used as monitoring airflow with thermistors.

What is the clinical significance of hypopneas? Hypopneas can result in hypoventilation, significant arterial oxygen desaturation, and arousal from sleep. Thus, hypopneas have the same clinical significance as apneas. Monitoring of most patients with obstructive apnea reveals some hypopneas. Some patients have hypopneas when sleeping in the lateral decubitus position and apneas when supine (gravity increases the tendency for the airway to collapse). An occasional patient has only hypopnea. Because hypopneas and apneas have similar clinical significance, the apnea + hypopnea index (AHI) generally is computed (number of apneas + hypopneas / hour of sleep). This index (also known as the respiratory disturbance index) is a more inclusive estimate of the severity of sleep-disordered breathing than the apnea index.

In the present case, the thermistor recording underestimates the reduction in airflow, and the flat shape of airflow is appreciated only in the pneumotachograph tracing. Note that the amount of respiratory effort (esophageal pressure deflection) *increases* during the event despite a decrease in airflow. Therefore, the hypopnea is obstructive. Within each breath, the pattern of a flat airflow curve (constant flow) despite increasing respiratory effort is consistent with airflow limitation in a collapsing upper airway.

## Clinical Pearls

1. The separation of events into apneas and hypopneas is imprecise and may depend on the sensitivity/calibration of the airflow recording system. Thus the AHI is a more accurate (and inclusive) estimate of the severity of sleep-disordered breathing than the apnea index.

2. Paradoxical motion of the chest or abdomen during hypopnea suggests an obstructive hypopnea.

3. Identification of hypopneas is important because these events may result in arterial oxygen desaturation and arousal from sleep.

## REFERENCES
1. Block AJ, Boysen PG, Wynne WJ, et al: Sleep apnea, hypopnea, and oxygen desaturation in normal subjects: A strong male predominance. N Engl J Med 1979; 300:513–517.
2. West P, Kryger MH: Sleep and respiration: Terminology and methodology. Clin Chest Med 1985; 6:691–712.
3. Gould GA, KF Whyte, GB Rhind, et al: The sleep hypopnea syndrome. Am Rev Respir Dis 1988; 137:895–898.

# PATIENT 28

### A 45-year-old man with a snoring problem

A 45-year-old man sought treatment of his snoring, which had been present for many years. His wife slept in another bedroom because the snoring "shook the walls." The patient denied symptoms of excessive daytime sleepiness, morning headache, or problems at work (he was a successful accountant). He did admit to drinking more than five cups of coffee daily. There was no history of recent weight gain or alcohol use.

*Physical Examination:*    Height 5 feet 10 inches, weight 190 pounds, blood pressure 150/90. Neck: 18-inch circumference, no jugular venous distention. HEENT: edematous uvula, dependent palate (see below). Chest: clear. Cardiac: normal. Extremities: no edema.

*Figure:*    Compare the typical adult with the individual presenting in this case.

*Question:*    What missing bit of historical information is essential to determining whether or not a sleep study should be performed to rule out obstructive sleep apnea?

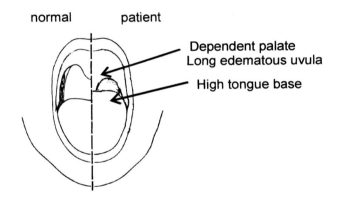

*Answer:* Question the spouse about observed apnea/gasping during sleep.

*Discussion:* Obstructive sleep apnea (OSA) is a common disorder occurring in about 4% of men and 2% of women. During sleep, closure of the upper airway results in cessation of airflow despite continued respiratory effort. The termination of apnea is associated with a brief awakening. The resulting sleep fragmentation reduces the amount of slow wave and REM sleep and causes varying degrees of daytime sleepiness.

The presence and severity of OSA can be precisely defined by sleep monitoring. However, because in-lab monitoring is expensive with limited availability, many investigators have applied selection and screening methods to patients considered for study. In a recent study examining the predictive value of a number of historical and physical findings, neck circumference, hypertension, habitual snoring, and bed partner reports of gasping/choking respirations were found to be the best predictors. Body weight, recent weight gain, and older age also were significant factors. Interestingly, the classic daytime symptoms said to be present in sleep apnea (daytime sleepiness, morning headaches, and cognitive impairment) were *not* predictive of the disorder. Unfortunately, many patients who deny symptoms of daytime sleepiness do have significant sleep apnea.

Once a patient has been selected for study, the physician decides between a full polysomnography (overnight) or a screening study (ambulatory). Initially, screening studies consisted of pulse oximetry. Later refinements added monitoring of respiration (airflow and inspiratory effort) and oxygen saturation. Today it is practical to gather the usual complete polysomnographic data on an ambulatory basis. How the data is analyzed is as important as which data is recorded. Full disclosure (a second-by-second view of the raw data rather than a simple overnight summary) is the optimal way to determine if the recording was technically adequate and to arrive at a correct diagnosis. False negative studies may occur for a number of reasons: inadequate sleep, no REM sleep recorded, no sleep in the supine position, respiratory events with minimal desaturation (oximetry screening), sleep disturbance for reasons other than apnea (periodic leg movements), respiratory-related arousals with minimal apnea/hypopnea. If the suspicion for OSA is high, a screening study will not save money if a subsequent nasal CPAP titration is required. Regardless of whether full polysomnography or a screening study is performed, it is critical that a physician knowledgeable in sleep medicine evaluate the technical adequacy of the study and correlate the findings with the patient's symptoms. For example, when the clinical suspicion of a sleep disorder is high (e.g., sleep apnea), a negative screening study should prompt more comprehensive sleep testing.

In the present case, the patient's wife reported hearing her husband stop breathing and then abruptly "snort and gasp for air." This history along with the presence of hypertension, a large neck, and habitual snoring suggested that a sleep study should be performed. The patient had an AHI of 60/hour. After nasal CPAP therapy he reported a much improved energy level, and he was more productive at work.

## Clinical Pearls

1. The presence or absence of excessive daytime sleepiness—the cardinal manifestation of OSA—is *not* a good predictor of OSA.

2. A large neck circumference, hypertension, habitual snoring, and witnessed choking/gasping during sleep are good predictors of the presence of sleep apnea.

3. Screening studies (depending on the data recorded) may have a high number of false negatives if mild-to-moderate cases of OSA are studied.

## REFERENCES

1. Young T, Palta M, Leder R, et al: The occurrence of sleep-disordered breathing among middle-aged adults. N Engl J Med 1993; 328:1230–1235.
2. Flemons WW, Whitelaw WA, Brant R, et al: Likelihood ratios for a sleep apnea clinical prediction rule. Am J Respir Crit Care Med 1994; 150:1279–1285.
3. Standards of Practice Committee, American Sleep Disorders Association: Portable recording in the assessment of obstructive sleep apnea. Sleep 1994; 17:378–392.

# PATIENT 29

## A 30-year-old woman with severe fatigue

A 30-year-old woman of normal body weight complained of severe fatigue and daytime sleepiness of 3-year duration. Her husband reported that she snored, especially during periods of nasal congestion. There was no history of symptoms characteristic of narcolepsy (cataplexy, sleep paralysis, or hypnogogic hallucinations). The patient reported getting at least 8 hours of sleep each night and denied feeling depressed. There was no history of alcohol or sedative use. An extensive medical examination found no cause for the patient's fatigue. A previous polysomnogram showed an AHI of 5/hr. Another polysomnogram and a multiple sleep latency test (MSLT) were performed.

**Physical Examination:** Normal.

**Sleep Study**

| Total sleep time | 406.55 min (394–457) | Sleep Stages | %SPT |
|---|---|---|---|
| Sleep period time (SPT) | 432.5 min (414–453) | | |
| Sleep latency | 2.5 min (0–19) | Stage Wake | 6 (0–6) |
| REM latency | 70.0 min (69–88) | Stage 1 | 8.8 (3–6) |
| AHI | 4.6/hour ($<$ 5/hr) | Stage 2 | 56.1 (46–62) |
| AHI, NREM/REM | 2.6 / 14.5 events/hr | Stages 3 and 4 | 13.8 (7–21) |
| AHI, Supine/Other | 5.3 / 4.8 events/hr | Stage REM | 15.3 (21–31) |
| | | Arousal index | 15/hr |
| | | PLM index | 0/hr |

( ) = normal values for age, AHI = apnea + hypopnea index, PLM = periodic limb (leg) movement

**MSLT:** Mean sleep latency 2 minutes, no REM periods in five naps.

**Figure:** A sample tracing from the polysomnogram is shown below.

**Question:** What is the cause of the patient's severe sleepiness?

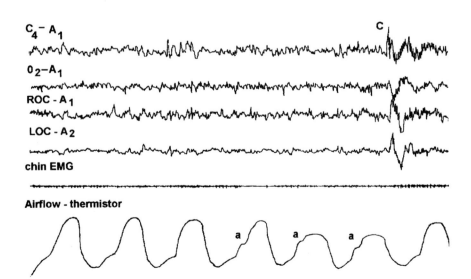

*Diagnosis:* Upper airway resistance syndrome.

*Discussion:* When symptoms or findings of daytime sleepiness are more severe than expected from the AHI on a sleep study, several possibilities must be considered. The sleep study may have underestimated the severity of illness (no supine monitoring, low amount of REM sleep). Additionally, a variety of disorders can cause daytime sleepiness, including: insufficient sleep, narcolepsy, depression, periodic leg movements in sleep, idiopathic hypersomnolence, drug abuse, and the upper airway resistance syndrome (UARS).

UARS is manifested by little or no discrete apnea or hypopnea but **repeated arousal** during periods of high upper airway resistance (increased inspiratory effort). **Fatigue** rather than daytime sleepiness can be the major complaint. While snoring is common in UARS, not all patients with this syndrome snore. This diagnosis may be missed with routine sleep monitoring unless the large number of unexplained arousals is noticed. On close examination, subtle changes in airflow or inspiratory effort precede the arousals. Monitoring of esophageal pressure in these patients reveals high esophageal pressure deflections preceding arousal. A progressive increase in respiratory effort—the **crescendo pattern**—may be seen prior to arousal. Other patients have a stable but high level of inspiratory effort associated with arousal.

An expert panel of sleep physicians recently suggested that UARS is not a separate syndrome, but simply part of the spectrum between simple snoring and obstructive apnea. It was also suggested that respiratory effort–related arousals (RERAs) be separately tabulated as part of polysomnography.

In the current case, the nocturnal sleep study provided no evidence for periodic limb movements in sleep. The amount of apnea was small and associated mainly with REM sleep. The arousal index was not high enough to explain the severity of daytime sleepiness documented on the MSLT (sleep latency 2 minutes). The MSLT showed no REM periods, and there were no symptoms of narcolepsy. The patient's sleep diary showed adequate sleep (no evidence for the insufficient sleep syndrome). Prior to a description and understanding of UARS, this patient may have been given the diagnosis of idiopathic hypersomnia. However, careful review of the polysomnogram revealed many similar episodes (see figure) recorded mainly when the patient was supine.

In this tracing, the EEG change (*C*) met standard criteria for an arousal. Note the subtle changes in the shape (*a, a, a*) and size of airflow prior to the EEG change. This construction was seen before each "unexplained" arousal. Many other episodes of such changes in airflow were followed by short bursts of slow waves or a K complex. When these were counted as arousals, the arousal index was 40/hour. This pattern and its repetition were unlikely to be coincidental. Thus, standard arousal criteria (which were designed to be conservative) may underestimate the frequency of cerebral activation. Indeed, there is a report of a group of sleepy women with high upper airway resistance and no evidence of arousal (at least by current criteria) who improved with nasal CPAP.

During a subsequent sleep study with esophageal pressure monitoring, the present patient exhibited a repeated pattern of increased esophageal pressure deflections over several breaths (crescendo pattern), followed by a sudden EEG change (not always meeting arousal criteria) and a subsequent abrupt decrease in esophageal pressure. This study confirmed the suspicion of UARS. The patient's symptoms of both fatigue and sleepiness improved dramatically after uvulopalatopharyngoplasty.

# Clinical Pearls

1. UARS (or RERAs) always should be considered in patients with unexplained, excessive daytime sleepiness.

2. Using standard monitoring, the only clue that UARS may be present is repetitive episodes of subtle changes in respiration followed by arousals (or transient EEG changes).

3. Monitoring of esophageal pressure can help diagnose UARS by documenting high levels of inspiratory effort (upper airway resistance) preceding EEG changes.

## REFERENCES

1. Guilleminault C, Stoohs R, Clerk A, et al: A cause of excessive daytime sleepiness: The upper airway resistance syndrome. Chest 1993; 104:781–787.
2. Guilleminault C, Stoohs R, Clerk A, et al: Excessive daytime somnolence in women with abnormal respiratory effort during sleep. Sleep 1993; 16:S137–138.
3. Guilleminault C, Stoohs R, Kim U, et al: Upper airway-sleep-disordered breathing in women. Ann Intern Med 1995; 122:493–501.

## Treatment of Obstructive Sleep Apnea

The first, essential determination in selecting appropriate treatment for obstructive sleep apnea (OSA) is the severity of illness. The AHI provides an overall index of the frequency of respiratory disturbance. Arbitrary but useful guidelines are: severe > 40/hr, moderate 20–40/hr, mild < 20/hr.

Factors in Assessing OSA Severity

Apnea + hypopnea index
Respiratory arousal index (sleep fragmentation)
Severity of daytime sleepiness/requirement for alertness
Severity of arterial oxygen desaturation
Comorbid illness (e.g., congestive heart failure)
Sleep-associated arrhythmias

It also is essential to consider factors that may have prevented a night of sleep recording from accurately estimating the usual severity of illness (e.g., minimal supine sleep, lack of REM sleep). The amount of sleep fragmentation (frequency of arousals) may correlate better with symptoms of daytime sleepiness than the AHI. The severity of arterial oxygen desaturation can have important consequences for the development of pulmonary hypertension and right heart failure. Some patients have minimal desaturation but are very sleepy. Other patients have mild symptoms of daytime sleepiness but severe signs of cor pulmonale. When assessing the severity of daytime sleepiness, question family members about their estimates. Additionally, consider the requirements for alertness: a professional truck driven has a more critical need for alertness than a retired, 80-year-old patient.

Generally, each category of severity in OSA is best managed by specific treatments (see table). However, a given treatment might work in other categories of disease as well. For example, a patient with severe OSA can have dramatic improvement with an oral appliance, or a patient with upper airway resistance syndrome may tolerate treatment with nasal continuous positive airway pressure. All of these treatments are discussed in the following cases.

### General Treatment Guidelines

| UARS | Mild OSA | Moderate OSA | Severe OSA |
|---|---|---|---|
| Weight loss | Weight loss | Weight loss-adjunctive | Weight loss-adjunctive |
| Position therapy | Position therapy | Oral appliances | Nasal CPAP |
| Oral appliances | Oral appliances | Nasal CPAP | Tracheostomy |
| Protriptyline + others | Protriptyline + others | UPPP | Maxillofacial surgery |
| UPPP/LAP | Nasal CPAP | Maxillofacial surgery | |
| | UPPP/LAP | | |

UARS = upper airway resistance syndrome, UPPP = uvulopalatopharyngoplasty, LAP = laser assisted palatoplasty, CPAP = continuous positive airway pressure

# PATIENT 30

## A 40-year-old woman with mild sleep apnea

A 40-year-old woman was referred by her internist for evaluation of daytime sleepiness. About a year ago he had ordered a screening sleep oximetry study, which showed minimal desaturation. The patient was labeled as having mild disease and told to lose weight. However, her daytime sleepiness persisted despite 10 pounds of weight loss. Her husband reported that she snored softly and frequently had a "pause" in breathing.

*Physical Examination:*    Mildly obese woman—weight 120 pounds, height 5 feet 2 inches. HEENT: edematous palate. Neck: 15 1/2–inch circumference. Chest: clear. Cardiac: normal. Extremities: no edema.

*Figure:*    The initial portion of the oximetry study is shown below.

*Question:*    Do you agree that this patient has mild sleep apnea?

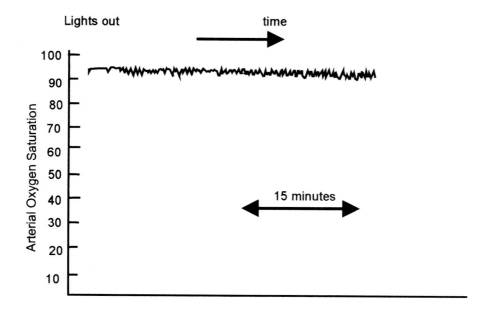

*Diagnosis:* Severe sleep apnea with minimal arterial oxygen desaturation.

*Discussion:* In determining the severity of obstructive apnea (OSA), several factors must be considered. Some patients with minimal desaturation have frequent events, a high arousal index, and severe daytime sleepiness. Thus, if an oximetry study is used to screen patients for OSA, the tracing should be scrutinized for evidence of the **saw-tooth pattern** of repeated changes in $SaO_2$. It is not sufficient to simply observe summary information. In fact, some patients have respiratory arousals without any changes in $SaO_2$. Alternatively, other patients with an AHI in the moderate range (20–40/hr) have impressive arterial oxygen desaturations and a low sleeping baseline $SaO_2$.

Studies of breath holding in normal subjects suggest that the rate of $SaO_2$ fall is inversely proportional to the baseline $SaO_2$ and to the lung volume (oxygen stores) at the start of breath hold. The rate of fall is disproportionately higher at low lung volumes secondary to increases in ventilation/perfusion mismatch. A study of OSA patients found that the severity of nocturnal arterial oxygen desaturation was related to several factors, including: the **awake supine $PaO_2$**, the percentage of **sleeptime spent in apnea,** and the **expiratory reserve volume.**

Patients with a baseline $PaO_2$ of 55–60 mmHg are on the steep part of the oxyhemoglobin saturation curve. A small fall in $PaO_2$ results in significant desaturation. While apnea duration is an obvious factor in the severity of desaturation, the length of the ventilatory period also is important. Some patients do not completely resaturate between events as they quickly return to sleep, and the airway closes again. Long event duration and short periods between apneas mean the percentage of sleeptime spent in apnea is high. The clinical significance of a low expiratory reserve volume (ERV) may be less obvious. The ERV is the difference between the functional residual capacity (FRC; end expiratory lung volume) and the residual volume (RV; volume at maximal exhalation). The FRC is reduced in obesity secondary to low compliance of the chest wall/abdomen. The residual volume is increased if patients have any degree of obstructive airway disease (airtrapping). Thus a low ERV means that the patient has low oxygen stores at the start of apnea (a low FRC) and significant ventilation/perfusion mismatch at low lung volumes (identified by a high RV).

Clinically, the groups of OSA patients with severe desaturation include patients with a low $PO_2$ for any reason (severe obesity, daytime hypoventilation, and chronic obstructive pulmonary disease [COPD]). In fact, some patients can have significant desaturation after events as short as 10–15 seconds. The severity of desaturation also depends on sleep stage. In most OSA patients, the longest apneas and most severe desaturations occur in REM sleep. Some studies also have suggested that at equivalent apnea length, the severity of desaturation is worse in obstructive than central apnea.

In the present case, a complete sleep study revealed an AHI of 60/hr. The events were short (mean duration 15 seconds), and the baseline sleeping $SaO_2$ was 95%. The patient was only mildly obese and had no evidence of COPD. Thus, it is not surprising that the arterial oxygen desaturation was mild. However, the arousal index was 55/hr—consistent with several sleep fragmentation. The patient was treated with nasal CPAP, and she experienced a rapid improvement.

## Clinical Pearls

1. Some patients with minimal arterial oxygen desaturation have severe OSA, indicated by a high AHI and severe sleep fragmentation.

2. The severity of arterial oxygen desaturation in patients with OSA depends on the baseline supine $PO_2$, the percentage of apnea time (apnea length), and the degrees of obesity (decreased FRC) and obstructive lung disease (increased RV).

3. Arterial oxygen desaturation usually is more severe in REM than NREM sleep and in obstructive rather than central apnea (equivalent length).

4. Screening for OSA for oximetry can result in false negatives in patients with mild arterial oxygen desaturation during apnea/hypopnea.

## REFERENCES

1. Findley LJ, Ries AL, Tisi GM: Hypoxemia during apnea in normal subjects: Mechanisms and impact of lung volume. J Appl Physiol 1983; 55:1777–1783.
2. Bradley TD, Martinez D, Rutherford R, et al: Physiological determinants of nocturnal arterial oxygenation in patients with obstructive sleep apnea. J Appl Physiol 1985; 59:1364–1368.
3. Series F, Cormier Y, La Forge J: Influence of apnea type and sleep stage on nocturnal postapneic desaturation. Am Rev Respir Dis 1990; 141:1522–1526.

# PATIENT 31

## A 55-year-old man with heavy nighttime snoring and daytime sleepiness

A 55-year-old obese man was evaluated for complaints of excessive daytime sleepiness of 4-year duration. He snored heavily and was observed by his wife to stop breathing during sleep. Because of a strong suspicion for obstructive sleep apnea (OSA), the patient underwent a partial or split-night study. The first portion of the night was a diagnostic study and the second portion a nasal continuous positive airway pressure (CPAP) titration. The test was terminated at the patient's request because he no longer felt sleepy. He had some initial difficulty tolerating CPAP at 10–12.5 cm $H_2O$.

*Physical Examination:*   Obese—weight 240 pounds, height 5 feet 11 inches. HEENT: long, dependent palate. Neck: 18-inch circumference. Chest: clear. Cardiac: normal. Extremities: no edema.

*Sleep Study*

| CPAP (cm $H_2O$) | 0 (diagnostic) | 5.0 | 7.5 | 10 | 12.5 |
|---|---|---|---|---|---|
| Monitoring time (min) | 240 | 60 | 60 | 60 | 40 |
| NREM (min) | 180 | 40 | 50 | 30 | 20 |
| REM (min) | 10 | 10 | 10 | 0 | 0 |
| AHI (/hr) | 75 | 60 | 50 | 40 | 10 |
| Body position | Supine | Supine | Lateral | Lateral | Lateral |

*Question:*   Why is this CPAP titration suboptimal?

*Answer:* The efficacy of nasal CPAP in the supine position during REM sleep has not been documented.

*Discussion:* Nasal CPAP is probably the treatment of choice for most patients with moderate-to-severe OSA. The mechanism of action is to provide a pneumatic splint to preserve upper airway patency. The pressure level required to maintain airway patency is determined by **CPAP titration:** pressure is incrementally increased to find the point at which apnea, hypopnea, snoring, desaturation, and respiratory effort–related arousals are prevented (the "**optimal pressure**"). This pressure varies 5–20 cm $H_2O$ between patients. The required pressure even varies in the same patient, depending on body posture (higher supine) and sleep stage (usually higher in REM). *Thus the optimal pressure for a patient is one that is effective in all body positions and stages of sleep.* To avoid the high cost of performing two separate sleep studies, many sleep centers perform partial or split-night studies. As in this case, the first portion of the night is diagnostic; the second portion is a CPAP titration. The length of time required for the diagnostic portion and the indications for initiating a CPAP titration vary between sleep centers.

There is a certain amount of art as well as science in the CPAP titration. For many patients the trial is also a desensitization exercise in which the patient becomes acclimated to the mask and pressure. Sometimes the level of pressure must be reduced (at least temporarily) even if it is not the optimal pressure. Patient education *before* the sleep study begins can help tremendously in the adjustment process. (Education about nasal CPAP at 3 AM tends to be poorly received by most patients.) The initial acceptance of CPAP depends on an adequate mask fit. Mask and headgear fit also is best determined prior to beginning the study. The art of dealing with patient concerns and determining when to increase the pressure (and when to back off for a while) is a challenging part of the sleep technician's job.

The proper endpoint for CPAP titration is still the subject of research. When initially introduced, the usual goal was prevention of apnea, hypopnea, and desaturation. Most centers continued to increase the CPAP level until snoring was eliminated. With the recognition that high upper airway resistance (high inspiratory effort) can induce arousals even if snoring is absent (upper airway resistance syndrome), upward titration of CPAP typically is continued if repiratory effort–related arousals are occurring. A few laboratories place esophageal catheters as part of routine sleep studies/CPAP titrations. Those centers titrate until esophageal pressure swings reach 5–10 cm $H_2O$. Other centers have used the shape of inspiratory airflow (flow limitation) to identify high upper airway resistance. Flow-limited breaths are characterized by a constant or decreasing flow despite increased respiratory effort (esophageal pressure deflection). The tracing of inspiratory airflow is flat and wide rather than rounded. The pattern of flow limitation usually is noted during periods of high inspiratory effort. This method requires more accurate airflow monitoring than possible with thermocouples. Monitoring must be performed with pneumotachographs or nasal cannula attached to pressure transducers. Fortunately, many diagnostic CPAP units have an analog output derived from a flow signal measured with an internal pneumotachograph. CPAP is titrated upward until evidence of flow limitation is eliminated. The best method of choosing the optimal CPAP pressure remains to be determined. Ultimately, the goal of CPAP titration is to produce high-quality, restorative sleep rather than endpoints related to upper airway function.

In the present case, the AHI was reduced to 10/hr—a fairly reasonable level—at a CPAP level of 12.5 cm $H_2O$. However, efficacy was not documented either in the supine position or in REM sleep. Thus, the true optimal pressure for this patient has not been determined. In retrospect, less time should have been spent on the diagnostic part of the study (a case of obvious severe OSA) and more time on the CPAP titration.

## Clinical Pearls

1. The goal of the CPAP titration is to determine the optimal pressure—one that is effective in all body positions and stages of sleep.

2. The optimal CPAP level should not only prevent sleep-disordered breathing, but allow for maintenance of high-quality, restorative sleep (reduced arousals, normal sleep architecture).

3. A split-night study is economical but reduces the time both for diagnosis and CPAP titration. Appropriate education pre-study is essential.

4. CPAP titration is an art as well as a science. The importance of education and technician-patient rapport cannot be overemphasized.

# REFERENCES

1. Sanders MH, NB Kern, JP Costantino, et al: Adequacy of prescribing positive airway pressure therapy by mask for sleep apnea on the basis of a partial-night trial. Am Rev Respir Dis 1993; 147:1169–1174.
2. American Thoracic Society: Indications and standards for use of nasal continuous positive airway pressure (CPAP) in sleep apnea syndromes. Am J Resp Crit Care Med 1994; 50:1738–1745.
3. Montserrat JM, Ballester E, Olivi H: Time course of stepwise CPAP titration. Am J Respir Crit Care Med 1995; 152:1854–1859.
4. Rapoport DM: Methods to stabilize the upper airway using positive pressure. Sleep 1996; 19:S123–S130.

# PATIENT 32

## A 45-year-old man with heavy snoring

A 45-year-old man was evaluated for complaints of heavy snoring for many years and daytime sleepiness of about 4-year duration. There was no history of cataplexy or sleep paralysis. The patient did not drink alcohol.

*Physical Examination:* Height 5 feet 10 inches, weight 180 pounds. HEENT: edematous uvula. Neck: 15-inch circumference. Otherwise normal exam.

### Sleep Study

| | | | |
|---|---|---|---|
| Time in bed | 480 min (390–468) | Sleep Stages | % SPT |
| Total sleep time | 350 min (343–436) | Stage Wake | 18 (1–12) |
| Sleep period time (SPT) | 425 min (378–452) | Stage 1 | 13 (5–11) |
| Sleep latency | 10 min (2–18) | Stage 2 | 49 (44–66) |
| REM latency | 90 min (55–78) | Stages 3 and 4 | 5 (2–15) |
| Arousal index (/hr) | 20/hr | Stage REM | 15 (19–27) |
| AHI | 12/hr (<5) | | |
| AHI, NREM sleep | 5/hr | PLM index | 0/hr |
| AHI, REM sleep | 50/hr | | |

( ) = normal values for age, PLM = periodic leg movement.

*Question:* For what disorder should this patient be treated?

***Answer:*** REM-related obstructive sleep apnea

***Discussion:*** Some patients have episodes of obstructive sleep apnea (OSA) primarily during REM sleep. Thus, the overall AHI may be low even if the AHI during REM sleep is fairly high. Many of these patients also may have a postural component to their apnea, with apnea occurring during NREM sleep only in the supine position. In the absence of other disorders to explain the excessive daytime sleepiness, many clinicians have empirically treated these patients, who have REM-specific sleep apnea, with usual treatments such as nasal continuous positive airway pressure (CPAP).

It is possible that some of these patients have upper airway resistance syndrome in NREM sleep—arousals secondary to high inspiratory effort without overt apnea. A recent study of a group of patients with a low overall AHI (<10/hr) but varying amounts of apnea-hypopnea during REM sleep found that 80% with a REM-specific AHI > 15/hr had a short sleep latency during daytime naps (evidence of excessive sleepiness). Thus, frequent apnea during REM sleep alone may justify treatment.

In the present case, the patient had a very high AHI in REM sleep and almost no apnea in NREM sleep. The REM-associated apneas were quite long and the desaturation impressive (see figure below). The patient underwent a nasal CPAP trial and was treated with 10 cm $H_2O$ with resolution of his symptoms. During the trial, he had a large rebound in the amount of REM sleep (30% of SPT).

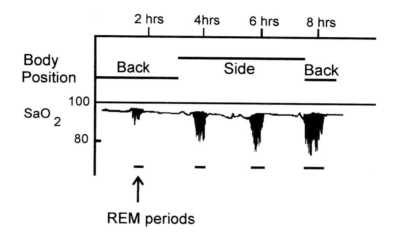

## Clinical Pearls

1. Some patients have OSA primarily during REM sleep, resulting in a low overall AHI despite frequent events and associated arousals in REM sleep.

2. In patients with excessive daytime sleepiness and significant, REM-specific sleep apnea, treatment may be indicated. Other possible causes of daytime sleepiness should be excluded.

## REFERENCES

1. Guilleminault C, Stoohs R, Clerk A, et al: A cause of excessive daytime sleepiness: The upper airway resistance syndrome. Chest 1993; 104:781–787.
2. Kass JE, Akers SM, Bartter TC, et al: REM-specific sleep-disordered breathing: A possible cause of excessive daytime sleepiness. Am J Respir Crit Care Med 1996; 154:167–169.

# PATIENT 33

## A 30-year-old man with heavy snoring and daytime sleepiness

A 30-year-old man was evaluated for complaints of heavy snoring, daytime sleepiness, and apnea (witnessed by his wife) of at least 5-year duration. The patient had gained about 30 pounds over this period. He admitted to drinking several cocktails nightly. There was no history of cataplexy or sleep paralysis.

*Physical Examination:* Blood pressure 160/88, pulse 88. General: obese—weight 210 pounds, height 5 feet 10 inches. HEENT: dependent, edematous uvula. Neck: 18-inch circumference. Chest: clear. Cardiac: normal. Extremities: no edema.

*Sleep Study*

| | |
|---|---|
| AHI | 12/hr |
| AHI, NREM sleep | 10/hr (80% of total sleep time) |
| AHI, REM sleep | 20/hr (20% of total sleep time) |
| PLM index | 5/hr |
| Arousal index | 20/hr |
| Minimum SaO$_2$ | 85% |
| Body position | 25% lateral decubitus, 75% supine |

*Question:* In view of the severe symptoms, why does the sleep study document only mild apnea?

**Answer:**    The patient was abstinent from alcohol at the time of the study.

**Discussion:**    The clinician often is faced with the problem of interpreting a sleep study that at first glance appears to show milder obstructive sleep apnea (OSA) than suspected on the basis of the history (significant daytime sleepiness). Rough guidelines for interpreting the apnea + hypopnea index (AHI) are: AHI < 20 mild, 20–40 moderate, > 40 severe. However, the AHI is only one means of assessing the severity of OSA. In fact, the correlation between AHI and symptomatic or MSLT measures of daytime sleepiness is low (but statistically significant). Two patients with the same AHI may have quite different amounts of daytime sleepiness. The arousal index also must be considered. Some patients with an AHI indicating mild apnea have considerably more respiratory arousals secondary to high respiratory effort (upper airway resistance syndrome).

Another explanation for a sleep study showing milder than expected OSA is the normal night-to-night variation in the AHI, which is due to different body positions, variations in nasal resistance, variable amounts of REM sleep, and the effects of medications and beverages. Some patients have apnea only while supine or in stage REM sleep. Therefore, in these patients the AHI depends on the amount of time spent sleeping supine or in REM sleep. Nasal congestion is a factor because increases in nasal resistance increase the amount of apnea.

The use of ethanol always should be considered in evaluation of patients with OSA. This drug has a powerful, preferential, inhibitory effect on upper airway muscle activity and increases snoring and apnea. In addition to increasing the AHI, ethanol impairs the arousal response to airway occlusion; thus, apneas tend to be longer and associated with more severe desaturations. Ethanol suppresses REM sleep. This usually results in an increase in the REM latency and a shift of REM toward the morning (as the ethanol level drops). Therefore, the regular use of ethanol worsens sleep apnea considerably. Conversely, abstinence from ethanol could reduce the AHI and apnea duration/degree of arterial oxygen desaturation recorded on a sleep study.

Some have hypothesized that ethanol might reduce the effectiveness of an optimal level of nasal CPAP. However, at least two studies have shown that this is not the case. The use of alcohol still should be discouraged in patients undergoing this treatment, because they may fall asleep without putting the nasal CPAP on, or they may remove the CPAP during the night.

In the present patient, the arousal index was only slightly higher than the AHI, and both REM sleep and the supine position were evaluated. However, the patient did not ingest his favorite alcoholic beverages before this sleep study. Repeat testing after the patient's usual intake of ethanol showed an AHI of 40 and an increase in mean apnea duration by 5 seconds.

## Clinical Pearls

1. When a sleep study reveals milder apnea than suspected on the basis of clinical symptoms, consider the effects of body position, the amount of REM sleep, and the possible presence of the upper airway resistance syndrome (arousal index much higher than the AHI).

2. The effects of ethanol use (or abstinence) on the severity of sleep apnea always should be considered.

3. Ethanol use increases the amount of apnea and the duration of obstructive events, as well as the severity of desaturation.

4. Ethanol increases the REM latency and decreases the amount of REM sleep.

## REFERENCES
1. Issa FG, Sullivan CE: Alcohol, snoring, and sleep apnea. J Neurol Neurosurg Psychiatry 1982; 45:353–359.
2. Remmers JE: Obstructive sleep apnea—A common disorder exacerbated by alcohol. (Editorial) Am Rev Respir Dis 1984; 130:153–155.
3. Berry RB, Desa MM, Light RW: Effect of ethanol on the efficacy of nasal continuous positive airway pressure as a treatment for obstructive sleep apnea. Chest 1991; 99:339–343.
4. Berry RB, Bonnet MH, Light RW: The effect of ethanol on the arousal response to airway occlusion during sleep in normal subjects. Am Rev Respir Dis 1992; 145:445–452.

# PATIENT 34

## A 30-year-old man with weight loss and sleep apnea

A 30-year-old man—height 5 feet 10 inches, weight 230 pounds—was diagnosed as having severe obstructive sleep apnea (AHI 60/hr). He underwent a nasal CPAP titration, and CPAP at a level of 12 cm $H_2O$ was found to reduce his AHI to < 5/hr. The patient underwent treatment and noted a rapid resolution in his daytime sleepiness. After 1 year of treatment he began a high-fiber, low-fat diet to reduce elevated cholesterol. Over the next 5 months he lost 30 pounds, and his cholesterol improved. He requested that another CPAP titration be performed. Encouraged by the results, he continued his weight loss program and dropped another 10 pounds. Since the original study, the patient's neck size had decreased from 18 to 15 ½ inches. He requested another sleep study off nasal CPAP to determine if treatment was still necessary.

### Sleep Studies

| | | | | |
|---|---|---|---|---|
| Weight (lbs.) | 230 | 230 | 200 | 190 |
| CPAP | None | 12 cmH$_2$O | 7.5 cm H$_2$O | None |
| AHI | 60/hr | 5/hr | 5/hr | 10/hr |
| Arousal index | 45/hr | 5/hr | 7/hr | 15/hr |

*Question:*  Should nasal CPAP treatment be discontinued?

*Answer:*  Nasal CPAP can be discontinued if weight loss is maintained.

*Discussion:*  Obesity is a major risk factor for the development of OSA. In some studies, approximately 66% of patients with OSA were obese (body weight > 120% of predicted). Neck circumference is a better predictor of OSA than body weight, indicating that nuchal obesity is more important than total body obesity. The mechanisms by which obesity causes OSA still are unknown.

Studies suggest that obesity has direct effects on upper airway function (changes in the nature of upper airway tissues) or indirect effects secondary to changes in lung volume. One magnetic resonance study of the upper airway in OSA suggested that fat deposition adjacent to the lateral pharyngeal walls reduced the upper airway size. Another study found thickened lateral pharyngeal walls, but these changes were not secondary to fat or edema. Patients with OSA tend to have small upper airways, although there is considerable overlap. Shape may be as important as size. The **shape of the upper airway** in OSA patients is different (see figure). How obesity and weight loss directly change the size of the upper airway remains to be determined.

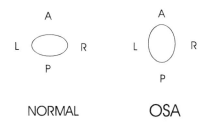

A = anterior,  P = posterior,  R ,L = right and left

The size of the upper airway varies with lung volume, probably secondary to the effects of tracheal displacement (tracheal tug). Obesity reduces supine lung volume and therefore upper airway size. Studies also have shown that the collapsibility of the upper airway is decreased by weight loss, implying that obesity increases the tendency of the upper airway to collapse.

Many studies have documented that weight loss of modest proportions (5–10%) can produce significant improvement in sleep apnea. Even patients with mild obesity (110–115% of ideal body weight) can benefit from weight reduction. The results vary among patients; for example, a given amount of weight loss may have more effect on upper body obesity in one individual than in another. Nevertheless, weight loss decreases both the AHI and the collapsibility of the upper airway in patients with OSA. The level of nasal CPAP required to maintain upper airway patency also may decrease following weight reduction. Surgical, behavioral, and pharmacologic approaches to weight loss have all been successful in select groups of patients. The major problem to date has been **maintenance of weight loss.**

In the present patient, weight reduction initially decreased the amount of nasal CPAP required to maintain airway patency. After additional weight reduction, the AHI off CPAP was near normal. The patient was anxious to stop CPAP and reported no relapse in symptoms when this treatment was discontinued. Unfortunately, 4 months later the patient's weight increased to 200 pounds. He still denied a return of excessive daytime sleepiness. The patient was counseled that resumption of treatment might be necessary if further weight gain occurred.

## Clinical Pearls

1. Weight reduction can significantly improve the severity of OSA. The amount of reduction required varies widely, but can be only 5–10% of body weight.

2. Weight reduction (weight gain) may decrease (increase) the level of nasal CPAP required to maintain upper airway patency.

3. The major challenge of weight reduction as a treatment for OSA is *maintaining* the weight loss.

## REFERENCES

1. Smith PL, Gold AR, Meyers DA, et al: Weight loss in mildly to moderately obese patients with obstructive sleep apnea. Ann Intern Med 1985; 103:850–855.
2. Schwartz AR, Gold AR, Schubert N, et al: Effect of weight loss on upper airway collapsibility in obstructive sleep apnea. Am Rev Respir Dis 1991; 144:494–498.
3. Shelton KE, Woodson H, Spencer G, et al: Pharyngeal fat in obstructive sleep apnea. Am Rev Respir Dis 1993; 148:462-466.
4. Schwab RJ. Functional properties of the pharyngeal airway: Properties of tissues surrounding the upper airway. Sleep 1996; 19:S170–S174.
5. Strobel RJ, Rosen RC: Obesity and weight loss in obstructive sleep apnea: A critical review. Sleep 1996; 19:104–115.

# PATIENT 35

**A 55-year-old man having difficulty with CPAP because of nasal congestion**

A 55-year-old man was diagnosed as having severe obstructive sleep apnea (AHI 55/hr). After CPAP titration, treatment with nasal CPAP was initiated. Unfortunately, the patient developed severe nasal congestion and was unable to continue treatment. He had a long history of mild nasal congestion that worsened during the spring. He was treated with a nonsedating antihistamine and nasal steroid medications without much improvement. He reported waking up several hours after starting nasal CPAP and being unable to breathe through his nose. A very dry mouth usually was noted at that time.

*Physical Examination:*  Nose: edematous mucosa, no polyps. HEENT: large tongue, edematous uvula. Neck: 18-inch circumference. Chest: clear. Cardiac: normal. Extremities: no edema.

*Question:*  What further therapy would you consider?

*Answer:*    Humidification and aggressive decongestant therapy may ease CPAP side effects.

*Discussion:*    Nasal symptoms are common in patients with OSA before treatment, and nasal obstruction itself may be a cause of sleep-disordered breathing. After starting treatment with nasal CPAP, many patients report new or increased nasal symptoms. Of patients using nasal CPAP, 30–50% experience nasal congestion, dry nose and throat, sore throat, and even bleeding from the nose. These side effects can dramatically reduce compliance and result in cessation of therapy.

It is unclear how nasal CPAP increases or causes nasal symptoms. In some patients, the necessity of nasal respiration draws attention to de novo nasal symptoms. In others, airway pressure on the nasal mucosa induces rhinitis by reflex mechanisms. These patients may respond to inhaled, anticholinergic medication (ipratropium bromide). However, in most patients nasal congestion rather than rhinitis is the major problem.

The etiology of worsening nasal congestion is not known with certainty but may be related to **mucosal drying.** Cold, dry air appears to induce release of mediators from mast cells. Some degree of mouth breathing may initiate a unidirectional airleak (out the mouth), and the loss of moisture from the system overwhelms the capacity of the nasal mucosa to humidify inspired air. Further drying of the nasal mucosa results in more nasal congestion and even higher nasal resistance, which, in turn, promotes more mouth breathing. Thus, a vicious cycle develops. In many patients, adequate **humidification** of air can break this cycle. It also can improve symptoms of nasal congestion. While pass-over humidification (air blown over water) may be adequate in mild cases, most patients with significant symptoms require heated humidification.

Another approach to **mouth leaks** is to use chin straps. Their efficacy has not been studied systematically, but some patients improve with their use. Interestingly, recent studies suggest that patients with a prior uvulopalatopharyngoplasty may have a greater tendency for mouth leaks. This finding seems reasonable, as the absence of a mouth leak in most patients using nasal CPAP probably is due to the forward movement of the palate against the tongue (sealing off the oral passages from flow). In patients with nasal congestion who fail a trial of humidification, topical or oral vasoconstrictors can be tried (at bedtime only). Most physicians are aware that topical nasal vasoconstrictors cannot be used continuously without inducing rebound nasal congestion.

In the present patient, heated humidification was added to the nasal CPAP circuit with improvement in the symptoms of nasal congestion. The patient resumed treatment and only rarely required a topical nasal vasoconstrictor at bedtime. He continued the use of an inhaled nasal steroid medication.

## Clinical Pearls

1. Nasal symptoms are a major cause of compliance problems with nasal CPAP therapy.

2. Mouth leaks may further increase nasal resistance by setting up a unidirectional flow out the mouth (leak) and drying the nasal mucosa.

3. If initial therapy for nasal congestion with nasal steroids and nonsedating antihistamines (if an allergic component is suspected) fails or the patient complains of dry nose/mouth, then humidification should be added to the CPAP circuit.

4. Topical vasoconstrictors can be used to treat nasal congestion as a last resort at bedtime only.

REFERENCES
1. Kribbs NB, Pack AI, Kline LR, et al: Objective measurement of patterns of nasal CPAP use by patients with obstructive sleep apnea. Am J Resp Crit Care Med 1993; 147:887–895.
2. Richards GN, Cistulli PA, Ungar RG, et al: Mouth leak with nasal continuous positive airway pressure increases nasal airway resistance. Am J Respir Crit Care Med 1996; 154:182–186.

# PATIENT 36

## A 30-year-old man unable to tolerate nasal CPAP

A 30-year-old man with severe obstructive sleep apnea stopped using nasal CPAP because the prescribed pressure of 10 cm $H_2O$ was "too high." He was unable to fall asleep using nasal CPAP and felt that the pressure level was more than he could tolerate. A summary of his original CPAP titration is shown below. When the patient changed from the left lateral to supine position, a CPAP level of 5 cm $H_2O$ was no longer adequate, and it was increased to 7.5 cm $H_2O$. At 7.5 cm $H_2O$ there were few events until the patient entered REM sleep. The CPAP level was increased to 9 and then to 10 cm $H_2O$ to maintain airway patency.

### Sleep Study—CPAP Titration

| Pressure (cm $H_2O$) | 0 | 5 | 5 | 7.5 | 10 |
|---|---|---|---|---|---|
| Body position | Left lateral | Left lateral | Supine | Supine | Supine |
| AHI (events/hr) | 55 | 10 | 50 | 15 | 5 |
| AHI, NREM | 60 | 10 | 50 | 5 | 0 |
| AHI, REM | — | — | — | 40 | 5 |

**Question:** What measures could make treatment with nasal CPAP acceptable to this patient?

***Answer:*** Measures include the ramp option, self-adjusting CPAP, bilevel pressure, postural changes, and lower prescription pressure.

***Discussion:*** Several approaches are available when patients have difficulty tolerating the prescribed CPAP pressure. The **ramp mode** on many commercial CPAP units allows a slow increase in airway pressure from a low setting (around 3 cm $H_2O$) to the prescribed pressure, so that the patient can fall asleep at lower pressures. The ramp period (time to reach set pressure) is adjustable on most units. If the patient awakens during the night, the ramp mode can be reinitiated. Two important points: (1) The mask seal must be tested at the final (prescribed) pressure before the ramp is initiated. If this is not done, mask leaks may appear as the pressure increases. (2) The low initial pressure is a problem for some patients. These patients may have trouble falling asleep due to difficulty breathing through the system even when awake. Some CPAP units allow an increase of the initial pressure in the ramp mode. If not, a short ramp period may be better tolerated than a long one.

Recently, "smart" CPAP units have been developed that allow **auto-titration** of the level of pressure. These units apply a variety of detection methods—searching for apnea and airway vibration and profiling inspiratory airflow—to ascertain whether airway pressure should be increased. When no events are detected, the units slowly lower the level of pressure. This continuous titration of pressures may lower the mean pressure required to maintain airway patency. For example, while sleeping in the lateral decubitus position a pressure level of 5 cm $H_2O$ is adequate. When supine (perhaps 40% of the night), the required pressure increases to 10 cm $H_2O$. Thus, the mean pressure is 7 cm $H_2O$ instead of a single setting of 10 cm $H_2O$. Whether such devices increase compliance remains to be determined. It is likely that selected patients will benefit from this new technology.

Another approach to intolerance of a level of CPAP is to switch to **bilevel pressure.** This method can allow maintenance of airway patency with a lower pressure during expiration and may be especially useful in patients who mainly complain of difficulty exhaling. Bilevel pressure is detailed in another case (see Patient 38, page 105).

Adjunctive therapy also may decrease the level of pressure required to maintain airway patency. Weight loss can minimize the tendency of the upper airway to collapse, and medications such as pro-triptyline can augment upper airway muscle tone. The simultaneous use of an oral appliance can sometimes improve the efficacy of a given level of CPAP. Aggressive treatment of nasal resistance (congestion) also can reduce the required mask pressure. Note that the pressure level at the mask is *not* the inspiratory pressure level in the oropharynx or hypopharynx, due to a pressure drop across the nose.

A recent study suggests that **postural change** can be beneficial in this situation, as well. However, although most people snore less when sleeping in the lateral decubitus position, this posture can be ineffective in very obese patients. Moreover, it is difficult to constrain patients to sleep on their sides. Alternatively, a recent study found that modest head elevation (30%) reduced the pressure required to maintain upper airway patency by almost 5 cm $H_2O$.

A final approach is simply to accept a lower pressure than the optimal pressure determined during the CPAP trial. For example, the present patient did well at 7.5 cm $H_2O$ in the supine position until he entered REM sleep. He may be better served by using nasal CPAP at a **lower-than-optimal pressure** than by stopping therapy altogether. Five events per hour in NREM sleep is much better than 55 per hour (no CPAP), even if maintenance of airway patency in REM is incomplete. With an AHI 5/hr in NREM and 40/hr in REM, the overall AHI is likely to be around 16/hr (assuming 20% REM sleep). In many other treatments for OSA, an AHI of 15/hr in a patient with 55/hr at baseline would be considered a good response. Accepting less-than-perfect treatment results is especially important for patients with severe OSA, in whom the only effective alternatives are tracheostomy or extensive upper airway surgery (not always available). Long-term use of CPAP can reduce airway edema in some patients, and a lower level of CPAP may be more efficacious with time.

In the present case, the patient was unable to tolerate 10 cm $H_2O$ despite use of the ramp system. He was able to tolerate a CPAP of 7.5 cm $H_2O$ and was told to elevate the head of his bed and lose weight. With this management, the patient had an acceptable resolution of symptoms. A repeat nasal CPAP titration 3 months later, after a 10-pound weight loss, showed an overall AHI of 10/hr in the supine position on 7.5 cm $H_2O$.

# Clinical Pearls

1. The ramp mode, self-adjusting CPAP, and bilevel pressure are treatment alternatives in patients unable to use nasal CPAP at the optimal pressure due to pressure intolerance.

2. Adjunctive measures such as postural changes, weight loss, decreased nasal resistance, and medications to increase upper airway tone can improve the efficacy of a given level of CPAP.

3. Many patients are better served by using a less-than-optimal CPAP pressure rather than no effective therapy at all. With chronic treatment the lower levels of CPAP may become more effective, possibly due to reduced airway edema.

## REFERENCES

1. Nino-Murcia G, Bliwise D, Keenan S, et al: Treatment of obstructive sleep apnea and protriptyline. Chest 1988; 94:1314–1315.
2. Schwartz AR, Gold AR, Schubert N: Effect of weight loss on upper airway collapsibility in obstructive sleep apnea. Am Rev Respir Dis 1991; 144:494–498.
3. Mortimore IL, Kochhar P, Douglas NJ: Effect of continuous positive airway pressure (CPAP) therapy on upper airway size in patients with sleep apnea/hypopnea syndrome. Thorax 1996; 51:190-192.
4. Rapoport DM: Methods of stabilize the upper airway using positive pressure. Sleep 1996; 19:S123–S130.
5. Neill AM, Angus S, Sajovo D, McEvoy RD: Effects of sleep posture on upper airway stability in patients with obstructive sleep apnea. Am J Resp Crit Care Med 1997; 155:199–204.

# PATIENT 37

**A 55-year-old man unable to use nasal CPAP due to intractable nasal congestion**

A 55-year-old man with a long history of nasal congestion was diagnosed as having severe obstructive sleep apnea (AHI 70/hr). He underwent a nasal CPAP titration but the procedure was terminated at the patient's request because he could not breathe thorough his nose. He already was being treated with a nonsedating antihistamine and a nasal steroid inhaler. In the past he reported improvement with oxymetazalone (a topical nasal vasoconstrictor), but he developed dependence on this medication (rebound). He refused to consider surgical treatments for OSA.

***Physical Examination:*** Nose: slightly deviated septum, moderate mucosal edema and erythema, no polyps. Tongue: large, difficult to see oropharyngeal aperture.

***Question:*** What treatment options are available for this patient?

*Answer:*    Consider full face mask CPAP, also called oronasal CPAP.

*Discussion:*    Occasionally a patient with OSA is unable to tolerate the initial CPAP titration due to difficulty with nasal breathing. While medical treatment of nasal congestion or surgical treatment of structural obstruction may ultimately improve the condition, the loss of a CPAP titration opportunity in the sleep laboratory is expensive. Other patients may complain of intractable nasal obstruction once CPAP treatment is initiated and are unable to continue treatment. In both cases, application of CPAP by a full face mask (oronasal CPAP) provides a useful treatment alternative, allowing patients to breathe through both the nose and mouth.

Two studies have shown that full face CPAP works in patients unable to tolerate nasal CPAP due to nasal obstruction. Full face masks, which became commercially available just recently, have some **unique features** compared to nasal masks. First, quick removal must be possible should the patient need to vomit. Second, there must be a valve to allow entry of room air in case the source of air fails (CPAP unit failure). Third, a good seal must be obtained with a full face mask. This is more difficult than with a nasal mask because there is a larger area to be covered and sealed. Many edentulous patients have a less rigid face, making a seal even more difficult. Nevertheless, the full face mask may be the only method some patients will tolerate.

After completion of CPAP titration in the laboratory, intensive treatment of the nose may allow some patients to be switched to nasal CPAP. However, there are a few patients for whom full face CPAP is the only truly effective, nonsurgical alternative.

Another group in whom full face masks can be useful are those patients with a large oral leak. Chin straps may work in a few of these patients. In others, the addition of humidification and treatment of nasal congestion may decrease the tendency to open the mouth during sleep. However, a patient not responding to these measures may benefit from oronasal CPAP.

The present patient underwent a repeat CPAP titration with a full face mask. At 15 cm $H_2O$ the AHI was reduced to 5/hr. The patient currently is using CPAP with a full face mask and is experiencing good improvement of symptoms.

## Clinical Pearls

1. When patients are unable to tolerate nasal CPAP titration due to nasal obstruction, titration with a full face mask should be tried to avoid losing a night in the sleep lab.

2. In cases of *intractable* nasal congestion, oronasal CPAP may be the only treatment option that is tolerated.

3. Nasal CPAP via a full face mask can be useful in patients with a large, oral air leak that does not respond to chin straps.

REFERENCES
1. Prosise GL, Berry RB: Oral-nasal continuous positive airway pressure as a treatment for obstructive sleep apnea. Chest 1994; 106:180–186.
2. Sanders MH, Kern NB, Stiller RA, et al: CPAP therapy via oronasal mask for obstructive sleep apnea. Chest 1994; 106:774–779.

# PATIENT 38

## A 45-year-old man with intolerance to nasal CPAP because of difficulty exhaling

A 45-year-old man was diagnosed as having severe obstructive sleep apnea (AHI 80/hr). He underwent a nasal CPAP titration, and the optimal pressure was determined to be 14 cm $H_2O$. Treatment with nasal CPAP at this pressure was initiated. However, the patient returned complaining that the pressure was too high. He stated that it was especially uncomfortable to exhale against the pressure. Review of the CPAP titration showed that at 13 cm $H_2O$ the patient still had 25 hypopneas per hour in NREM sleep. Rather than lower the pressure, the patient underwent a trial with bilevel pressure.

*Figure:* Events such as this were common at an expiratory positive airway pressure (EPAP) of 10 cm $H_2O$ and an inspiratory positive airway pressure (IPAP) of 12 cm $H_2O$. This level of pressure can be designated as 12/10 cm $H_2O$. Bands around the patient's chest and abdomen were used to detect respiratory effort.

*Question:* What adjustment would you make to the pressure levels?

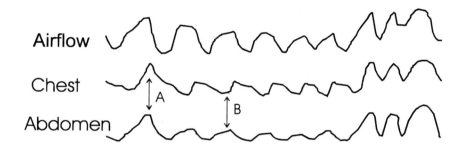

*Answer:*    Increase inspiratory positive airway pressure.

*Discussion:* Separately adjustable IPAP and EPAP (bilevel pressure) was introduced with the goal of being able to use lower expiratory pressures and still maintain upper airway patency during sleep. Some patients with OSA who are treated with nasal CPAP complain of great difficulty breathing out against the expiratory pressure. With bilevel pressure, airway patency usually can be maintained with a lower level of expiratory pressure. As CPAP is titrated upward, upper airway occlusion (apnea) typically converts to upper airway narrowing (hypopnea). Further increases in pressure distend the airway until significant upper airway narrowing is prevented (no hypopnea or snoring). The usual paradigm for bilevel pressure titration is to increase both pressures (IPAP=EPAP) until apnea is prevented. Then the IPAP is increased until hypopnea and snoring are prevented. With bilevel pressure, the EPAP must be high enough to prevent airway collapse during expiration, and the higher IPAP must sufficiently open the airway during inspiration to prevent hypopnea (airway narrowing).

When originally introduced, bilevel pressure units were much more expensive than CPAP units. The first units were introduced with the trade name BIPAP, and this term is commonly (but incorrectly) used to refer to the bilevel pressure treatment modality. Today several bilevel units are marketed, and the cost—while still high—has decreased. Should all OSA patients be treated with bilevel pressure? One study of patient preferences found no significant advantage to bilevel pressure over traditional CPAP. In this study, the mean difference between IPAP and EPAP was about 4 cm $H_2O$.

Probably the most cost-effective approach is to begin treatment with CPAP, and if patients are unable to tolerate the device and complain of high pressure, then bilevel pressure can be tried. Such a plan assumes that the different between IPAP and EPAP is likely to be significant ($> 2$ cm $H_2O$) at the optimal pressure settings.

Another group of patients in whom bilevel pressure may be useful are those with hypoventilation secondary to muscle weakness, lung disease, or abnormal ventilatory control. Some patients with the obesity hypoventilation syndrome (OSA plus hypoventilation) also may have better nocturnal gas exchange with bilevel pressure than CPAP. The IPAP-EPAP pressure difference is equivalent to pressure-support ventilation by nasal mask. Thus, a bilevel pressure setting of 15/5 is equivalent to ventilating a patient with a positive end expiratory pressure of 5 and a pressure support of 10 cm $H_2O$. Obviously, some patients with hypoventilation still require traditional ventilatory support and intubation/tracheostomy. In patients with milder, more stable illness, however, bilevel pressure may work quite well and can prevent the need for mechanical ventilation.

In the present patient, hypopnea was present at a bilevel pressure of 12/10. Note that chest and abdominal movements are in-phase before (see figure; *A*) and out-of-phase during (*B*) the event. Hypopnea resolved after the IPAP was increased to 16 cm $H_2O$. Treatment was begun with bilevel pressure of 16/10 rather than a CPAP at 14 cm $H_2O$. The patient tolerated this therapy and noted an improvement in daytime sleepiness.

## Clinical Pearls

1. Bilevel pressure treatment allows separate adjustment of the IPAP and EPAP pressure levels; thus, upper airway patency can be maintained with an EPAP level lower than the required level of CPAP.

2. The level of EPAP is titrated to prevent apnea; the level of IPAP is titrated to prevent hypopnea and snoring.

3. Despite theoretical advantages, bilevel pressure has not been demonstrated to improve compliance over traditional nasal CPAP in unselected patients. In individual cases, some patients tolerate bilevel pressure and not CPAP.

4. Bilevel pressure can provide a form of pressure support ventilation, which is useful in patients with hypoventilation.

## REFERENCES

1. Sanders MH, Kern N: Obstructive sleep apnea treated by independently adjusted inspiratory and expiratory positive airway pressures via nasal mask. Chest 1990; 98:317–324.
2. Reeves-Hoché MK, DW Hudgel, R Meck, et al: Continuous versus bilevel positive airway pressure for obstructive sleep apnea. Am J Respir Crit Care Med 1995; 151:443–449.

# PATIENT 39

## A 55-year-old obese man with desaturation during a nasal CPAP trial

A 55-year-old, very obese man was suspected of having severe obstructive sleep apnea. He underwent a partial night study, and an AHI of 80/hr was noted during the initial 2-hour diagnostic portion (CPAP = 0). The patient underwent a nasal CPAP titration. At 16 cm $H_2O$, apnea and hypopnea were absent and repetitive arousals did not occur. The arterial oxygen saturation was slightly reduced (to approximately 92%). However, further increases in the level of CPAP produced mask leaks and were not tolerated by the patient. Subsequently, moderate arterial oxygen desaturation developed, despite uninterrupted sleep and no apnea or hypopnea.

*Figure:* Tracing on nasal CPAP at 16 cm $H_2O$.

*Question:* What is occurring?

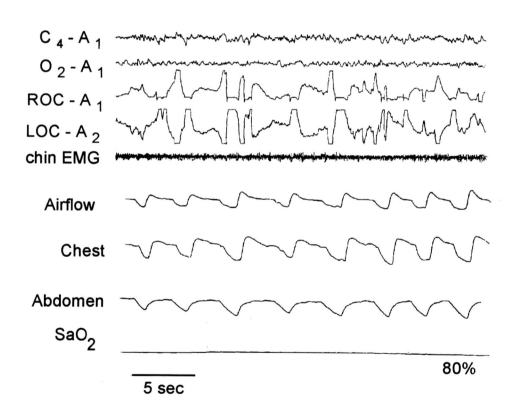

*Answer:* This is an episode of nonapneic hypoventilation in REM sleep exacerbated by REM rebound.

*Discussion:* Early in the clinical use of nasal CPAP in patients with severe OSA it was appreciated that periods of hypoventilation and desaturation could occur during REM sleep despite a patent upper airway. The first night the upper airway is stabilized, long periods of REM sleep (REM rebound) and high REM density are noted. These features of REM rebound occur because the patient has been REM-deprived as a consequence of repeated arousals. Thus, prevention of upper airway obstruction prevents arousal—despite the presence of severe hypoxia and hypercapnia. This fact demonstrates that stimuli involved with airway obstruction play a significant role in the arousal process.

Deterioration in gas exchange during REM periods with a high REM density represents an exaggeration of normal changes that occur in ventilation during REM sleep. In normal individuals, tidal volume falls during bursts of eye movements in REM sleep because of associated reductions in phrenic nerve activity (less diaphragmatic activity) and loss of intercostal muscle respiratory pump function (REM-associated skeletal muscle hypotonia). Periods of REM sleep with the most eye movements are associated with the greatest changes in ventilation. Obese patients with a large mechanical load on the respiratory pump and/or daytime hypoxia and hypercapnia may develop significant hypoventilation and hypoxia during these periods of high REM density. The failure to arouse despite severe hypoxemia is probably secondary to an increased arousal threshold (prior sleep fragmentation) and the lack of stimuli associated with increased respiratory effort during apnea (the airway is patent on CPAP).

There are limited treatment options for these REM-rebound–associated periods of severe desaturation. A further increase in CPAP pressure can be attempted, but it may not be tolerated by the patient, or it may be associated with increased mask leaking. Another option is to add supplemental oxygen to the nasal CPAP treatment. The oxygen flow is titrated to obtain an $SaO_2 > 85–90\%$. Alternatively, bilevel pressure support may be a solution. Unfortunately, in severely ill patients the expiratory positive airway pressure (EPAP) may have to be quite high to maintain upper airway patency. As increases in inspiratory positive airway pressure (IPAP) are limited by mask leaks, patient tolerance, or the maximum pressure the devices can deliver, a high EPAP reduces the amount of pressure support (IPAP-EPAP) that can be provided. Finally, volume-cycled ventilation via nasal or full face mask can be attempted. This has been reported to work in patients with severe hypercapnia and OSA.

Fortunately, after several days of treatment, respiration during REM sleep on nasal CPAP usually improves. The reduction in REM rebound may reduce the REM density, and baseline gas exchange (daytime and sleeping $PCO_2$) may improve in hypercapnic patients. For example, there is a parallel shift of the ventilatory response curve to $PCO_2$ to the left during wakefulness (higher ventilation at the same $PCO_2$) after days to weeks of CPAP treatment. Thus, patients started on both nasal CPAP and oxygen may no longer need the oxygen after several weeks of treatment.

In the present case, the figure on page 107 shows a high REM density and a low $SaO_2$ despite regular airflow. The figure on page 109 shows a plot of $SaO_2$ during the diagnostic and CPAP = 16 cm $H_2O$ portions of the study. Note that with the onset of REM sleep on CPAP, desaturation occurred until supplemental oxygen was added at 2 L/min. The patient was discharged on nasal CPAP and 2 L/min oxygen via the nasal mask at night. After 2 months, a repeat sleep study showed adequate nocturnal saturations ($> 88\%$) during REM sleep using only nasal CPAP.

## Clinical Pearls

1. During initial nasal CPAP treatment of patients with OSA, there usually is a dramatic REM rebound associated with long periods of REM and a high REM density.

2. Severe hypoxemia and hypercapnia may be associated with REM periods during initial nasal CPAP treatment—despite maintenance of upper airway patency—in patients with severe OSA who are obese and/or have daytime hypercapnia.

3. Treatment of these episodes may require addition of supplemental oxygen, a switch to bilevel pressure, or, in extreme cases, volume-cycled positive pressure ventilation via nasal (or full face) mask.

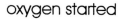

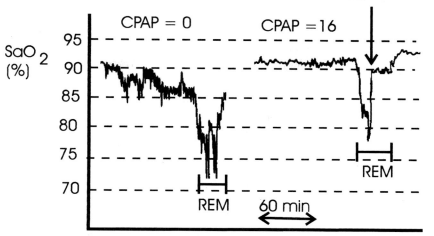

## REFERENCES

1. Krieger J. Weitzenblum E, Monassier JP, et al: Dangerous hypoxemia during continuous positive airway pressure treatment of obstructive sleep apnea. Lancet 1983; 2:1429–1430.
2. Gould GA, Gugger M, Molloy J, et al: Breathing pattern and eye movement density during REM sleep in humans. Am Rev Respir Dis 1988; 138:874–877.
3. Waldhorn RE. Nocturnal nasal intermittent positive pressure ventilation with bi-level pressure in respiratory failure. Chest 1992; 101:516–521.
4. Piper AJ, Sullivan CE: Effects of short-term NIPPV in the treatment of patients with severe obstructive sleep apnea and hypercapnia. Chest 1994; 105:434–440.

# PATIENT 40

## A 30-year-old woman with fatigue and mild daytime sleepiness

A 30-year-old woman complained of fatigue and mild daytime sleepiness of 2-year duration. Her general internist was unable to find an explanation for her fatigue. The patient's husband reported that she snored heavily, especially in the supine position. She had gained 20 pounds over the last 2 years.

The diagnosis is determined to be mild-to-moderate obstructive sleep apnea. Nasal CPAP titration is recommended to the patient, but she refuses this treatment.

***Physical Examination:***   Height 5 feet 3 inches, weight 135 pounds. HEENT: dependent palate, long edematous uvula, tongue normal, prominent pharyngeal tonsils. Neck: 14-inch circumference. Chest: clear. Cardiac: normal. Extremities: trace edema.

### Sleep Study

| | | | |
|---|---|---|---|
| AHI | 30/hr | Arousal index | 35/hr |
| Supine | 40/hr | PLM index | 0/hr |
| Lateral decubitus | 15/hr | | |

***Question:***   What treatment options would you consider?

*Answer:* Consider weight loss, uvulopalatopharyngoplasty, and oral appliances as alternatives to nasal CPAP.

*Discussion:* Uvulopalatopharyngoplasty (UPPP) is an operation that removes residual tonsillar tissue, the uvula, a portion of the soft palate, and redundant tissue from the pharyngeal area. Its disadvantages include the need for general anesthesia and some postoperative discomfort. The most frequent complication is velopharyngeal insufficiency, which is manifested as some degree of nasal reflux when drinking fluids. This usually resolves within a month of surgery. Other potential complications include voice change, postoperative bleeding, and nasopharyngeal stenosis (secondary to scarring). A few cases of severe postsurgical bleeding or upper airway obstruction requiring reintubation have been reported. It is prudent to admit patients to the intensive care unit after surgery for close observation. Significant apnea and desaturation can occur during the recovery period in patients with severe obstructive sleep apnea (OSA). These problems often can be managed with nasal CPAP.

However, the major problem with UPPP is less-than-perfect efficacy as a treatment for OSA. UPPP does not address airway narrowing behind the tongue or in the hypopharynx; therefore, it is not universally effective in preventing sleep apnea. It is much more effective in decreasing the incidence or loudness of snoring (vibration of the soft palate). In general, 40–50% of all patients undergoing UPPP have about a 50% decrease in their AHI, to less than 20/hour. Frequently, the number of apneas decreases, and the number of hypopneas increases. One study reported that a significant number of initial responders to UPPP may later relapse, especially if there is weight gain. Thus, patients treated with UPPP should be restudied if symptoms or signs of sleep apnea return.

Several methods have been studied to determine if responders can be identified preoperatively. These methods include cephalometric radiographs, computerized axial tomography, fluoroscopy, fiber optic endoscopy of the upper airway during Mueller maneuvers (precipitating airway collapse), and upper airway pressure monitoring during sleep. In some of these methods the patient is upright, and in most the patient is awake; therefore, it is not surprising that predictions of what happens during sleep are less than perfect. Patients with obstruction only in the palatal area are the most likely to respond to UPPP.

However, no method can predict with certainty which patients will benefit from this surgery. Interestingly, a few studies have determined that the site of greatest upper airway narrowing in UPPP failures is the retropalatal area. Presumably, postsurgical changes secondary to either palatal edema or scarring are to blame.

Laser assisted palatoplasty (LAP) has been introduced recently as a treatment for snoring. In this procedure only a small portion of the uvula/soft palate is removed. This procedure can be done on an outpatient basis using local anesthesia. It is generally considered a treatment for snoring but has been used for the upper airway resistance syndrome (UARS) and milder cases of sleep apnea when suitable upper airway anatomy exists. The long-term efficacy of LAP remains to be established. In general, LAP is not an effective treatment for most patients with OSA. Somnoplasty (radiofrequency energy ablation), another relatively new outpatient method of palatoplasty for treatment of snoring (and possibly UARS), appears to be well tolerated, but requires more documentation of efficacy.

UPPP is considered less effective than nasal CPAP because it is less likely to eliminate apnea and normalize sleep. However, when nasal CPAP is refused or not tolerated, UPPP can be a treatment alternative—especially in mild-to-moderate apnea. With disease of this severity, there usually is a reasonable chance of obtaining a postoperative AHI less than 15/hr. If UPPP fails, there is always the option of again trying nasal CPAP. However, one study suggested that when nasal CPAP is used after UPPP, air leak via the mouth may be more likely.

The present patient had mild-to-moderate sleep apnea, and she refused a trial of nasal CPAP. Weight loss may dramatically reduce the severity of apnea in this patient, but weight loss is difficult to achieve and even more difficult to maintain. Oral appliances are an option (see Patients 41 and 42). However, when the patient performed a Müller maneuver nasopharyngoscopy revealed collapse mainly in the retropalatal area; thus, the patient was considered a reasonable candidate for UPPP. A polysomnogram 3 months after UPPP showed an AHI 15/hr with an arousal index of 10/hr. The patient reported a great improvement in symptoms. Weight loss has been attempted unsuccessfully.

# Clinical Pearls

1. UPPP has roughly a 40–50% chance of reducing the AHI by 50%, to less than 20/hr.

2. Patients with obstruction only in the retropalatal area are more likely to respond to UPPP.

3. As subjective improvement exceeds objective response, a repeat polysomnogram several months postoperative is needed to document efficacy.

4. An experienced surgeon and careful monitoring during the postoperative period are essential to reduce immediate complications of this procedure.

5. A significant number of initial responders to UPPP may relapse, especially if weight gain occurs. Patients should be restudied if signs or symptoms of sleep apnea return.

## REFERENCES

1. Hudgel DW, Harasick T, Katz RL, et al: Uvulopalatopharyngoplasty in obstructive apnea: Value of preoperative localization of site of upper airway narrowing during sleep. Am Rev Respir Dis 1991; 143:942–946.
2. Larsson LH, Carlsson-Norlander B, Svanborg E: Four year follow-up after uvulopalatopharynoplasty in 50 unselected patients with obstructive sleep apnea syndrome. Laryngoscope 1994; 104:1362–1368.
3. American Sleep Disorders Association, Standards of Practice Committee: Practice parameters for the treatment of obstructive sleep apnea in adults: The efficacy of surgical modifications of the upper airway. Sleep 1996; 19:152–155.
4. Sher AE, Schechtman KB, Piccirillo JF: The efficacy of surgical modifications of the upper airway in adults with obstructive sleep apnea syndrome. Sleep 1996; 19:156–177.
5. Powell NB, Riley RW, Troell RJ, et al: Radiofrequency volumetric tissue reduction of the palate in subjects with sleep-disordered breathing. Chest 1998; 113:1163–1174.

# PATIENT 41

## A 40-year-old man with sleep apnea unable to tolerate nasal CPAP

A 40-year-old man was evaluated for complaints of loud snoring and daytime sleepiness. Although he was able to function fairly well, he sometimes fell asleep in large business meetings. His work required him to travel frequently. The patient reported only occasional ethanol use. He had lost 15 pounds on a diet. This improved his snoring and sleepiness somewhat. After examination, the diagnosis is determined to be mild-to-moderate sleep apnea.

The patient had read extensively about sleep apnea and wanted to avoid nasal CPAP if possible. He was recently divorced and feared use of this device would impair his social life. In addition, he wanted to avoid surgery if possible.

*Physical Examination:*   Height 5 feet 10 inches, weight 220 pounds. Blood pressure: normal. HEENT: slight retrognathia, palate edematous but other wise normal. Neck: 16-inch circumference. Cardiac: normal. Extremities: no edema.

*Sleep Study:*   AHI 30/hr, PLM index 0/hr.

*Question:*   What treatment option is illustrated below?

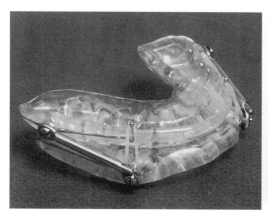 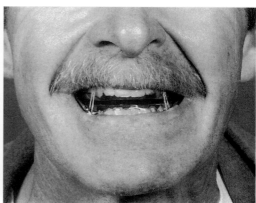

*Answer:*  An oral appliance

*Discussion:*  Oral appliances can be effective treatment in patients with snoring or mild-to-moderate obstructive sleep apnea (OSA). An occasional patient with severe apnea also will respond. The devices work either by retaining the tongue in a forward position (tongue-retaining device) or by moving the mandible forward (thereby indirectly moving the tongue). Patients with a posteriorly placed mandible might be expected to improve the most. However, the amount of forward movement of the tongue (supine position) probably is the most critical element in determining effectiveness.

A fairly large number of oral appliances is available. The effectiveness of several has been confirmed by well-designed studies. The tongue-retaining devices secure the tongue in a forward position by holding the tongue tip in a soft bulb (with negative pressure). The bulb is held anterior to the lips and teeth by a flange on the mouthpiece behind the bulb portion of the device. Most dental devices require fitting by a trained dentist to obtain the dental impression and bite registration, and the device is fabricated in a dental laboratory. A few devices composed of thermolabile material can be molded to the patient's teeth in the office. However, the involvement of a dentist is recommended because if the mandible is moved too far forward, temporomandibular joint (TMJ) problems can occur. With careful fitting of oral appliances, TMJ problems should not be common. However, these devices generally are *not* recommended for patients with *preexisting* TMJ problems.

Oral devices frequently induce excess salivation, at least initially, as well as some mild discomfort in the morning. Thus, compliance is a problem with oral devices as with nasal CPAP. Studies in which both nasal CPAP and oral appliances were effective have revealed that many patients prefer treatment with an oral appliance. Costs are roughly comparable, though device and dental expenses usually are slightly less than the fee for an economical nasal CPAP unit. Unlike nasal CPAP, a sleep study is not needed for initial titration. However, once the device has been optimally adjusted, a sleep study is recommended for those with moderate OSA to ensure effectiveness. Rarely, oral appliances worsen the severity of sleep apnea. The patient should be followed by a dentist to ensure that TMJ or occlusion problems do not develop.

In the present case, nasal CPAP would be effective but was not acceptable to the patient. Other suitable treatment options included uvulopalatopharyngoplasty and other types of upper airway surgery, or oral appliances. Respecting the patient's wish to avoid surgery if possible, he was referred to a dentist experienced in using oral appliances. An impression of the patient's teeth was made, a bite registration was taken, and a dental laboratory prepared a Herbst device. This device allows forward movement of the jaw. It is attached to the teeth on both maxilla and mandible and is unlikely to fall out during the night. The patient reported reduction in both his snoring and amount of daytime sleepiness, and planned to continue a weight-loss program.

## Clinical Pearls

1. An oral appliance can be effective treatment in mild-to-moderate OSA.
2. Patients with TMJ problems are poor candidates for oral appliances.
3. Involvement of a dentist is crucial in preventing complications of oral appliances.

## REFERENCES

1. Lowe AA: Dental appliances for treatment of snoring and obstructive sleep apnea. *In* Kryger M, Roth T, Dement W (eds): Principles and Practice of Sleep Medicine. 2nd edition. Philadelphia, WB Saunders Co, 1994, pp 722–735.
2. American Sleep Disorders Association: Practice parameters for the treatment of snoring and obstructive sleep apnea with oral appliances. Sleep 1995; 18:511–513.
3. Schmidt-Nowara W, Lowe A, Wiegand L, et al: Oral appliances for the treatment of snoring and obstructive sleep apnea: A review. Sleep 1995; 18:501–510.

# PATIENT 42

## A 45-year-old man still experiencing daytime sleepiness after uvulopalatopharyngoplasty

A 45-year-old man was diagnosed with severe sleep apnea (AHI 60/hr). He underwent a nasal CPAP titration but did not tolerate this treatment. After several treatment options were discussed, the patient decided to have uvulopalatopharyngoplasty (UPPP). This was performed, and the patient initially noted improvement in snoring and daytime sleepiness. However, 4 months after the UPPP, he began to have increased symptoms of daytime sleepiness and fatigue. The patient admitted that he had gained about 20 pounds since surgery. A repeat sleep study was ordered.

*Physical Examination:* Blood pressure 160/90, pulse 88, respirations 16. HEENT: well-healed UPPP palatal defect, moderate-size tongue. Chest: clear. Cardiac: normal. Extremities: no edema.

*Sleep Study*

|  | Before UPPP | 6 Months After UPPP |
|---|---|---|
| Total sleep time | 340 min | 360 min |
| AHI | 60/hr | 40/hr |
| Type of events |  |  |
| Obstructive/mixed apnea | 100% | 40% |
| Central apnea | 0% | 0% |
| Hypopnea | 0% | 60% |

*Question:* What treatment would you recommend?

*Answer:* Consider an oral appliance and weight loss for persistent obstructive sleep apnea.

*Discussion:* The sleep physician frequently is confronted with the problem of treatment in patients who experience inadequate improvement after UPPP. If the initial procedure was conservative, then one option is to increase the size of the palatal defect. If the UPPP was aggressive, lack of improvement may be due to an increase in side effects such as velopharyngeal insufficiency. Another option is to try nasal CPAP. Unfortunately, many patients undergo UPPP because they declined CPAP. However, some will reconsider this decision and submit to a nasal CPAP titration. While one study has suggested that mouth leaks are more common on nasal CPAP following UPPP, nasal CPAP may work—especially if the required pressure is not high. A third alternative is to proceed to more advanced surgical treatment, such as inferior sagittal mandibular osteotomy or genioglossus advancement with hyoid suspension (see Patient 45). This procedure usually is available only in tertiary referral centers.

Oral appliances may be useful in some patients who have not improved after UPPP: the UPPP should have improved upper airway narrowing at the palatal area, and an oral appliance can improve the posterior airspace behind the tongue. At least one study has reported success in a few patients for whom UPPP failed.

Weight loss of just 10–20% of body weight can dramatically reduce the AHI in some patients (see Patient 34). Certainly weight gain should be avoided in any patient undergoing UPPP. Because weight loss is difficult (and often slow) to achieve and maintain, it should not be relied upon as the sole treatment for obstructive sleep apnea except in the mildest cases.

In the present patient, a sleep study 6 months after UPPP showed persistent, significant sleep apnea. In the table, note that the amount of apnea decreased, and the amount of hypopnea increased. The patient declined nasal CPAP treatment and was referred to a dentist. A Herbst appliance (see Patient 41) was constructed. Using this device, the patient's symptoms improved. A repeat sleep study with the device in place showed an overall AHI of 15/hr. While this was not a perfect result, the patient felt better and still declined a trial of nasal CPAP. He was referred to a dietician and started a structured weight-loss program.

## Clinical Pearls

1. Patients who undergo UPPP should be followed closely. In some patients, symptoms of obstructive sleep apnea return after an initial improvement.

2. Nasal CPAP treatment may be more difficult in patients with a previous UPPP due to an increased tendency for mouth leaks.

3. Oral appliances may be a satisfactory treatment for some patients in whom UPPP failed.

4. Weight loss can be a useful adjunctive therapy no matter which mode of treatment is selected in patients with even mild obesity.

REFERENCES
1. Calderelli DD, Cartwright RD, Lilie JK: Obstructive sleep apnea: Variations in surgical management. Laryngoscope 1985; 95:1070–1073.
2. Mortimore IL, Bradley PA, Murray JAM, et al: Uvulopalatopharyngoplasty may compromise nasal CPAP therapy in sleep apnea syndromes. Am J Respir Care Med 1995; 154:1759–1762.

# PATIENT 43

## A 50-year-old man with a return of snoring 6 months after uvulopalatopharyngoplasty

A 50-year-old man underwent uvulopalatopharyngoplasty (UPPP) as treatment for severe snoring. A sleep study presurgery showed an AHI of 10/hr, but the patient denied any symptoms of excessive daytime sleepiness. After surgery, the patient initially reported a considerable decrease in the loudness of his snoring. However, over the next 4 months he began to feel increasingly sleepy during the day. The patient also reported a sore throat and problems breathing through his nose. His wife stated that his snoring had returned and that she noticed some periods of time when he did not breathe followed by "gasping for air."

**Physical Examination:** Vital signs: normal. HEENT: see figure. Note the patient's palatal area (*A*) and a more typical UPPP result (*B*).

### Sleep Study

| | Before UPPP | After UPPP |
|---|---|---|
| Total sleep time | 420 min | 430 min |
| AHI | 10/hr | 50/hr |
| Type of events | | |
|   Obstructive/mixed apnea | 10 | 60 |
|   Central apnea | 0 | 0 |
|   Hypopnea | 90 | 40 |

*Question:* What is causing the worsening symptoms after UPPP?

A

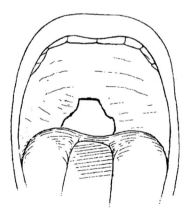

B

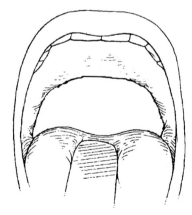

*Diagnosis:*  Nasopharyngeal stenosis has worsened the patient's sleep apnea.

*Discussion:*  It appears that patients with upper airway narrowing localized to the retropalatal area have the best results with UPPP. Thus, in patients for whom UPPP has failed, the most prominent areas of obstruction would be expected in the hypopharynx. A few studies have found, however, that the most common major site of narrowing postsurgery in failed UPPP cases is still the retropalatal area. This **recurrence of narrowing** may be secondary to edema-swelling of the palatal edge at the surgical site.

A less common but severe complication of UPPP is the formation of **nasopharyngeal inlet stenosis,** which can markedly worsen airway obstruction during sleep. The time it takes for stenosis to develop is variable. Causes are believed to include technique (e.g., simultaneous adenoidectomy, ex-cessive removal of the posterior tonsillar pillars), scarring in keloid-forming patients, wound dehiscence, wound infection, or treatment of postsurgical bleeding with electrocautery. The best way to treat this problem is unclear. However, repair with a **$CO_2$ laser** has been reported. The laser causes less damage to deeper tissues and hopefully less chance of repeat scarring.

The present patient was referred to an ENT surgeon for evaluation. Treatment was performed with a $CO_2$ laser, and the involved area opened. At 3 months the patient's symptoms of sleepiness had improved, and a repeat sleep study showed a reduction of the AHI to 20/hr (still worse than presurgery). The patient has declined treatment with nasal CPAP or oral appliances.

## Clinical Pearls

1. The severity of obstructive sleep apnea can worsen after UPPP. Close follow-up by both the surgeon and the sleep specialist is essential.
2. Nasopharyngeal inlet stenosis is a rare but severe complication of UPPP. Recurrence of retropalatal narrowing probably is a more common problem.

## REFERENCES
1. Fairbanks DNF: Uvulopalatopharyngoplasty complications and avoidance strategies. Otolaryngol Head Neck Surg 1990; 102:239–245.
2. Van Duyne J, Coleman JA: Treatment of nasopharyngeal Inlet stenosis following uvulopalatopharyngoplasty with $CO_2$ laser. Laryngoscope 1995; 105:914–918.

# PATIENT 44

## A 45-year-old man who snores when sleeping on his back

A 45-year-old man of average weight was referred for symptoms of daytime sleepiness. His wife reported that he snored heavily when sleeping on his back. She also recalled seeing periods of apnea. There was no history of the patient's legs jerking during sleep. After the sleep study the patient was offered a nasal CPAP trial, but he declined. In addition, he refused surgical options.

*Physical Examination:*    Vital signs: unremarkable. Neck: 17 inch-circumference. HEENT: edematous palate and uvula. Chest: clear. Cardiac: normal. Extremities: no pedal edema.

### Sleep Study

| Total sleep time | 406.5 min (343–436) | Sleep Stages | % SPT |
|---|---|---|---|
| Sleep period time (SPT) | 432.5 min (378–452) | | |
| Sleep latency | 2.5 min (2–18) | Stage Wake | 6 (1–12) |
| REM latency | 70 min (55–78) | Stage 1 | 14 (5–11) |
| AHI | 30/hr ($< 5$) | Stage 2 | 55 (44–66) |
| AHI, NREM/REM | 30/35 | Stages 3 and 4 | 10 (2–15) |
| AHI, Supine/lateral decubitus | 45/10 | Stage REM | 15 (19–27) |
| | | Arousal index | 15/hr |
| | | PLM index | 5/hr |

( ) = normal values for age, PLM = periodic leg movement

*Question:*    What other treatment option is suggested by the results of the sleep study?

*Answer:* Position therapy should be considered for this patient's positional sleep apnea.

*Discussion:* Some patients with obstructive sleep apnea (OSA) have a significant worsening of apnea in the supine position. In this position, gravity tends to pull the tongue backward and narrow the airway. Thus, an overall apnea index may reflect moderate-to-severe apnea when the patient is supine and minimal apnea in the lateral decubitus body position. In one study, approximately 55% of a large group of patients with sleep apnea had AHIs at least two times higher in the supine than in the lateral decubitus position. The patients with positional apnea tended to be younger and thinner. Sleep architecture was better preserved in this group. Unfortunately, many obese patients with severe sleep apnea still have severe apnea in the lateral decubitus position. In these patients, studies have suggested that elevation of the head of the bed (30 degrees) may be a more effective postural maneuver.

It is essential to note if a patient has positional apnea for several reasons. Knowing the amount of time the patient slept in the supine position is critical to correct assessment of the overall AHI. Moreover, if the sleep study contains little monitoring in this position, the overall AHI may underestimate the severity of the patient's disease. Patients with mild-to-moderate AHI are said to have more night-to-night variability in the severity of apnea. A large part of this variability may be due to differences in the amount of time spent in the supine position. Consideration of body position also is essential when comparing the effects of treatments such as UPPP and nasal CPAP. The amount of supine sleep on the treatment night should be equivalent to that on the control night. If not, the results in each body position could be compared (control supine versus treatment supine). Finally, body position may affect the level of CPAP needed to maintain upper airway patency during nasal CPAP titration. An adequate CPAP titration always records sleep in the supine position at the optimal pressure level.

Body position is a potential treatment for some patients with OSA. It is under-utilized as such because no commercial devices are available to prevent patients from sleeping in the supine position. One simple method is to place a hard rubber ball into a pocket sewn on the back of the patient's night shirt. The ball makes the supine position uncomfortable. Alternatively, elevating the head of the bed might improve the efficacy of a suboptimal level of CPAP in patients with severe OSA who are unable to tolerate a higher, more effective pressure. A lower level of pressure may be adequate in this position.

The present patient did not want either nasal CPAP or surgery. As he had a low AHI in the lateral position, positional treatment was attempted. The patient's wife gladly assisted with the ball-and-pocket approach. Using this treatment, the patient noted improvement in his symptoms, and his wife noted much less snoring. The long-term benefits of this treatment remain to be determined. The patient also was directed to lose weight.

## Clinical Pearls

1. Body position has an important effect on the severity of OSA in more than 50% of patients. These effects always should be considered in assessing the results of polysomnography.

2. Position therapy can be effective in select patients. Long-term effectiveness and compliance have not been well documented.

3. Elevating the head of the bed may be a more effective postural maneuver in very obese patients.

REFERENCES
1. Carwright RD, Lloyd S, Lilie J, et al: Sleep position training as treatment for sleep apnea syndrome: A preliminary study. Sleep 1985; 8:87–94.
2. McEvoy RD, Sharp DJ, Thornton AT: The effects of posture on obstructive sleep apnea. Am Rev Respir Dis 1986; 133:662–666.
3. Neill AM, Angus SM, Sajkov D, McEvoy RD: Effects of sleep posture on upper airway stability in patients with obstructive sleep apnea. Am J Respir Crit Care Med 1997; 155:199–204.
4. Oksenberg A, Silverberg DS, Arons E, Radwan: Positional vs nonpositional obstructive sleep apnea patients. Chest 1997; 112:629–639.

# PATIENT 45

## A 55-year-old man with severe daytime sleepiness and limited treatment options

A 55-year-old man was referred for severe daytime sleepiness of at least 3-year duration. He had been previously evaluated and found to have severe obstructive sleep apnea (OSA). At that time he was started on nasal CPAP, but he could not tolerate this treatment. The patient subsequently underwent a uvulopalatopharyngoplasty (UPPP) with limited improvement in his symptoms. He was unable to lose weight but did discontinue drinking alcohol. He fell asleep at work and was fired. His driver's license had been suspended after two sleep-associated traffic accidents.

*Physical Examination:* Height 5 feet 8 inches, weight 220 pounds. HEENT: large tongue, well-healed palatal defect. Neck: short, 17-inch circumference. Chest: clear. Cardiac: distant heart sounds. Extremities: 1+ pedal edema. Neurologic: patient asleep in the waiting room.

*Sleep Study:* AHI 80/hr, no position dependence. Type of events: mixed/obstructive apnea 50%, central apnea 5%, hypopnea 45%. Aterial oxygen saturation: 200 desaturations to < 80%, 50 desaturations to < 60%. Cardiac: sinus arrhythmia, rare premature ventricular contractions.

*Question:* What treatment do you recommend?

*Answer:*    Tracheostomy is recommended.

*Discussion:* Patients with severe sleep apnea who do not tolerate nasal CPAP are a difficult problem for the sleep physician. UPPP may be tried, but it has only a 40–50% chance of reducing the AHI by 50%. Thus, many patients with severe OSA will continue to have an AHI > 20/hr after UPPP. Weight loss can be prescribed but this treatment takes time, and successful maintenance of weight loss is uncommon. An occasional patient responds to treatments for mild-to-moderate sleep apnea, such as position therapy or oral appliances.

Tracheostomy is a highly effective treatment for OSA. However, it is cosmetically unacceptable to many patients. The indications used in one large series included: (1) disabling sleepiness with severe consequences, (2) cardiac arrhythmias with sleep apnea, (3) cor pulmonale, (4) AHI > 40/hr, (5) frequent desaturations below 40% and (6) no improvement after other therapy. Tracheostomy has significant complications in patients with OSA. For example, anesthesia and intubation tend to be more difficult. Postoperative complications include stoma infection/granulation tissue, accidental decannulation, obstruction of the tube when the head is turned or hyperextended, recurrent purulent bronchitis, and psychosocial difficulties (depression).

Noncuffed, size 6 French tubes usually suffice. A longer-than-usual tracheostomy tube may be needed for very obese patients with thick necks. The end of the tracheostomy tube typically is plugged during the day and, because of its small size, air flows around it between the lungs and the upper airway. If resistance to flow around the tube is a problem, a fenestrated tube (hole at bend of the superior end of the tube) may be used. During sleep the tracheostomy tube is unplugged to bypass the upper airway obstruction.

Because of the ineffectiveness of UPPP in many patients with OSA and the morbidity involved with tracheostomy, several other surgical approaches have been developed to target retroglossal and hypopharyngeal obstruction. In one approach, patients are classified preoperatively on the basis of fiberoptic examination as having type 1 (retropalatal), type 3 (retrolingual), or type 2 (both) upper airway compromise. UPPP is ideal for patients with type 1 occlusion. The procedures targeting the retrolingual area are added to UPPP for patients with type 2 occlusions or used alone for type 3 occlusions. In some centers a retrolingual procedure is done at the time of UPPP; in others, the additional procedures are added after UPPP failure.

Laser midline glossectomy (LMG) and lingualplasty (LP) increase the retroglossal airway by removing tongue tissue. When combined with UPPP, the procedures are known collectively as UPPGP. UPPP + LP appears to be the most effective. Postoperative bleeding and odynophagia are potential complications.

Another procedure consists of inferior sagittal mandibular osteotomy with genio-glossal advancement and hyoid myotomy (GAHM) with suspension. In the first component, the attachment of the genioglossus at the genioid tubercle of the mandible is advanced by a limited mandibular osteotomy. In the second component, the hyoid is released from its inferior muscular attachments and suspended from the anterior mandible. This does not require any change in dental occlusion. Complications of GAHM include transient anesthesia of the lower anterior teeth (all) and, rarely, tooth injury. In a later modification of the hyoid suspension, the hyoid is attached to the thyroid cartilage rather than suspended from the anterior mandible. This modification has increased the response rate to around 80%.

The next level of complexity is maxillomandibular osteotomy and advancement (MMO). The maxilla and mandible are advanced together, and both upper and lower teeth are moved to maintain occlusion. The procedure increases the retrolingual and, to a small extent, the retropalatal segments of the upper airway. The maxilla is moved by a Le Fort I osteotomy and the mandible by a sagittal-split osteotomy. Numbness of the chin and cheek areas is an expected complication that resolves in 6–12 months in most patients. In some institutions, MMO is performed only after UPPP + GAHM (whether performed simultaneously or sequentially) fails. In others, MMO + adjunctive procedures is the first surgery offered. Response rates up to 90% have been published. Obviously, GAHM and MMO should be done by maxillofacial surgeons with considerable experience in these operations. Such procedures are usually available only at large tertiary-referral hospitals.

The present patient had persistent, disabling daytime sleepiness and moderate-to-severe oxygen desaturations after UPPP. When presented with the options of tracheostomy at a local hospital or referral for an alternative procedure, he chose tracheostomy. After this procedure he noted rapid improvement in daytime sleepiness. Other than minor inflammation at the tracheal stoma site, he has not developed major complications.

# Clinical Pearls

1. The most reliable treatment for severe OSA in patients refusing or not tolerating nasal CPAP is tracheostomy.

2. Unless upper airway obstruction is localized to the retropalatal area, UPPP alone often is ineffective in severe OSA.

3. GAHM may increase the effectiveness of UPPP by preventing obstruction in the retroglossal hypopharyngeal region.

4. MMO is an extensive procedure available only in a few specialized centers.

## REFERENCES

1. Guilleminault C, Simmons B, Motta J, et al: Obstructive sleep apnea syndrome and tracheostomy. Arch Intern Med 1981; 141:985–988.
2. Riley RW, Powell NB, Guilleminault C: Obstructive sleep apnea and the hyoid: A revised surgical procedure. Otolaryngol Head Neck Surg 1994; 111:717–721.
3. American Sleep Disorders Association: Practice parameters for the treatment of obstructive sleep apnea in adults: The efficacy of surgical modifications of the upper airway. Sleep 1996; 19:152–155.

# PATIENT 46

## A 50-year-old man needing objective confirmation of his ability to stay awake

A 50-year-old man was suspended from his job as a truck driver when he was diagnosed as having severe obstructive sleep apnea (OSA). A multiple sleep latency test performed at that time showed a mean sleep latency of 4.5 minutes. Following treatment with nasal CPAP, the patient noted marked symptomatic improvement. However, his company required that he have repeat testing before reinstatement.

***Sleep Study*** (on prescribed level of nasal CPAP)

| | | Sleep Stages | % SPT |
|---|---|---|---|
| Time in bed | 440 min (378–468) | | |
| Total sleep time | 404 min (340–439) | Stage Wake | 5 (2–7) |
| Sleep period time (SPT) | 425 min (414–453) | Stage 1 | 13 (4–12) |
| Sleep efficiency | .92 (.88–.96) | Stage 2 | 49 (51–72) |
| Sleep latency | 10 min (0–19) | Stages 3 and 4 | 15 (0–13) |
| REM latency | 80 min (69–88) | Stage REM | 18 (17–25) |
| Arousal index | 10/hr | | |
| | | AHI | 3/hr ($< 5$) |
| | | PLM index | 0/hr |

( ) = normal values for age, PLM = periodic leg movement

***MSLT:*** Mean sleep latency 8 minutes (still in the abnormal range); no REM sleep in five naps.

***Question:*** What would you recommend to document an adequate ability to stay awake?

*Answer:*   The maintenance of wakefulness test documents ability to stay awake.

*Discussion:*   The multiple sleep latency test (MSLT) is a measure of the tendency to fall asleep during normal waking hours. However, the patient being tested is not trying to stay awake. When the MSLT is performed on patients with OSA before and after treatment, the mean sleep latency usually shows only modest improvement and still may not be in the normal range ($> 10$ minutes), despite dramatic symptomatic improvement. Similarly, patients with narcolepsy who are treated with stimulants tend to have only modest improvements in mean sleep latency. Thus it was appreciated that the MSLT may not be a sensitive measure of ability to maintain wakefulness nor of improvement in this ability after treatment.

The maintenance of wakefulness test (MWT) was designed to test the patient's ability to stay awake. The patient is seated upright in bed in a dimly lighted room and asked to remain awake for 40 minutes. The usual EEG, EOG, and EMG monitoring is performed to detect sleep. The test is terminated if sleep is noted or after 40 minutes if the patient maintains wakefulness. The test is repeated four to five times across the day, and the mean sleep latency is determined (40 minutes if no sleep is recorded).

When both the MSLT and MWT were administered to a group of patients with excessive daytime sleepiness, the correlation was significant but low. Several individuals did not fall asleep during the MWT, but had some degree of daytime sleepiness as assessed by the MSLT. In another study, the MWT sleep latency increased from 18 to 31 minutes in a group of patients with OSA after adequate treatment. One normative study has suggested that a normal MWT latency should be greater than 19 minutes on a 40-minute test (or 11 minutes on an abbreviated 20-minute MWT).

The MWT latency required for a person to safely pursue an occupation critically dependent on alertness has not been standardized. Furthermore, the ability to stay awake is not the same as maintaining alertness. Studies using driving simulators have attempted to provide a performance-based test of alertness. Test results showed decreased alertness in patients with OSA and in patients with narcolepsy, as compared to a control group. However, these results did not correlate with MSLT results, and half of each group performed as well as controls. While these studies are important first steps, they have not been validated by performance tests of the real thing. Thus, for now, clinical judgement still is required.

The present patient remained awake over four MWT tests (40 minutes). He was reinstated with the provision that he must comply with the nasal CPAP therapy that was prescribed and undergo repeat testing in 6 months.

# Clinical Pearls

1. The maintenance of wakefulness test (MWT) is a more sensitive measure of improvement in the ability to stay awake after treatment in patients with disorders of excessive daytime sleepiness than the MSLT.

2. The MWT and MSLT, although correlated, give discordant results in an appreciable number of patients.

3. MWT criteria for clearance for occupations requiring alertness have yet to be established.

REFERENCES

1. Poceta, JS, Timms RM, Jeong D, et al: Maintenance of wakefulness test in obstructive sleep apnea syndrome. Chest 1992; 101:893–902.
2. Sangal RB, Thomas L, Mitler MM: Maintenance of wakefulness test and multiple sleep latency test: Measurements of different abilities in patients with sleep disorders. Chest 1992; 101:898–902.
3. George CFP, Boudreau AC, Smiley A: Comparison of simulated driving performance in narcolepsy and sleep apnea patients. Sleep 1996; 19:711–717.
4. Doghramji K, Mitler MM, Sangal RB, et al: A normative study of the maintenance of wakefulness test (MWT). Electroencephalogr Clin Neurophysiol 1997; 103:554–562.

# PATIENT 47

## A 45-year-old man falling asleep at the wheel while driving

A 45-year-old man was evaluated for complaints of excessive daytime sleepiness. He had a long history of heavy snoring. Recently, he had fallen asleep several times while stopped at traffic lights and stop signs. He admitted to having a recent auto accident, but claimed this was not secondary to his sleepiness.

A partial night study (diagnostic/nasal CPAP titration) was planned. Nasal CPAP titration was attempted after 2 hours of monitoring, but the patient refused to continue. The study was completed as a diagnostic study.

***Physical Examination:*** Height 5 feet 8 inches, weight 230 pounds. Blood pressure 150/80, pulse 88. HEENT: large tongue. Neck: 17-inch circumference. Chest: clear. Cardiac: $S_4$ gallop. Extremities: trace edema. Neurologic: oriented to person, place, and time (but asleep in the waiting room).

### Sleep Study

| | | Sleep Stages | % SPT |
|---|---|---|---|
| Time in bed (monitoring time) | 426 min (390–468) | | |
| Total sleep time (TST) | 369 min (343–436) | Stage Wake | 10 (1–12) |
| Sleep period time (SPT) | 410 min (378–452) | Stage 1 | 20 (5–11) |
| WASO | 41 min | Stage 2 | 60 (44–66) |
| Sleep efficiency | .87 (.85–.97) | Stages 3 and 4 | 0 (2–15) |
| Sleep latency | 1 min (2–18) | Stage REM | 10 (19–27) |
| REM latency | 120 (55–78) | | |
| | | AHI | 80/hr |
| | | PLM index | 10/hr |

( ) = normal values for age, PLM = periodic leg movement

***Question:*** Should this patient be reported to the appropriate licensing agency as having a medical condition making driving hazardous?

***Answer:*** This patient has severe OSA, and he should not drive until adequately treated.

***Discussion:*** The question of whether or not to report a patient to state authorities as having a medical condition making driving hazardous is one of the most difficult problems facing sleep physicians. The patient has a right to confidentiality, but the physician has ethical and legal obligations to the driving public. Large financial tort settlements have been brought successfully against some physicians for failure to report a person with a medical condition who was subsequently involved in a serious traffic accident. Each state has its own laws, and local medical societies have guidelines. However, in the end, the decision rests with the judgement of the treating physician. In some states, such as California, reporting is done to a health agency rather than directly to the motor vehicle licensing agency. Note that reporting does not always result in the loss of the patient's license.

What is the increase in risk of having an automobile accident for the patient with OSA? This is difficult to estimate, but one study found a two to three times greater risk. Clearly, not all patients with sleep apnea are at high risk of having an auto accident. It appears that the presence of sleep apnea plus a history of a previous accident (or frequent falling asleep at the wheel) identifies a group of patients with especially high risk. A committee of the American Thoracic Society has issued the following reasonable recommendations: "In those jurisdictions in which conditions such as excessive daytime sleepiness caused by sleep apnea may be construed as reportable events, we recommend reporting to licensing bureaus if: (a) the patient has excessive daytime sleepiness, sleep apnea, and a history of a motor vehicle accident or equivalent level of clinical concern; *and* (b) one of the following circumstances exists: (i) the patient's condition is untreatable or is not amenable to expeditious treatment (within 2 months of diagnosis); or (ii) the patient is not willing to accept treatment or is unwilling to restrict driving until effective treatment has been instituted."

The committee also noted that it is the physician's responsibility to notify every patient with sleep apnea that driving when sleepy is risky. Some form of written documentation that the patient understands this warning is prudent.

To date there is no objective test that can quantify a patient's degree of driving impairment. The multiple sleep latency test quantifies sleepiness, but does not predict the patient's ability to stay awake. One study did not find a correlation between MSLT results and reported accidents. The maintenance of wakefulness test is a better test of the ability to remain awake, but it does not assess alertness or the ability to drive. There have been promising attempts at developing driving simulators, but the results of these performance tests have not correlated with actual driving ability. The risk of traffic accidents does appear to be reduced with nasal CPAP therapy (if patients are compliant).

In the present case, the sleep study showed severe OSA. Note the absence of stages 3 and 4 sleep and the decrease in REM sleep. Unfortunately, the patient did not tolerate a nasal CPAP titration. After being confronted with the sleep study results, he still declined CPAP and other effective treatments. He said he would try to lose weight. The patient was asked to sign a document confirming that it was recommended that he not drive until adequately treated. His condition was reported to the local health department for eventual submission to the appropriate agency.

## Clinical Pearls

1. Patients with OSA who fall asleep at the wheel or have had previous accidents are at increased risk of having a sleep-related automobile accident.

2. Patients at risk should be advised not to drive until adequate treatment has begun.

3. Reporting of patients to appropriate state authorities is prudent when they refuse to comply with effective therapy or restrict their driving until adequately treated.

## REFERENCES

1. Findley LJ, Unverzagt ME, Suratt PM: Automobile accidents involving patients with obstructive sleep apnea. Am Rev Respir Dis 1988; 138:337–340.
2. American Thoracic Society Official Statement: Sleep apnea, sleepiness, and driving risk. Am J Respir Crit Care Med 1994; 150:1463–1473.
3. Cassel W, Ploch C, Becker D, et al: Risk of traffic accidents in patients with sleep disordered breathing: Reduction with nasal CPAP. Eur Respir J 1996; 9:2602–2611.
4. George CFP, Boudreau AC, Smiley A: Simulated driving performance in patients with obstructive sleep apnea. Am J Respir Crit Care Med 1996; 154:175–181.

# PATIENT 48

## A 30-year-old man with mild daytime sleepiness

A 30-year-old man was evaluated for mild symptoms of daytime sleepiness that had been present for several years. His wife reported that he snored and sometimes stopped breathing. The patient denied symptoms of nasal congestion and did not drink ethanol. There was no history of cataplexy or sleep paralysis. When the results of the sleep study and treatment alternatives were discussed with the patient, he expressed a desire to avoid surgery and appliances if possible.

*Physical Examination:* General: thin; good physical condition. Vital signs: unremarkable. HEENT: dependent palate, long uvula. Neck: 15½-inch circumference. Chest: clear. Cardiac: normal. Extremities: no edema.

### Sleep Study

| | | Sleep Stages | % SPT |
|---|---|---|---|
| Time in bed (monitoring time) | 435 min (414–455) | | |
| Total sleep time (TST) | 411.5 min (400–443) | Stage Wake | 5 (0–3) |
| Sleep period (SPT) | 410 min (405–451) | Stage 1 | 10 (2–9) |
| Wake after sleep onset | 20.5 min | Stage 2 | 60 (50–64) |
| Sleep efficiency | .94 (.95–.99) | Stages 3 and 4 | 10 (7–18) |
| Sleep latency | 2 min (2–10) | Stage REM | 15 (20–27) |
| REM latency | 95 (70–100) | | |
| | | AHI | 20/hr |
| | | PLM index | 5/hr |

( ) = normal values for age, PLM = periodic leg movement

*Question:* What treatment options are available?

***Diagnosis:*** Simple snoring

***Discussion:*** While snoring is a cardinal symptom of obstructive sleep apnea (OSA), not all snorers have a significant number of apneas and hypopneas nor the upper airway resistance syndrome (UARS). In fact, most snoring patients have minimal apnea, normal sleep architectures, and no daytime sleepiness. They are said to have simple snoring.

Snoring may be defined as a vibratory, sonorous noise made during inspiration and, less commonly, expiration. It is associated with a vibration (fluttering) of the soft palate and other pharyngeal structures. Snoring is difficult to quantify but may be described on the basis of intensity or vibratory qualities. It is associated with a narrowing of the upper airway. Anything that narrows the upper airway, increases nasal resistance, or decreases upper airway muscle tone worsens snoring. Thus, nasal congestion, the supine posture, and ethanol or hypnotics may have this effect.

There is a definite male predominance, although a considerable number of women also snore. Simple snoring is common and tends to increase with age. Some studies have suggested that up to 60% of men and 40% of women over the age of 40 are habitual snorers.

Snoring intensity is loudest in slow wave sleep and softest in REM sleep. During snoring the esophageal pressure can be quite negative, and systemic blood pressure may increase (or not fall as it normally does in NREM sleep). A possible association between snoring and hypertension is still debated; to date, simple snoring does not appear to be associated with an increased risk of hypertension. However, patients with heavy snoring are at risk for developing UARS or frank OSA.

On routine polysomnography, increases in chin EMG activity during inspiration may be seen during snoring episodes. Many sleep laboratories find it useful to record snoring on the polygraph tracings by using a microphone near the patient's neck. If a pneumotachograph is used to monitor airflow,

vibrations in the airflow tracing during snoring may be seen—provided the proper amplifier filter settings are used. If thermistors or thermocouples are used to detect airflow, these vibrations will not be seen. In the figure below, snoring (*S*) is noted in the pneumotachograph but not the thermistor tracing. Note that during airflow (*pneumotach*) tracings show a flat profile when snoring is present and higher esophageal pressure deflections (compared to initial nonsnoring breath). Snoring vibrations also can be seen in esophageal pressure tracings.

Before attempting to treat snoring, first assess whether significant sleep apnea is present. Although patient assessment of daytime sleepiness is a poor predictor of OSA, it is not economically feasible to study every patient with snoring. A large neck circumference and bedmate-witnessed gasping or apnea are the best historical predictors of OSA. If either of these is present or the patient reports significant daytime sleepiness, a sleep study is indicated. Some have suggested that any case of snoring serious enough to warrant surgery deserves an objective evaluation. If significant sleep apnea is present, other treatment options may be more effective.

In the present case, the wife's observations were not helpful as she slept in another bedroom. The history of heavy habitual snoring prompted a sleep study. Large phasic increases in the chin EMG and smaller tidal volumes were seen during snoring (see figure on page 130). However, the patient had a normal AHI, arousal index, and sleep architecture. Therefore, he was diagnosed as having simple snoring. It is possible that the sleep study underestimated the severity of sleep apnea because the patient did not drink his usual alcoholic beverages beforehand. In any case, because he desired "to get this problem fixed quickly," he was treated with a laser-assisted palatoplasty and counseled to avoid weight gain and abstain from ethanol. (See Patient 50 for a discussion of treatment for snoring.)

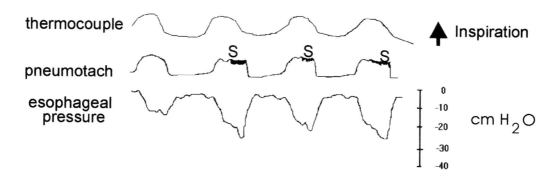

# Clinical Pearls

1. Snoring patients without the symptoms and signs of OSA or UARS are classified as having simple snoring.

2. Patients with simple snoring may be at risk for eventual development of frank OSA and therefore should be educated about the symptoms and signs of OSA.

3. Snoring severe enough to warrant surgical intervention probably deserves evaluation with a sleep study.

## REFERENCES

1. Lugaresi E, Cirignotta F, Coccanga G, et al: Some epidemiological data on snoring and cardiorespiratory disturbances. Sleep 1980; 3:221–224.
2. Stoohs R, Guilleminault C: Snoring during NREM sleep: Respiratory timing, esophageal pressure and EEG arousal. Respir Physiol 1991; 85:151–167.
3. Hoffstein V: Snoring. Chest 1996; 109:201–222.

# PATIENT 50

## A 30-year-old choir singer with heavy snoring

A 30-year-old woman was evaluated for complaints of heavy snoring that had been present for several years. She had originally seen an ENT surgeon who offered her laser-assisted palatoplasty. However, the patient sang in her church choir and was hesitant to undergo the operation because of the possibility of a change in her singing voice. The patient denied drinking alcohol and had no history of nasal congestion.

Snoring was noted during the sleep study in all body positions.

***Physical Examination:*** General: mildly obese. Vital signs: normal. HEENT: large uvula. Neck: 15-inch circumference. Chest clear. Cardiac: normal. Extremities: no edema.

### Sleep Study

| | | | |
|---|---|---|---|
| Time in bed (monitoring time) | 440 min (425–462) | Sleep Stages | % SPT |
| Total sleep time | 411.5 min (394–457) | Stage Wake | 2 (0–6) |
| Sleep period time (SPT) | 420 min (414–453) | Stage 1 | 8 (3–6) |
| WASO | 8.5 min | Stage 2 | 50 (46–52) |
| Sleep efficiency | .94 (90–100) | Stages 3 and 4 | 15 (7–21) |
| Sleep latency | 2.5 min (0–19) | Stage REM | 25 (21–31) |
| REM latency | 90 min (69–88) | | |
| | | Arousal index | 10/hr |
| | | AHI | 4/hr |

( ) = normal values for age

***Question:*** What treatment would you recommend?

***Answer:*** An oral appliance or CPAP can be offered to this patient with simple snoring.

***Discussion:*** Possible treatments of simple snoring are much the same as those appropriate for mild obstructive sleep apnea (OSA) or upper airway resistance syndrome (UARS). These include treatment of nasal disease (medical or surgical), weight loss, position treatment (avoiding the supine posture), oral appliances, avoidance of alcohol and sedatives, and possibly a trial of medications that increase upper airway muscle tone (protriptyline). More severe cases of snoring that do not respond to these measures may warrant laser-assisted palatoplasty (LAP) or traditional uvulopalatopharyngoplasty (UPPP). While both of these are effective for snoring in the short term, no long-term study of their effectiveness exists.

Nasal CPAP also is an effective treatment for snoring, but it is rarely tolerated unless OSA or UARS is present (see figure below). The vibrations in the inspiratory limb are eliminated by an increase in pressure. The presence of snoring ($S$) while patients are on CPAP is an important clue that the pressure needs to be increased. Patients using CPAP at home should be told to notify their sleep physician if snoring occurs while they are sleeping with CPAP.

The present patient had moderate snoring without a significant alteration in her sleep architecture or arousal index. As she had been unable to lose weight and did not desire surgery, she was offered an oral appliance or nasal CPAP. However, an oral appliance failed to substantially relieve her snoring. She underwent a nasal CPAP titration, and at 5 cm $H_2O$ snoring was eliminated in all body positions. The patient reported increased energy and satisfaction with nasal CPAP treatment.

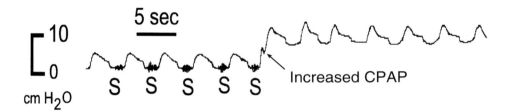

## Clinical Pearls

1. Treatment of simple snoring includes weight loss, avoidance of alcohol, treatment of nasal congestion, medications increasing upper airway muscle activity, oral appliances, and LAP or UPPP. Rarely, a patient accepts nasal CPAP as a treatment for severe snoring.

2. Snoring while using nasal CPAP treatment is a clue that the prescribed pressure needs to be increased.

## REFERENCES
1. Berry RB, Block AJ: Positive nasal airway pressure eliminates snoring as well as obstructive sleep apnea. Chest 1984; 85:15–20.
2. American Sleep Disorders Association: Practice parameters for use of laser-assisted uvulopalatoplasty Sleep 1994; 17:44–48.
3. Krespi YP, Pearlman SJ, Keidar A: Laser-assisted uvulopalatoplasty for snoring. J Otolaryngol 1994; 17:744–748.
4. Rauscher H, Formanek D, Zwick H: Nasal continuous positive airway pressure for non-apneic snoring? Chest 1995; 107:58–61.

# PATIENT 51

## A 45-year-old man with unexplained daytime sleepiness

A thin, 45-year-old man was referred for evaluation of excessive daytime sleepiness of at least 3-year duration. In a prior sleep study, AHI was 5/hr. No evidence of periodic leg movement (PLM) was reported, and arousals were not quantified. There was no history of cataplexy or sleep paralysis. The patient was diagnosed as having idiopathic hypersomnia and treated with stimulants. However, the stimulants made him jumpy, and he had persistent sleepiness.

*Physical Examination:*   General: thin. HEENT: edematous palate. Otherwise unremarkable.

*Sleep study:*   AHI 5/hr, PLM index 0/hr, arousal index 30/hr. No desaturations noted.

*Figure:*   A typical segment associated with arousal is shown below. The event was not associated with a change in arterial oxygen saturation.

*Question:*   What is causing the arousals and daytime sleepiness?

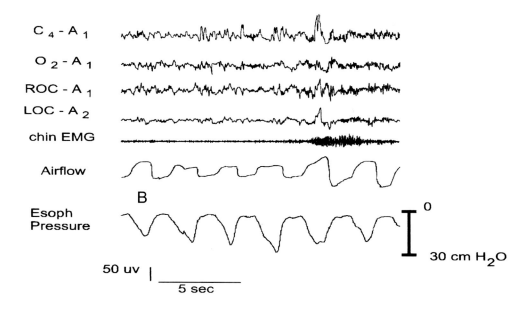

*Diagnosis:*    Upper airway resistance syndrome

*Discussion:*    Recent studies of the mechanisms by which respiratory stimuli induce arousal from sleep have suggested that the arousal stimulus during upper airway narrowing or closure may be related to the **level of inspiratory effort** (airway suction pressure, esophageal pressure deflection), at least during NREM sleep. Some snorers are able to maintain adequate ventilation (and oxygen saturation) despite long periods of upper airway narrowing and arouse intermittently during very high levels of inspiratory effort. Other patients arouse after only a few breaths of high inspiratory effort (not meeting criteria for hypopnea) before substantial desaturation can occur. Thus, apnea, hypopnea, and desaturation are not required for respiratory arousal from sleep. A high upper airway resistance with the associated increase in respiratory effort can trigger arousal even if the decrease in airflow is brief or minimal. Many normal people experience this type of sleep disturbance during nasal congestion secondary to viral illness.

During experimental mask occlusion in normal subjects, arousal usually occurs when suction pressure reaches 20–30 cm $H_2O$. However, snorers and patients with OSA may not arouse until pressures reach 40–80 cm $H_2O$. This implies a decrease in arousability in these groups. During obstructive apnea, the arousal response and apnea termination are associated with a preferential increase in upper airway muscle activity and restoration of airway patency. Thus, while frequent arousals cause excessive daytime sleepiness in patients with OSA, the arousal response is believed essential for termination of the apnea.

The fact that not all event terminations are associated with clear-cut cortical EEG changes may represent a lack of sensitivity of routine monitoring methods (limited montage) or arousal on a subcortical level. However, in most cases of moderate-to-severe OSA, the majority of obstructive events are associated with clear-cut arousal. When the AHI is $\geq 80/hr$, counting arousals probably is unnecessary. However, determination of arousal is definitely useful in milder cases of sleep-disordered breathing. When no other apparent reason is found for multiple arousals during sleep, consider the upper airway resistance syndrome (UARS).

Diagnosis of UARS is not always possible during routine monitoring methods. Sometimes subtle changes in airflow or respiratory effort can be detected prior to arousals. A more sensitive and direct method is to monitor pressure changes across the upper airway by **measuring esophageal pressure** during sleep. While esophageal pressure changes reflect both upper and lower airway resistance, the latter component is smaller and changes minimally during the night in most patients. Measurement with small, fluid-filled catheters is technically easier and more comfortable for the patient than the traditional esophageal balloon catheters. An alternative approach is to measure airflow using a pneumotachograph and face mask. A flattened airflow profile correlates well with increased upper airway resistance in many patients. The flat airflow profile (constant flow) despite an increasing pressure gradient across the airway is consistent with airflow limitation. Unfortunately, thermocouples (the standard method of detecting airflow) do not sufficiently quantify airflow to reliably detect such patterns. A reasonably accurate airflow profile can be produced by connecting a nasal cannula ($CO_2$- monitoring or oxygen-delivery cannula) to a pressure transducer to measure the pressure drop (related to flow) across the nasal orifice.

In the present patient, the sample tracing (see figure) showed a short period of change in airflow profile (flattened) and a crescendo pattern of esophageal pressure deflections associated with arousal. Such events were frequent throughout the study. Note that airflow is reduced only slightly below baseline (breath *B*); thus the event does not meet the definition of hypopnea. The diagnosis was corrected from idiopathic hypersomnia to UARS, and treatment with stimulants was discontinued. Treatment methods for UARS are the same as those for mild-to-moderate OSA. After a uvulopalatoplasty, the patient noted considerable improvement in his daytime sleepiness.

# Clinical Pearls

1. Increased inspiratory effort can trigger arousal from sleep in the absence of apnea, hypopnea, or desaturation.

2. Frequent, unexplained arousals in a patient with daytime sleepiness suggests UARS.

3. Esophageal pressure monitoring with soft, fluid-filled catheters can provide a good estimate of respiratory effort during sleep and help identify UARS.

4. Identification of a pattern of airflow limitation (pneumotachograph or nasal cannula–pressure transducer) also may identify periods of high upper airway resistance and respiratory effort.

# REFERENCES

1. Flemale A, Gillard C, Dierckx JP: Comparison of central venous, esophageal and mouth occlusion pressure with water-filled catheters for estimating pleural pressure changes in healthy adults. Eur Resp J 1988; 1:51–57.
2. Condos R, Norman RG, Krishanan I, et al: Flow limitations as a noninvasive assessment of residual upper airway resistance during CPAP therapy of obstructive sleep apnea. Am Rev Respir Dis 1994; 150:475–480.
3. Berry RB, Gleeson K: Respiratory arousal from sleep: Mechanisms and significance. Sleep 1997; 20:654–675.
4. Monserrat JP, Farré R, Ballester E, et al: Evaluation of nasal prongs for estimating nasal flow. Am J Respir Crit Care Med 1997; 155:211–215.

# PATIENT 52

## A 40-year-old woman with sleep apnea and fatigue

A 40-year-old woman was referred for a sleep study because of symptoms of daytime sleepiness. On questioning she admitted to being drowsy during the day and fatigued even when feeling alert. She had noted about 10 pounds of weight gain over 1 year, constipation, and dry skin.

*Physical Examination:*   Blood pressure 130/80 mmHg, pulse 70, temperature 37°C. General: obese with a hoarse voice. HEENT: large tongue, edematous palate. Neck: possible thyromegaly, 14-inch circumference. Chest: clear. Cardiac: normal. Abdomen: obese. Extremities: trace pedal edema. Neurologic: slow relaxation phase of deep tendon reflexes in ankle.

*Sleep Study:*   AHI 35/hr: 50% hypopneas, 50% obstructive apneas. PLM index 0/hr.

*Question:*   What medical condition may be exacerbating the patient's sleep apnea?

***Diagnosis:*** Hypothyroidism

***Discussion:*** Hypothyroidism has been demonstrated to cause or exacerbate **obstructive sleep apnea** (OSA). While some sleep centers routinely obtain thyroid studies on all patients with suspected OSA, a recent study found hypothyroidism in less than 1% of these screened patients. Therefore, routine thyroid studies probably are indicated only if symptoms and signs are suggestive of hypothyroidism. Thyroid studies also may be indicated if the subsequent sleep study provides no explanation for sleepiness and fatigue, or if patients with OSA do not respond to treatment.

The group of OSA patients at highest risk for coexistent hypothyroidism is **older women**. While hypothyroidism is present in a low percentage of patients with OSA, a much higher percentage of patients with known hypothyroidism have OSA. One study of patients newly diagnosed with hypothyroidism revealed OSA in nine of eleven patients.

Treatment of hypothyroidism may dramatically improve OSA. In one study, the mean AHI fell from 78/hr to 12/hr after patients became euthyroid. However, restoration of the euthyroid condition in patients with OSA does not reliably reverse sleep apnea in all patients. Moreover, initiation of even low doses of thyroid replacement in untreated patients with OSA and coronary artery disease has been reported to cause nocturnal angina. Therefore, *treatment of OSA should be begun when thyroid replacement is initiated.* After the euthyroid state is attained, a repeat sleep study can determine if continued treatment of OSA (other than thyroid replacement) is required. Some patients do, in fact, experience complete reversal of sleep apnea following adequate treatment of hypothyroidism, even if body weight remains constant.

The reason hypothyroidism exacerbates OSA is unclear and possibly multifactorial. Upper airway muscle myopathy, narrowing of the upper airway by mucoprotein deposition in the tongue (macroglossia), and abnormalities in ventilatory control are possible mechanisms.

In the present patient, an elevated thyroid-stimulating hormone of 18 mIU/L ($<$ 6 is normal) and a low free T4 documented primary hypothyroidism. Treatment was begun with low doses of thyroid replacement and nasal CPAP. The thyroid replacement was gradually increased until the euthyroid state was attained. A repeat sleep study (off nasal CPAP) several months later revealed an AHI $<$ 5/hr. Nasal CPAP therapy was discontinued, and the patient remained alert during the day and felt well.

## Clinical Pearls

1. Hypothyroidism is a predisposing condition for the development of OSA and should be considered in all patients with OSA.

2. Routine thyroid screening may not be cost-effective in all patients with suspected OSA.

3. Restoration of the euthyroid state does not eliminate sleep apnea in all patients with OSA and hypothyroidism.

4. Treatment of both OSA and hypothyroidism should be initiated. A repeat sleep study several months after the euthyroid state is restored determines if continued OSA treatment (other than thyroid replacement) is necessary.

## REFERENCES

1. Rajagopal KR, Abbrecht PH, Derderian SS, et al: Obstructive sleep apnea in hypothyroidism. Ann Intern Med 1984; 101:491–494.
2. Grunestein RR, Sullivan CE: Sleep apnea and hypothyroidism: Mechanisms and management. Am J Med 1988; 85:775–779.
3. Winkelman JW, Goldman H, Piscatelli N, et al: Are thyroid function studies necessary in patients with suspected sleep apnea? Sleep 1996; 19:790–793.

# PATIENT 53

## A 50-year-old man with severe hypertension

A 50-year-old-man with a history of severe hypertension (previous systolic blood pressure 180–190 mmHg) was admitted to the intensive care unit (ICU) when his physician noted a blood pressure of 230/130 mmHg in the office. At the time of admission the patient was being treated with benazapril and amlodipine for his hypertension, but he had run out of medication. During the first night in the ICU the patient was noted to have periods of obvious obstructive apnea and swings in blood pressure. He adamantly denied symptoms of daytime sleepiness.

*Physical Examination:* Height 5 feet 11 inches, weight 220 pounds. Blood pressure 180/95 mmHg. HEENT: edematous soft palate and uvula. Neck: 16-inch circumference. Chest: clear. Cardiac: $S_4$ gallop. Extremities: 1+ edema, right arterial line in place.

*Laboratory Finding:* EKG: left ventricular hypertrophy.

*Figure:* Airflow and arterial blood pressure were recorded on a two-channel chart during the night in the ICU.

*Question:* Should this patient be treated for a sleep disorder even though he denies daytime sleepiness?

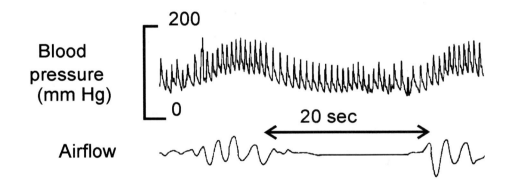

*Diagnosis:*    Obstructive sleep apnea and nocturnal worsening of systemic hypertension

*Discussion:* Reversal of excessive daytime sleepiness is not the only reason patients with significant obstructive sleep apnea (OSA) should be treated. Retrospective studies have suggested that when the apnea index is greater than 20/hr, untreated OSA is associated with a decreased survival rate. Further, this decrease is not secondary to links with other disorders, such as obesity and hypertension: effective treatment of OSA is associated with a normal cumulative 5-year survival. While prospective studies of the impact of OSA on life expectancy are needed, it seems likely that untreated, significant OSA does shorten survival. The question is: How?

One possibility is that OSA causes or worsens the known morbidity and mortality associated with systemic hypertension. In normal subjects, heart rate and systemic blood pressure fall during NREM sleep. Patients with OSA have cyclic increases in heart rate and systemic and pulmonary arterial blood pressure following apnea termination during sleep. Depending on the frequency of apnea during the night, many patients with OSA (with and without daytime hypertension) fail to show a mean fall in blood pressure during the night ("non-dippers"). The etiology of the post-apnea surges in blood pressure is complex, but activation of the autonomic nervous system (increased sympathetic activity) and arousal probably are the major causes.

While some epidemiologic studies have linked daytime hypertension to OSA, others have not. The biggest problem is separating out the coexisting factors of age and obesity. Certainly there is a 50–60% incidence of hypertension in most series of patients with OSA. However, even if OSA does not cause systemic hypertension, it may worsen the consequences. Most hypertensive patients *without*

OSA still have a dip in blood pressure during sleep. Conversely, many hypertensive and nonhypertensive patients *with* OSA are non-dippers (no sleep-associated fall in blood pressure). Studies have suggested that patients with both daytime and nocturnal hypertension (non-dippers) appear to have an increased risk of developing left ventricular hypertrophy. Thus, **OSA may worsen the impact of hypertension** on the heart and perhaps the peripheral vasculature.

Can treatment of OSA favorably alter the impact of hypertension? Several studies have shown a reduction in *nocturnal* blood pressure on nasal CPAP in OSA patients with daytime hypertension. In some patients, daytime blood pressure also may improve, although most patients still require treatment of hypertension with medication. Whether nasal CPAP treatment favorably alters the development of left ventricular hypertrophy remains to be determined. Of note, while nasal CPAP prevents nocturnal rises in blood pressure in patients with OSA, many still fail to have the normal nocturnal dip in blood pressure.

In the present case, the chart recorder documented numerous apneas associated with a surge in blood pressure after apnea termination. The patient initially refused a complete sleep study. However, after discussion about the cardiovascular consequences and increased mortality associated with untreated sleep apnea, he agreed. A split-night study showed an AHI of 80/hr. Treatment with nasal CPAP at 12 cm $H_2O$ reduced the AHI to 8/hr. After a month of treatment with nasal CPAP, the patient reported an improved energy level. While antihypertensive therapy was still needed, improved control was noted, with systolic blood pressures in the 140–150 mmHg range.

## Clinical Pearls

1. Reversal of daytime sleepiness is not the only reason patients with significant OSA should be treated.

2. OSA prevents the normal sleep-associated fall in systemic blood pressure.

3. While OSA *may* be an association with rather than a cause of systemic hypertension, it likely worsens the severity or the consequences of hypertension in many patients.

4. Effective treatment of OSA prevents the cyclic nocturnal increases in blood pressure and may improve daytime blood pressure control and/or the long-term consequences of hypertension.

## REFERENCES

1. He J, Kryger MH, Zorick FJ, et al: Mortality and apnea index in obstructive sleep apnea. Chest 1988; 94:9–14.
2. Verdecchia P, Schiallica G, Guerrier M, et al: Circadian blood pressure changes and left ventricular hypertrophy in essential hypertension. Circulation 1990; 81:528–536.
3. Shephard JW Jr: Hypertension, cardiac arrhythmias, myocardial infarction, and stroke in relation to obstructive sleep apnea. Clin Chest Med 1992; 13:437–458.
4. Fletcher EC: Can treatment of sleep apnea syndrome prevent the cardiovascular consequences? Sleep 1996; 19:S67–S70.
5. Weiss JW, Remsburg S, Garpestad E, et al: Hemodynamic consequences of obstructive sleep apnea. Sleep 1996; 19:388–397.

# PATIENT 54

## A 55-year-old man with premature ventricular contractions during sleep

A 55-year-old man was undergoing coronary angiography. Before the procedure he was given mida-zolam (a potent benzodiazepine), and he fell asleep. During this time, heavy snoring and pauses in breathing were noted. The patient was referred for sleep evaluation. His angiogram had shown significant three-vessel coronary artery disease.

*Physical Examination:*   Blood pressure 135/88 mmHg, pulse 80 and regular. HEENT: large uvula, edematous pharynx. Neck: 16-inch circumference. Chest: clear. Cardiac: $S_4$ gallop. Extremities: no edema.

*Sleep Study:*   AHI 40/hr. Minimum arterial oxygen saturation: 85% during NREM, 75% during REM.

*Figure:*   A sample tracing from the sleep study is shown.

*Question:*   Are the premature ventricular contractions (PVCs) being caused by obstructive sleep apnea?

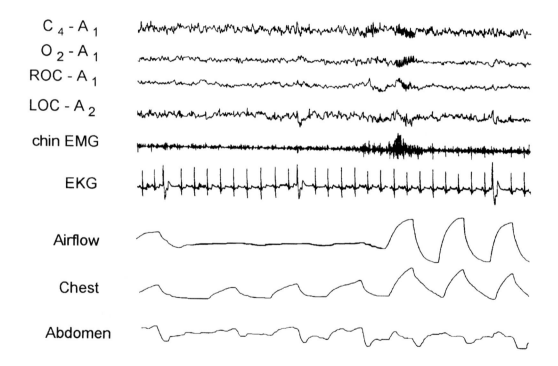

*Diagnosis:*   Severe obstructive sleep apnea is present, but frequent unifocal PVCs are unrelated.

*Discussion:*   In normal individuals, the heart rate falls during NREM sleep. This is thought to be due to parasympathetic predominance during sleep. In patients with OSA, the heart rate varies in cycles: slowing with apnea onset, increasing slightly during apnea, and increasing more dramatically in the post-apneic period. These changes are illustrated below in a tracing from another patient. The numbers under the EKG tracing are the instantaneous heart rates. Although these cycles are referred to as bradytachyarrhythmia, the heart rate often remains between 60 and 100 in many patients (sinus arrhythmia). In one series, 25% of OSA patients showed true bradycardia ($< 60$ bpm) and tachycardia ($> 100$ bpm). Bradyarrhythmias including heart block (2nd degree–mobitz types 1 and 2, and 3rd degree) occur in a minority of OSA patients (usually $\leq 10\%$).

Early studies attributed the slowing of heart rate during apnea to increased vagal tone and hypoxia. The slowing was diminished by atropine and supplemental oxygen. More recent studies have not consistently found a reduction in heart rate in the last part of apnea. Instead, they have focused on **tachycardia as the primary event at apnea termination**, with a subsequent fall in heart rate as sympathetic activity diminishes after the initial burst. Some have suggested that cyclic variability in heart rate might allow detection of sleep apnea by heart rate monitoring alone; however, any sleep disorder causing periodic arousals from sleep is associated with periodic variation in heart rate.

The cycles of heart rate slowing may have little significance, except in cases of significant bradycardia or heart block. However, the periods of tachycardia and elevated blood pressure post-apnea increase myocardial oxygen demand at the same time that hypoxemia exists, predisposing to ischemia and possibly tachyarrhythmias. In normal individuals, sleep usually is a time of reduced tachyarrhythmias and ischemia. Patients with OSA may not enjoy the same protection. While PVCs are not uncommon in patients with OSA, they typically are unrelated to apnea or desaturation. In one series of 400 patients with OSA, PVCs were more frequent during sleep in only 14% of patients. In another study, a clear association between PVC frequency and the severity of nocturnal desaturation was found only when the $SaO_2$ was less than 60%.

In the present patient, PVCs were noted during the middle of apnea rather than during periods of desaturation and arousal post-apnea. A 24-hour Holter monitor showed that the PVC rate was *lower* during the nocturnal hours. The patient underwent a nasal CPAP titration and was treated with 10 cm $H_2O$ pressure. He reported less daytime sleepiness. A coronary bypass surgery has been scheduled.

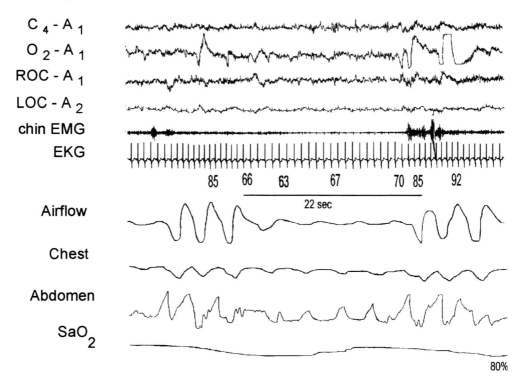

# Clinical Pearls

1. PVCs in patients with OSA usually are unrelated to sleep apnea unless the $SaO_2$ is less than 60%.

2. The most common cardiac rhythm during sleep in patients with OSA is a sinus arrhythmia, with slowing at apnea onset and an increase in heart rate following apnea termination.

## REFERENCES

1. Zwillich C, Devlin T, White D, et al: Bradycardia during sleep apnea. Characteristics and mechanisms. J Clin Invest 1982; 69:1286–1292.
2. Guilleminault C, Connoly SJ, Winkle RA: Cardiac arrhythmia and conduction disturbances during sleep in 400 patients with sleep apnea syndrome. Am J Cardiol 1983; 52:490–494.
3. Shepard JW, Jr. Garrison MW, Grither DA, et al: Relationship of ventricular ectopy to oxyhemoglobin desaturation in patients with obstructive sleep apnea. Chest 1985; 88:335–340.
4. Becker H, Brandenburg U, Peter JH, et al: Reversal of sinus arrest and atrioventricular conduction block in sleep apnea during nasal continuous positive airway pressure. Am J Resp Crit Care Med 1995; 151:215–218.

# PATIENT 55

## A 30-year-old pregnant woman with onset of snoring

A 30-year-old woman in the third trimester of her first pregnancy was noted by her husband (a physician) to snore heavily during the night. This occurred although she spent nearly all of the night sleeping in the lateral decubitus position. The patient had gained about 25 pounds during the pregnancy. During regular visits with her obstetrician, all fetal monitoring indicated a healthy pregnancy. There was no history of snoring prior to the pregnancy. Because the patient had been complaining of fatigue and was taking frequent naps, her husband was concerned that she might have obstructive sleep apnea (OSA). He had not heard any pauses in breathing during sleep. The patient denied falling asleep while watching television or reading during the day.

*Physical Examination:* General: healthy, gravid appearance. HEENT: moderately congested nasal mucosa; edematous palate and uvula. Neck: 15-inch circumference. Extremities: trace edema.

*Question:* Should a sleep study be performed?

*Answer:* A sleep study is unnecessary for snoring associated with pregnancy.

*Discussion:* Pregnancy is associated with a number of physiologic changes that affect respiration during wakefulness and sleep. A high level of progesterone (a respiratory stimulant) in the third trimester is associated with a lowering of the arterial $PCO_2$. Growing abdominal girth results in an upward displacement of the diaphragm. In addition, edema develops in the nasal passages and pharynx. These last two changes result in snoring in up to 30% of all pregnant women.

Although snoring is common in pregnant women, overt OSA is uncommon. A few cases of severe OSA have been reported. Some of these patients continued to have sleep apnea after delivery; thus, pregnancy probably worsened but did not cause sleep apnea in these patients. If sleep apnea is present, therapeutic options are somewhat limited. Severe cases probably should be treated with nasal CPAP. Close monitoring of both fetus and patient is essential. There is some evidence to suggest that severe OSA in the mother causes retardation of infant fetal growth, but this has not been determined conclusively.

In the present patient, the absence of respiratory pauses and symptoms of daytime sleepiness suggested that simple snoring was present. Regular obstetric care showed no evidence of fetal compromise. Therefore, the patient and husband were reassured and informed that if snoring persisted after delivery or if symptoms of daytime sleepiness were noted, then a sleep study would be performed.

## Clinical Pearls

1. Snoring during pregnancy (especially in the last trimester) is common.
2. Development of overt sleep apnea during pregnancy is uncommon.
3. If patients with OSA become pregnant, potential harm to the developing fetus is possible, and these patients warrant a sleep evaluation. Limited data suggests that nasal CPAP is the treatment of choice during pregnancy. Close fetal monitoring is essential.

## REFERENCES

1. Charbonneau M, Falcone T, Cosio, MG, et al: Obstructive sleep apnea during pregnancy. Am Rev Respir Dis 1991; 144:461–463.
2. Feinsilver SH, Hertz G: Respiration during sleep in pregnancy. Clin Chest Med 1992; 13:637–644.
3. Loube DI, Poceta JS, Morales MC, et al: Self-reported snoring during pregnancy: Association with fetal outcome. Chest 1996; 109:885–889.

# PATIENT 56

## A 45-year-old man with snoring and hypercapnia

A 45-year old obese man was evaluated for severe, bilateral, pedal edema of 1-year duration. The patient had smoked one pack of cigarettes per day for 10 years, but he denied a history of cough or wheezing. There was no history of hypertension, chest pain, or myocardial infarction. The patient's wife reported that he snored heavily. However, the patient denied excessive daytime sleepiness.

*Physical Examination:* Height 5 feet 9 inches, weight 275 pounds. Blood pressure 130/85 mmHg, pulse 80 and regular. Neck: short, 18-inch circumference. Chest: clear to auscultation. Cardiac: distant heart sounds, no murmurs. Extremities: 3+ pedal edema.

*Laboratory Findings:* Spirometry: $FEV_1$ 3.0 L (77% of predicted), FVC 3.4 L (70% of predicted), $FEV_1$/FVC 0.88. Arterial blood gas (room air): pH 7.35, $PCO_2$ 52 mmHg, $PO_2$ 55 mmHg, $HCO_3$ 33 mmol/L. Chest radiograph: borderline cardiomegaly.

*Sleep Study:* AHI 66/hr. Minimum oxygen saturation 40%. Number of desaturations to < 85%: 300.

*Questions:* What is the diagnosis? What treatment will reduce the level of hypercapnia?

***Diagnosis:*** Obesity hypoventilation syndrome. Nasal CPAP or tracheostomy reduces hypercapnia.

***Discussion:*** The diagnosis of obesity hypoventilation syndrome (OHS) requires that the patient be obese and hypoventilate for reasons other than lung disease or neuromuscular weakness. Most patients with OHS have obstructive sleep apnea (OSA). An occasional patient experiences worsening of daytime hypoventilation during sleep *without* discrete apneas or hypopneas. Patients with OHS sometimes are called Pickwickian. This term is best avoided because some physicians use it to refer to all patients with OSA.

The combination of **obesity, snoring,** and **unexplained $CO_2$ retention** always suggests the possibility of OHS. The absence of a history of severe daytime sleepiness does not rule out this diagnosis. Many patients underestimate the severity of their daytime sleepiness. Note that only about 15% of patients with OSA have significant daytime $CO_2$ retention, and these patients in whom $CO_2$ retention occurs form two groups: those with OHS and those with overlap syndrome (OSA + chronic obstructive pulmonary disease). These groups tend to have especially severe nocturnal oxygen desaturation and evidence of cor pulmonale.

The etiology of $CO_2$ retention in OHS is multifactorial. Patients with OHS have reduced ventilatory responses to hypercapnia and hypoxia. In addition, they have a lower chest wall compliance (increased work of breathing) than patients with a similar amount of obesity without hypoventilation. After adequate therapy of the OSA with tracheostomy or nasal CPAP, the hypercapnic ventilatory response changes. There is a parallel shift of the ventilation versus $PCO_2$ curve to the left, reflecting a higher ventilation at a given $PCO_2$ (slope unchanged). This type of alteration in the hypercapnic ventilatory response is probably due to prevention of nocturnal worsening of $CO_2$ retention and the associated retention of $HCO_3$. Removal of the depressant effects of chronic hypoxia on ventilatory drive also may be a factor. In any case, daytime $PCO_2$ usually decreases after treatment.

Adequate treatment of patients with OHS usually requires **nasal CPAP** or **tracheostomy**. In cases of severe daytime hypoxia, daytime oxygen and the addition of oxygen to nasal CPAP at night may be required until clinical improvement occurs. Although diuretic therapy often is prescribed, the cornerstone of treatment for cor pulmonale is relief of hypoxia (and the associated pulmonary capillary vasoconstriction). Medroxyprogesterone (Provera), a respiratory stimulant that takes several days to reach maximal effect, has been used to treat patients with OHS. Treatment usually improves the level of daytime $CO_2$ retention, nocturnal oxygenation, and signs of cor pulmonale. However, this agent does not reduce the AHI nor improve symptoms of daytime sleepiness. Side effects of medroxyprogesterone include decreased libido (decreased testosterone levels), alopecia, and hyperglycemia. For these reasons, it is no longer the treatment of choice in these patients.

In the present patient, the spirometric results (mild restrictive pattern) made $CO_2$ retention secondary to lung disease unlikely. The presence of obesity, severe sleep apnea, and high daytime $PCO_2$ is consistent with OHS. After several weeks of treatment with 14 cm $H_2O$ of nasal CPAP, the daytime $PCO_2$ fell to 45 mmHg.

# Clinical Pearls

1. Unexplained $CO_2$ retention and obesity suggest OHS.
2. Patients with OHS may present with signs of cor pulmonale rather than major complaints of excessive daytime sleepiness.
3. Adequate treatment of OSA frequently reduces the level of daytime $CO_2$ retention and improves the nocturnal arterial oxygen saturation and cor pulmonale.

## REFERENCES

1. Sullivan CE, Berthon-Jones M, Issa FG: Remission of severe obesity-hypoventilation syndrome after short-term treatment during sleep with nasal continuous positive airway pressure. Am Rev Respir Dis 1983; 128:177–81.
2. Rajagopal KR, Abbrecht PH, Jabbari B: Effects of medroxyprogesterone acetate in obstructive sleep apnea. Chest 1986; 90:815–821.
3. Rapoport DM, Garay SM, Epstein H, et al: Hypercapnia in the obstructive sleep apnea syndrome. Chest 1986; 89:627–635.
4. Berthon-Jones M, Sullivan CE: Time course of change in ventilatory response to $CO_2$ with long-term CPAP therapy for obstructive sleep apnea. Am Rev Respir Dis 1987; 135:144–147.

# PATIENT 57

## A 55-year-old man with hypercapnic respiratory failure

A 55-year-old man was admitted to the intensive care unit (ICU) with hypercapnic respiratory failure. The patient's wife reported that he snored heavily, had apneic episodes at night, and had been sleepy during the day for several years. Prior to admission, he had become increasingly somnolent and his ankles had swollen. There was no history of chest pain or fever. A previous pulmonary function test revealed only mild restrictive ventilatory dysfunction: $FEV_1$ 2.56 L (70% of predicted), FVC 3.33 L (72% of predicted), $FEV_1$/FVC 0.77.

*Physical Examination:* Height 5 feet 9 inches, weight 250 pounds. HEENT: large tongue, dependent palate. Neck: 18-inch circumference. Chest: a few rales at the bases, no wheezes. Cardiac: distant heart sounds. Abdomen: very obese. Extremities: 3+ pedal edema. Neurologic: easily arousable, but very sleepy.

*Laboratory Findings:* Chest radiograph: enlarged pulmonary arteries, no evidence of pulmonary edema. EKG: sinus rhythm, right axis deviation. Echocardiogram: normal left ventricular function, dilated right ventricle, increased estimated pulmonary arterial pressure (40 mmHg). Arterial blood gas (room air): pH 7.24, $PCO_2$ 70 mmHg, $PO_2$ 45 mmHg, $HCO_3$ 30 mmol/L.

*Question:* What is the cause of the patient's respiratory failure?

***Diagnosis:*** Obesity hypoventilation syndrome with acute worsening of chronic respiratory failure

***Discussion:*** Patients with the obesity hypoventilation syndrome (OHS) or the overlap syndrome (OSA + chronic obstructive pulmonary disease [COPD]) sometimes present with hypercapnic respiratory failure. There usually is evidence of a chronic component and a history of slow deterioration with increasing somnolence and evidence of right heart failure. The diagnosis should be suspected in any obese hypercapnic patient or in any hypercapnic patient with COPD who has an $FEV_1$ > 1 L. With COPD alone, hypercapnia is unusual until the $FEV_1$ falls below 1 L (40% of predicted). It is important to recognize the existence of OSA in patients with OHS or overlap syndrome because adequate treatment of the sleep apnea (usually tracheostomy or nasal CPAP) results in a reduction of daytime $PCO_2$ and an improvement in oxygenation and cor pulmonale.

When sleep monitoring equipment is available in the ICU, the presence of sleep apnea can be precisely documented in stable patients. Sometimes simple observation confirms the diagnosis, but more often empiric treatment is begun, and a confirmatory sleep study is obtained after the patient's condition improves. There are several therapeutic approaches. If the patient is alert, **controlled oxygen therapy** can be employed during the day, and empiric treatment with **nasal CPAP plus oxygen** can be used during sleep. The level of CPAP is titrated until obstructive apnea is prevented. Oxygen is added as needed to keep the oxygen saturation above 90%. If the patient is somnolent on admission, nasal CPAP and oxygen should commence immediately.

An alternative approach is to employ **bilevel pressure** via nasal mask (with added oxygen) to provide upper airway patency and some degree of assisted ventilation. In general, the level of end-expiratory positive airway pressure (EPAP) is titrated to prevent upper airway closure. When the patient is awake, a low level of EPAP usually suffices. During sleep, the level can be increased until airway obstruction is prevented. The inspiratory pressure (IPAP) level is titrated above the EPAP level to prevent hypopnea and to assist ventilation. The IPAP-EPAP difference is the level of pressure support. As in any chronically hypoventilating patient, the immediate goal of noninvasive ventilation is to stabilize the pH and $PO_2$ rather than normalize the $PCO_2$.

Another alternative is to use **positive pressure volume-cycled ventilation** (assist control mode) via nasal or full-face mask. The ventilator must be leak-tolerant; chin strips may be needed with a nasal mask to reduce mouth leak. Positive end-expiratory pressure is added to prevent upper airway closure. The $FiO_2$ (inspired oxygen concentration) is increased to maintain adequate oxygenation.

Treatment with **diuretics** also may be employed; however, the main goal in treating cor pulmonale is prevention of hypoxemia (pulmonary arterial vasoconstriction). Of course, obtunded or rapidly deteriorating patients are best treated with endotracheal intubation and mechanical ventilation.

In the present patient, the restrictive pattern on spirometry was not severe enough to account for $CO_2$ retention. The history was highly suggestive of OHS. The patient was alert enough to attempt nasal ventilation, and he was started on bilevel pressure via nasal mask at an IPAP/EPAP of 10/3 cm $H_2O$, with the addition of oxygen titrated to keep the $SaO_2$ above 90%. IPAP/EPAP was increased to 15/5 cm $H_2O$ over the first hour. The $PCO_2$ stabilized at 65 mmHg with the $SaO_2$ above 90%. Treatment included diuretics.

Over the next 3 days, edema decreased and the $PCO_2$ gradually improved to 50 mmHg; supplemental oxygen was no longer required during the day. A partial-night sleep study revealed an AHI of 80/hr and demonstrated that bilevel pressure of 17/12 was needed to maintain upper airway patency during sleep when the patient was supine. Supplemental oxygen at 1 L/min was required to maintain an oxygen saturation > 90%. The patient eventually was discharged on this treatment. When seen in clinic 3 weeks later, the daytime $PCO_2$ had improved to 45 mmHg.

# Clinical Pearls

1. Patients with OHS or the overlap syndrome may present with a mixture of acute and chronic ventilatory failure.

2. Conservative therapy with oxygen and nasal CPAP, bilevel pressure, or volume-cycled positive pressure ventilation (by mask) may avoid the need for intubation.

3. During sleep, the level of nasal CPAP or bilevel pressure can be titrated to prevent upper airway closure and hypopnea. A formal sleep study and pressure titration can be performed once the patient's condition stabilizes.

# REFERENCES

1. Sullivan CE, Berthon-Jones M, Issa FG: Remission of severe obesity-hypoventilation syndrome after short-term treatment during sleep with nasal continuous positive airway pressure. Am Rev Respir Dis 1983; 128:177–181.
2. Shivaram U, Cash ME, Beal A: Nasal continuous positive airway pressure in decompensated hypercapnic respiratory failure as a complication of sleep apnea. Chest 1993; 104:770–774.
3. Piper AJ, Sullivan CE: Effects of short-term NIPPV in the treatment of patients with severe obstructive sleep apnea and hypercapnia. Chest 1994; 105:434–440.

# PATIENT 58

## A 57-year-old man with severe obstructive sleep apnea treated with oxygen

An obese 57-year-old man was admitted to the intensive care unit twice in the same year for hypercapnic respiratory failure and congestive heart failure. Mechanical ventilation was required on one occasion, and on the other he was treated with bilevel pressure and oxygen by nasal mask. A sleep study performed after one admission showed an AHI of 80/hr and severe arterial oxygen desaturation. The patient responded to nasal CPAP but refused treatment with this therapy. He was treated with nocturnal oxygen at 3 L/min.

However, 3 months after his last admission, the patient was again admitted with hypercapnic respiratory failure and a weight gain of 30 pounds over 2 months. His wife had problems waking him up during the week prior to admission.

*Physical Examination:*  Blood pressure 160/90 mmHg, pulse 88. Height 5 feet 10 inches, weight 300 pounds. HEENT: massive tongue. Neck 18-inch circumference. Chest: rales at bases. Cardiac: $S_4$ gallop. Extremities: massive edema to upper thigh.

*Laboratory Findings:*  Arterial blood gas: pH 7.30, $PCO_2$ 80 mmHg, $PO_2$ 55 mmHg, $HCO_3$ 38.4 mmol/L on 4 L/min oxygen. Thyroid studies: normal. Spirometry: $FEV_1$ 2.5 L (66% predicted), FVC 3.0 L (62% predicted), $FEV_1$/FVC 0.83.

*Question:*  What long-term treatment do you recommend?

*Answer:* Tracheostomy and oxygen are recommended for this patient with obesity hypoventilation syndrome.

*Discussion:* Oxygen is not the treatment of choice in patients with OSA, because while oxygen may decrease the severity of nocturnal desaturation, it has only a minor impact (slight decrease) on the frequency of apnea and therefore the severity of daytime sleepiness. In severe cases, nocturnal desaturation may persist despite oxygen administration. In addition, oxygen induces modest increases in apnea duration and may induce a slight increase in daytime $PCO_2$ in nonhypercapnic OSA patients. Interestingly, oxygen tends to decrease central and mixed apneas and increase obstructive apneas.

In patients with cor pulmonale secondary to OSA who refuse more effective therapy, oxygen sometimes can result in clinical improvement. In patients with the overlap syndrome (OSA + COPD), oxygen can considerably worsen nocturnal hypercapnia. However, even in these patients, oxygen treatment may be the only alternative if nasal CPAP or other effective treatment for OSA is refused.

Tracheostomy, although rarely used today, still has a place in the treatment of patients with severe OSA. When such patients refuse other treatment, tracheostomy is preferable to an early death or repeated bouts of severe cor pulmonale and respiratory failure.

In some patients with OHS or the overlap syndrome, nocturnal desaturation persists during sleep even if upper airway obstruction is abolished. These patients have low baseline $PO_2$ values in the supine position and may hypoventilate during sleep even with a patent upper airway. In such patients, treatment with both tracheostomy (or nasal CPAP) and oxygen may be necessary, at least initially. The level of hypercapnia and oxygenation may subsequently improve with adequate treatment of the cor pulmonale and OSA. Thus, not all patients require long-term oxygen therapy.

After the third visit in the ICU in 1 year, the present patient was advised to have a tracheostomy or face possible early death. He underwent the procedure and was treated with nocturnal oxygen after a nocturnal oximetry study showed persistent desaturation post-tracheostomy. Over the subsequent month, the patient's daytime $PCO_2$ fell to 45 mmHg, and his edema improved tremendously. Two years have passed since his last bout of respiratory failure.

## Clinical Pearls

1. Oxygen treatment in patients with OSA may improve nocturnal desaturation but does not significantly decrease the AHI or the severity of daytime sleepiness. Therefore, it should be used as a treatment of last resort.

2. Patients with severe obesity, OHS, or the overlap syndrome may still have nocturnal desaturation even if upper airway patency is restored.

3. Tracheostomy still is a valid treatment for patients with severe OSA who refuse other effective therapy.

REFERENCES
1. Smith PL, Haponik EF, Bleecker ER: The effects of oxygen in patients with sleep apnea. Am Rev Respir Dis 1984; 130:958–963.
2. Fletcher EC, Brown DL: Nocturnal oxyhemoglobin desaturation following tracheostomy for obstructive sleep apnea. Am J Med 1985; 79:35–42.
3. Gold AR, Schwartz AR, Bleecker ER, et al: The effect of chronic nocturnal oxygen administration upon sleep apnea. Am Rev Respir Dis 1986; 134:925–929.
4. Fletcher EC, Munafo DA: Role of nocturnal oxygen therapy in obstructive sleep apnea. Chest 1990; 98:1497–1504.

# PATIENT 59

## A 10-year-old boy with large tonsils

A 10-year-old boy was referred for evaluation of heavy snoring at night of 2-year duration. His parents had not noted apnea, but were concerned that he seemed to be "working hard to breathe during sleep" and was often sweaty during the night. While he was not sleepy during the day, he had trouble concentrating and was doing poorly in school. In the past the patient had been well-behaved, but he had become irritable and emotionally labile.

*Physical Examination:* HEENT: bilateral, large tonsils (almost "kissing") with obstructed pharyngeal airway; boggy mucosa in nose. Otherwise unremarkable.

*Sleep Study:* AHI 5/hr, long periods of increased end-tidal $PCO_2$ to 55 mmHg, $SaO_2$ 92–93%.

*Figure:* A sample tracing from a period of heavy snoring is shown below.

*Question:* Should this patient have a tonsillectomy?

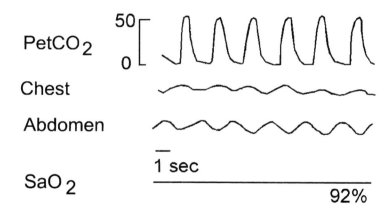

*Answer:* A tonsillectomy plus adenoidectomy should be performed.

*Discussion:* While many sleep physicians deal mainly with adults, sleep disorders such as sleep apnea also can affect children. Therefore, it is important to know some of the differences in presentation, diagnosis, and treatment of OSA in children versus adults. While excessive daytime sleepiness was the main presenting complaint in several initial studies of children with OSA, more recent studies have found this complaint in only a minority of patients. Snoring is common in children with OSA, although it is not universally present. As in adults, simple snoring is much more common than OSA. Parents may notice the child with OSA to have restless sleep with increased inspiratory effort and diaphoresis. Daytime symptoms of mouth breathing, behavioral problems, or poor progress in school may be noted. Rarely, developmental delay occurs.

With the exception of children with craniofacial abnormalities, most OSA in children is secondary to **obstruction from adenoid-tonsillar hypertrophy**. Interestingly, the severity of the disorder does not correlate with tonsil size. Some children have large tonsils and snoring, yet little impairment in breathing.

Polysomnographic findings in children with sleep apnea also can differ from those in adults. In adults, apnea in defined as a cessation of airflow for 10 seconds or more, and the normal AHI is considered to be ≤ 5/hr. In children, any cessation in airflow greater than two normal respiratory cycles is considered an apnea, and an **AHI ≥ 1/hr is considered to be abnormal**. Many children with OSA exhibit relatively few discrete apneas or hypopneas; instead they show long periods of hypoventilation and desaturation. For this reason, pediatric sleep laboratories often use end tidal $PCO_2$ monitoring to assess the periods of hypoventilation. An increase in end tidal $PCO_2$ to > 55 mmHg of any duration and > 50 mmHg for longer than 10% of the total sleep time (or > 45 mmHg for longer than 60%) is considered abnormal.

In most children with OSA, the treatment of choice is removal of enlarged adenoids and tonsils. Tonsillectomy generally is considered a routine surgery in children. Although usually effective, some patients continue to have problems after surgery. In children with OSA, postoperative complications such as upper airway obstruction can occur. Thus, **special postoperative care** often is indicated for children with OSA who undergo tonsillectomy; many hospitals routinely monitor them in an ICU setting overnight. One study suggests that presence of any of the following is an indication for postoperative ICU monitoring: age < 2 years, craniofacial abnormalities, failure to thrive, morbid obesity, cor pulmonale, AHI > 10/hr, nadir $SaO_2$ < 70%, daytime hypoventilation. Nasal CPAP has been used in the postoperative setting to help maintain upper airway patency and in patients not responding to adenotonsillectomy. In severe cases of childhood OSA with hypoventilation and craniofacial abnormalities, tracheostomy may be indicated.

In the present patient, despite an AHI of only 5/hr, there were long periods of snoring, shallow breathing, and increased end tidal $PCO_2$, as well as desaturation. The patient was referred to an ENT surgeon, and tonsillectomy plus adenoidectomy was performed. After surgery, the patient was monitored in an ICU overnight, but there were no signs of desaturation. Within days his disposition, behavior, and school work improved, and he slept better.

## Clinical Pearls

1. In children, the most common cause of OSA is hypertrophy of the adenoids and tonsils. Tonsillectomy plus adenoidectomy is the treatment of choice in most cases.
2. High-risk patients should be monitored in an ICU setting after surgery.
3. In children, an AHI ≥ 1/hr is considered abnormal.
4. Children with OSA may not complain of excessive daytime sleepiness.
5. In a pediatric study, the sleep environment should be suitable for children. Arrange for a parent to sleep in the same room with younger children.

## REFERENCES

1. Rosen GM, Muckle RP, Mahowald MW, et al: Postoperative respiratory compromise in children with obstructive sleep apnea syndrome: Can it be anticipated? Pediatrics 1994; 93:784–788.
2. Carroll JL, Loughlin GM: Obstructive sleep apnea in infants and children: Diagnosis and management. *In* Ferber R, Kryger M (eds): Principles and Practice of Sleep Medicine. Philadelphia, WB Saunders, 1995; pp 193–230.
3. American Thoracic Society: Standards and indications for cardiopulmonary sleep studies in children. Am J Respir Crit Care Med 1996; 153:866–878.

# PATIENT 60

## A 55-year-old man with chronic obstructive pulmonary disease and nocturnal desaturation

A 55-year-old man with severe chronic obstructive pulmonary disease (COPD) underwent nocturnal oximetry monitoring to determine if nocturnal desaturation might explain the presence of cor pulmonale. He admitted to snoring but denied daytime sleepiness.

*Physical Examination:* Height 5 feet 10 inches, weight 180 pounds. Blood pressure 130/90 mmHg, pulse 85, temperature 37°C, respirations 20/min. HEENT: edentulous, otherwise normal. Neck: 15½-inch circumference. Chest: decreased breath sounds. Cardiac: no murmurs or gallops. Extremities: 1+ pedal edema.

*Laboratory Findings:* Spirometry: $FEV_1$ 1.1 L (29% of predicted), FVC 2.5 L (52% of predicted), $FEV_1/FVC$ 0.44. Arterial blood gas (room air): pH 7.43, $PCO_2$ 38 mmHg, $PO_2$ 65 mmHg, $HCO_3$ 25 mmol/L.

*Figure:* A tracing from the nocturnal oximetry monitoring is shown below.

*Question:* What is causing the nocturnal arterial oxygen desaturation?

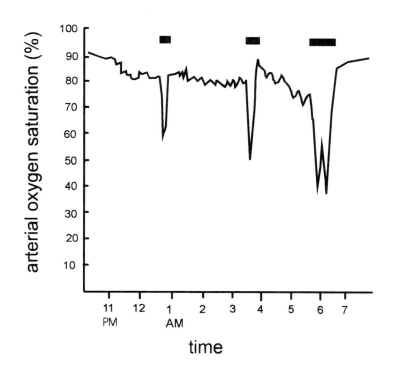

***Diagnosis:***   Chronic obstructive pulmonary disease.

***Discussion:***   Patients with COPD can have arterial oxygen desaturation during sleep for several reasons. First, the normal sleep-associated 8–10 mmHg fall in $PO_2$ has much greater significance if the baseline presleep $PO_2$ value is on the steep part of the oxyhemoglobin saturation curve ($PO_2$ 50–60 mmHg). At this point, a normal fall in $PO_2$ during NREM sleep results in significant arterial oxygen desaturation. Second, periods of sleep apnea of varying significance may occur. (See Patient 64 for a discussion of the overlap syndrome [COPD + OSA]). Third, nonapneic arterial oxygen desaturation can be abrupt and severe during REM sleep in patients with COPD.

The **REM-associated desaturations** are believed to be secondary to hypoventilation during periods of hypopnea, as well as to an **increase in ventilation-perfusion (V/Q) mismatch**. Often, the hypopneic periods are not well-defined and consist of small, variable tidal volumes over periods of time as long as several minutes. During REM sleep, the diaphragm is the only active muscle of inspiration (REM-associated skeletal muscle hypotonia). In patients with COPD, diaphragmatic function often is compromised secondary to hyperinflation. In addition, neural drive to the diaphragm may fall during bursts of eye movements in REM sleep, producing hypopnea (or central apnea). An increase in V/Q mismatch during these episodes also may contribute to hypoxemia. The increase in V/Q mismatch is believed to be secondary to a decrease in functional residual capacity during these REM-related hypopneic episodes.

Patients with COPD may have REM-associated desaturations without having sleep apnea even if their daytime $PO_2$ is $> 60$ mmHg. As expected, these REM-associated desaturations occur every 90–120 minutes during the night. The most severe and longest periods of desaturation typically occur in the early morning hours when REM periods are longer and the REM density (number of eye movements per minute) is greater. In contrast, the pattern of arterial oxygen desaturation on an all-night plot in patients with OSA shows a saw-tooth pattern consistent with repetitive, discrete episodes of desaturation. Several studies have determined equations to predict the severity of nocturnal desaturation in COPD patients based on awake measurements. In general, patients with lower $SaO_2$ and higher $PCO_2$ are more likely to have significant nocturnal desaturation. However, there is considerable individual variation.

In the present patient, the nocturnal oximetry showed a fall in $SaO_2$ to below 85% (see figure, page 157), with further episodes of steep desaturation (*bars*) probably associated with REM sleep. A complete sleep study was performed because of the history of snoring (despite the fact that the oximetry was not suggestive of sleep apnea). The dramatic falls in $SaO_2$ were associated with hypopneic breathing during REM sleep. The baseline $SaO_2$ again fell to less than 85% for the majority of NREM sleep. The AHI was only 10/hr. In the tracing from NREM sleep at right, note the low $SaO_2$ despite regular airflow. In contrast, a tracing from REM sleep shows irregular, small tidal volumes, reduced chest wall motion (chest wall muscle hypotonia), and a lower $SaO_2$. The patient was treated with nocturnal oxygen, and improvement in pedal edema was noted. (See Patient 61 for a discussion of the treatment of nocturnal oxygen desaturation associated with COPD.)

## Clinical Pearls

1. The usual pattern of nocturnal desaturation due to COPD is a fall in baseline $SaO_2$ during NREM sleep with more dramatic falls occurring during episodes of REM sleep. A saw-tooth pattern in the $SaO_2$ tracing suggests that substantial sleep apnea is present.

2. REM-associated desaturation in patients with COPD usually is secondary to periods of hypoventilation (hypopnea) rather than apnea.

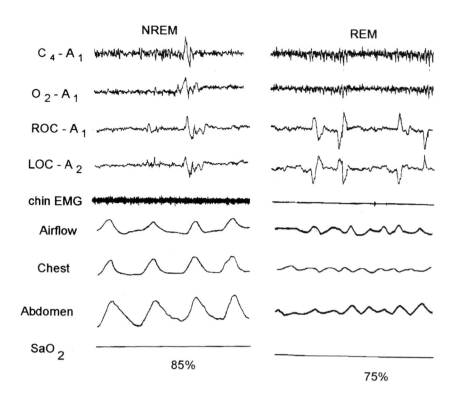

## REFERENCES

1. Fletcher EC, Gray BA, Levin DC: Nonapneic mechanisms of arterial oxygen desaturation during rapid-eye-movement sleep. J Appl Physiol 1983; 54:632–639.
2. Hudgel DW, Martin RJ, Capehart M, et al: Contribution of hypoventilation to sleep oxygen desaturation in chronic obstructive pulmonary disease. J Appl Physiol 1983; 55:669–677.
3. Douglas NJ, Flenley DC: Breathing during sleep in patients with obstructive lung disease. Am Rev Respir Dis 1990; 141:1055–1069.

# PATIENT 61

## A 60-year-old man with leg swelling

A 60-year-old man with a long history of heavy smoking and chronic obstructive pulmonary disease (COPD) was referred for evaluation. He had failed to qualify for home oxygen therapy on a recent examination. The patient had bouts of mild pedal edema during courses of steroid therapy for exacerbations of COPD. These bouts responded to diuretics. There was no history of snoring, and the patient denied daytime sleepiness. He used inhaled bronchodilators only on an as-needed basis.

*Physical Examination:* Height 5 feet 8 inches, weight 160 pounds. Blood pressure 140/89 mmHg, pulse 78. HEENT: edentulous. Neck 15½-inch circumference. Chest: bilateral wheezing. Cardiac: distant sounds. Extremities: 1+ pedal edema.

*Laboratory Findings:* ABG (room air): pH 7.42, $PCO_2$ 38 mmHg, $PO_2$ 62 mmHg, $HCO_3$ 23 mmol/L. Spirometry: $FEV_1$ 1.6 L (46% of predicted), FVC 3.2 L (73% of predicted), $FEV_1$/FVC 0.50. Chest radiography: possible mild enlargement of the pulmonary arteries.

*Question:* Should this patient have polysomnography or nocturnal oximetry?

**Answer:**    Nocturnal oximetry suffices in this case.

**Discussion:**    Some degree of nocturnal arterial oxygen desaturation is common in patients with moderate-to-severe COPD. One study found that daytime measurements of lung function could predict nocturnal desaturation. Although there was considerable variability, the lower the $SaO_2$ and the higher the $PCO_2$, the more likely nocturnal desaturation was to occur. The study also found that the survival of patients with greater-than-predicted nocturnal desaturation was no worse than that of patients with less nocturnal desaturation. The authors concluded that sleep studies were not useful in patients with COPD unless sleep apnea was suspected.

Another study of COPD patients with daytime $PO_2 > 60$ mmHg found that 27% showed some desaturation during sleep, although most of the desaturations were during REM sleep and often brief. Desaturation could not be predicted on the basis of daytime studies. In a subsequent investigation, modest improvements in daytime pulmonary artery pressures were documented in a group of patients with daytime $PO_2 > 60$ mmHg and nocturnal oxygen desaturation who received oxygen treatment. However, it is not clear that these improvements are clinically significant. To date, there appears to be no clear benefit to diagnosing or treating isolated periods of REM-associated nocturnal desaturation.

With the current state of knowledge, the clinician must **individualize the need for sleep studies and nocturnal oxygen treatment** in patients with COPD not qualifying for 24-hour oxygen treatment on the basis of daytime $PO_2$. A sleep study is indicated if obstructive sleep apnea (or another cause of excessive daytime sleepiness) is suspected. Patients with significant cor pulmonale *might* benefit from some type of sleep study.

The usual criteria for continuous oxygen therapy are a daytime $PO_2 < 55$ mmHg or 55–60 mmHg plus evidence of end-organ damage (cor pulmonale). Patients who qualify for oxygen on the basis of these criteria do not need a sleep study unless sleep apnea is suspected or they have failed to respond to oxygen treatment. For patients with a daytime $PO_2 > 60$ mmHg and evidence of significant cor pulmonale, a sleep study could provide documentation of significant nocturnal desaturation. However, there are no clear criteria for what constitutes significant nocturnal desaturation, and the optimal type of sleep study is not known.

It probably is reasonable to use nocturnal oxygen in treating COPD patients with significant desaturation ($< 85\%$) in both NREM and REM sleep and cor pulmonale. However, no clear benefit of doing so has been documented. The type of sleep study often depends on local resources. Oximetry alone may suffice in many cases. However, if the tracings suggest the presence of sleep apnea, a full sleep study (and nasal CPAP titration) may be required. The clinician should remember that oxygen is not the only treatment for nocturnal desaturation. In the original Nocturnal Oxygen Treatment Trial, 21% of the patients screened no longer met criteria when they were placed on intensive bronchodilator therapy. Some patients with minimal changes in the $FEV_1$ and FVC have steady improvement in oxygenation when treated with **smoking cessation** and **bronchodilator therapy**.

In the present patient, sleep apnea was not suspected, and nocturnal oximetry revealed only brief periods of mild desaturation (to 85%) probably associated with stage REM sleep. The baseline $SaO_2$ remained above 92% for the majority of the night. The patient was treated with more aggressive bronchodilator therapy, including sustained-action theophylline.

# Clinical Pearls

1. The clinical suspicion of sleep apnea is the main indication for a sleep study in patients with COPD.

2. In patients not qualifying for continuous oxygen treatment, sleep monitoring may be indicated if significant, unexplained cor pulmonale is present.

3. The criteria for what constitutes significant nocturnal desaturation and the benefits of treating such desaturation remain to be demonstrated.

## REFERENCES

1. Nocturnal oxygen Therapy Trial Group: Continuous or nocturnal oxygen therapy in hypoxemic chronic obstructive lung disease. Ann Intern Med 1980; 93:391–398.
2. Cannaughton JJ, Catterall JR, Elton RA: Do sleep studies contribute to the management of patients with severe chronic obstructive pulmonary disease? Am Rev Respir Dis 1988; 138:341–344.
3. Fletcher EC, Luckett RA, Goodnight-White S, et al: A double-blind trial of nocturnal supplemental oxygen for sleep desaturation in patients with chronic obstructive pulmonary disease and a daytime $PO_2$ above 60 mmHg. Am Rev Respir Dis 1992; 145:1070–1076.

# PATIENT 62

## A 55-year-old man with chronic obstructive pulmonary disease and severe pedal edema

A 55-year-old man with severe COPD was referred for evaluation of cor pulmonale. He did not qualify for home oxygen on a recent examination. The patient denied daytime sleepiness, but complained of frequent awakenings. His wife noted that he frequently snored, but she had never observed episodes of apnea.

**Physical Examination:** Pulse 90, blood pressure 130/90 mmHg. Height 5 feet 8 inches, weight 170 pounds. Chest: bilateral wheezing. Cardiac: regular rate and rhythm. Extremities: 3+ pedal edema.

**Laboratory Findings:** Spirometry: $FEV_1$ 1.0 L (27% of predicted), FVC 3.0 L (64% of predicted), $FEV_1$/FVC 0.33 (80–120% of predicted). Chest radiograph: hyperinflation, large pulmonary arteries. Arterial blood gas (room air): pH 7.42, $PCO_2$ 45 mmHg, $PO_2$ 62 mmHg, $HCO_3$ 25 mmol/L.

### Sleep Study

| | | Sleep Stages | % SPT | |
|---|---|---|---|---|
| Time in bed | 445 min (378–468) | | | |
| Total sleep time | 350 min (340–439) | Stage Wake | 18 (2–7) | |
| Sleep period time (SPT) | 425 min (361–453) | Stage 1 | 13 (4–12) | |
| Sleep efficiency | .79 min (.88–.96) | Stage 2 | 49 (51–72) | |
| Sleep latency | 10 min (1–22 min) | Stages 3 and 4 | 5 (0–13) | |
| REM latency | 2.5 min (65–104) | Stage REM | 15 (17–25) | |
| AHI | 4/hr (< 5) | | | |
| | | Mean $SaO_2$ | NREM | 84% |
| | | | REM | 70% |

( ) = normal values for age

*Question:* What treatment do you recommend?

**Answer:** Optimize treatment of COPD and initiate low-flow nocturnal oxygen.

**Discussion:** Low-flow oxygen by nasal cannula can prevent the typical, nonapneic arterial oxygen desaturation manifested by patients with COPD, without substantially increasing the nocturnal $PCO_2$. However, oxygen is expensive and therefore should be prescribed only when it is likely to be worth the cost. The benefits of chronic 24-hour oxygen therapy in patients with COPD have been well documented by the Nocturnal Oxygen Treatment Trial (NOTT) and other studies of patients meeting the standard criteria of a daytime $PO_2 < 55$ mmHg breathing room air. The value of 55 mmHg was chosen because below this point pulmonary arterial pressure starts to increase significantly secondary to hypoxic vasoconstriction. In the NOTT study, patients also received oxygen if the $PO_2$ was 55–60 mmHg and evidence of end organ damage was present (edema, hematocrit $> 55\%$, or P pulmonale on EKG). Today most physicians would consider evidence of **significant cor pulmonale** or **neurologic dysfunction** an indication for oxygen treatment in this group with borderline oxygenation.

In the group of patients meeting criteria for 24-hour oxygen, sleep studies are not indicated unless sleep apnea is suspected. However, the clinician often is faced with the difficult question of what to do about patients not meeting any of the above criteria (daytime $PO_2 > 60$ mmHg). Some patients may benefit from nocturnal oxygen therapy if significant and prolonged nocturnal desaturation is present. Criteria for what constitutes significant nocturnal desaturation have not been standardized (see Patient 61).

While low-flow supplemental oxygen induces little increase in $CO_2$ in most stable COPD patients during sleep, this is not the case if significant sleep apnea also is present (**the overlap syndrome**). When such patients are treated with oxygen, varying amounts of desaturation persist, the apneas tend to lengthen, and the nocturnal $PCO_2$ may increase significantly. Patients with the overlap syndrome also may complain of a morning headache after oxygen is initiated. Oxygen alone is not the optimal treatment for this group of patients. (See Patient 64 for a detailed discussion of the overlap syndrome.)

In the present patient, a sleep study was ordered because of the history of snoring (to rule out OSA). The study revealed a low AHI and relatively few discrete desaturations (changes in $SaO_2 > 4\%$). However, the baseline $SaO_2$ during NREM sleep was below 85% and even lower in REM sleep (64 min). An echocardiogram was consistent with cor pulmonale (right ventricle dilation, normal left ventricle function). Therefore, it was believed that the patient would benefit from nocturnal oxygen therapy. A separate oximetry study documented that oxygen at a flow rate of 2 L/min maintained a saturation above 90% for all but a few brief desaturations (probably in REM sleep). The patient was begun on nocturnal oxygen therapy and his pedal edema improved. He also reported improved sleep quality.

# Clinical Pearls

1. The criteria for treatment of COPD with a daytime $PO_2 > 60$ mmHg and nocturnal desaturation are not well defined. Patients with significant desaturation in both NREM and REM sleep probably should be treated, especially if evidence of significant cor pulmonale is present.

2. Low-flow oxygen treatment for COPD-associated nocturnal desaturation usually does not cause significant increases of nocturnal $CO_2$ unless significant sleep apnea is present.

## REFERENCES

1. Nocturnal Oxygen Therapy Trial Group: Continuous or nocturnal oxygen therapy in hypoxemic chronic obstructive lung disease. Ann Intern Med 1980; 93:391–398.
2. Goldstein RS, Ramcharan V, Bowes G, et al: Effect of supplemental nocturnal oxygen on gas exchange in patients with severe obstructive lung disease. N Engl J Med 1984; 310:425–429.
3. Douglas NJ, Flenley DC: Breathing during sleep in patients with obstructive lung disease. Am Rev Respir Dis 1990; 141:1055–1069.

# PATIENT 63

## A 60-year-old "pink puffer" with insomnia

A 60-year-old man with severe chronic obstructive pulmonary disease (COPD) was referred for complaints of poor sleep. He had difficulty falling asleep and then awakened several times during the night. Sometimes the awakenings were associated with dyspnea. There was no history of snoring or daytime sleepiness. The patient's medications included theophylline 300 mg bid and albuterol by metered-dose inhaler.

*Physical Examination:*   Height 5 feet 10 inches, weight 150 pounds. Blood pressure 150/80 mmHg, pulse 95. General: thin, nervous; no acute distress. HEENT: unremarkable. Neck: 15-inch circumference. Chest: hyperresonant to percussion, diminished breath sounds. Cardiac: distant heart sounds. Extremities: no edema.

*Laboratory Findings:*   Spirometry: $FEV_1$ 1.5 L (40% of predicted), FVC 2.8 L (59% of predicted), $FEV_1$/FVC 0.54, DLCO 15 ml/min/mmHg (44% of predicted). Chest radiograph: hyperinflation. ABG (room air): pH 7.43, $PCO_2$ 38 mmHg, $PO_2$ 65 mmHg. Theophylline level: 11.5 μg/ml.

*Question:*   What treatment do you recommend?

*Answer:* Try a long-acting inhaled bronchodilator.

*Discussion:* The sleep of patients with COPD is poor, with low sleep efficiencies and, often, reduced amounts of slow wave and REM sleep. Patients may complain of frequent awakenings. Many different approaches have been tried to improve sleep in these patients, but all of the approaches share one limitation: no one actually knows what is waking patients up. For example, isolated hypoxemia is a poor arousal stimulus. One study suggested that supplemental oxygen improves sleep, while another did not find an improvement. Cough or wheezing also could awaken patients. However, cough usually does not occur during sleep.

Nocturnal dyspnea is another possible cause of disturbed sleep. Patients with COPD have an exaggeration of the normal diurnal variation in lung function, with $FEV_1$ worsening around 6 AM. Many bronchodilators taken at bedtime may have worn off by the time they are most needed. Sustained-action **theophylline** might have an advantage; however, this drug's stimulant properties could disturb sleep. Studies have suggested that the advantages may balance the side effects in some patients. Moreover, the stimulatory side effects vary in severity among individuals. **Salmeterol**, a long-acting beta-agonist, has the potential of being an effective bronchodilator with less central nervous system stimulation. The effects of theophylline and salmeterol on sleep quality have not been directly compared in COPD patients, but one study of patients with asthma showed only a minimal advantage with salmeterol (not clinically significant). Thus, both of these medications may be useful in patients with COPD and nocturnal/early morning dyspnea. Another alternative is to use an increased dose of **ipratropium bromide** at bedtime (4 puffs qhs). This medication has few systemic side effects, and the higher dose may give a longer duration of effective bronchodilation.

Some patients with COPD may still complain of disturbed sleep despite optimal medical management. They often request sleeping pills, and many take over-the-counter medications. The question arises: are **hypnotics** safe in these patients? Numerous studies of hypnotic medications have found minimal worsening of nocturnal saturation. One important caveat is that most of the patients in these studies were stable (no acute exacerbations) and nonhypercapnic. Hypnotics can worsen obstructive sleep apnea; therefore, recipients should not have the overlap syndrome. This said, one would probably want to use shorter-acting benzodiazepines (**triazolam, temazepam**) or the nonbenzodiazepine **zolpidem**. The latter drug may suppress respiration less because it acts selectively at BZ-1 receptors. Other alternatives would be to use sedating tricyclic antidepressants (Sinequan and others) in low doses. Certainly each case must be individualized. Question patients carefully about morning confusion or memory loss.

In the present case, the patient reported that theophylline made him "jumpy." He was switched from theophylline to salmeterol (2 puffs every 12 hours). He also was given a limited supply of zolpidem 5 mg to use on occasional nights when he was unable to fall asleep. On this regimen the patient noted improved sleep most nights.

## Clinical Pearls

1. Patients with COPD have poor sleep quality with a low sleep efficiency and reductions in REM and slow wave sleep.

2. There is conflicting evidence about whether oxygen therapy improves sleep quality in hypoxemic patients.

3. In many patients the benefits of long-acting bronchodilator medications may balance potential side effects secondary to central nervous system stimulation.

4. Short- or intermediate-duration benzodiazepine hypnotics and the nonbenzodiazepine zolpidem usually result in only minimal worsening in breathing during sleep in stable nonhypercapnic patients with COPD. *Caution still is indicated.*

## REFERENCES

1. Calverly PMA, Brezinova V, Douglas NJ, et al: The effect of oxygenation on sleep quality in chronic bronchitis and emphysema. Am Rev Respir Dis 1982; 126:206–210.
2. Berry RB, Desa MM, Branum JP, et al: Effect of theophylline on sleep and sleep-disordered breathing in patients with chronic obstructive pulmonary disease. Am Rev Respir Dis 1991; 143:245–250.
3. Girault C, Muir JF, Mihaltan F, et al: Effects of repeated administration of zolpidem on sleep, diurnal and nocturnal respiratory function, vigilance, and physical performance in patients with COPD. Chest 1996; 110:1203–1211.
4. Selby C, Engleman HM, Fitzpatrick MF, et al: Inhaled salmeterol or oral theophylline in nocturnal asthma. Am J Respir Crit Care Med 1997; 155:104–108.

# PATIENT 64

## A 55-year-old man with chronic obstructive pulmonary disease and pedal edema

A 55-year-old man was being treated for severe COPD with bronchodilators and continuous oxygen therapy at 1 L/min. Despite this treatment he had severe, persistent pedal edema and $CO_2$ retention. Large doses of diuretics had not improved the pedal edema. His wife reported that he snored and fell asleep in front of the television during the day. The patient attributed this to poor sleep at night.

*Physical Examination:* Height 5 feet 9 inches, weight 200 pounds. Blood pressure 150/90 mmHg, pulse 88. HEENT: edematous uvula, dependent palate. Neck: 17-inch circumference. Chest: bilateral wheezes. Cardiac: distant heart sounds. Extremities: 3+ pedal edema.

*Laboratory Findings:* Spirometry: $FEV_1$ 1.7 L (46% of predicted), FVC 3.0 L (64% of predicted). ABG: pH 7.36, $PCO_2$ 55 mmHg, $PO_2$ 58 mmHg on 1 L/min of oxygen by nasal cannula. Chest radiograph: large pulmonary arteries, no pulmonary edema.

*Figure:* Below is a trace of the initial part of a nocturnal recording of $SaO_2$ (on oxygen at 1 L/min by nasal cannula).

*Question:* Would complete polysomnography be useful?

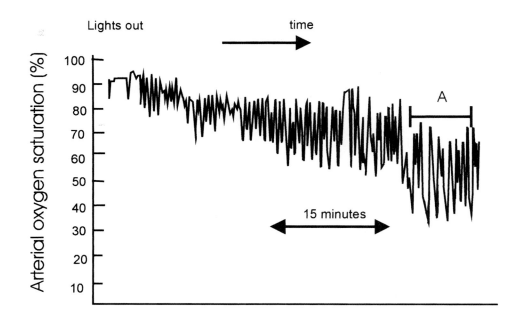

**Answer:** A sleep study (diagnostic/nasal CPAP titration) is indicated in this patient with the overlap syndrome.

**Discussion:** This patient fits the classic description of the **"blue bloater" variant of COPD** (hypercapnia plus cor pulmonale). Recently, it has been appreciated that many such COPD patients also have obstructive sleep apnea (OSA). Such patients are said to have the overlap syndrome (COPD + OSA). This combination has important consequences in terms of morbidity and treatment. A low baseline $PO_2$ and/or ventilation-perfusion mismatch secondary to COPD results in more significant oxygen desaturation during apnea. Thus, OSA patients with COPD tend to have more severe arterial oxygen desaturation and cor pulmonale.

Most OSA patients do not have daytime $CO_2$ retention. Those that do usually have a component of COPD or the obesity hypoventilation syndrome. However, the presence of OSA may impair ventilatory drive, so that while patients with hypercapnic COPD usually have an $FEV_1 < 1$ L, overlap patients may retain $CO_2$ with more moderate degrees of airflow obstruction.

The amount of $CO_2$ retention in overlap patients does not necessarily correlate with the AHI. One study comparing hypercapnic and nonhypercapnic patients with the overlap syndrome found no difference in the $FEV_1$ and AHI between the two groups. The hypercapnic group was heavier and had a history of heavy ethanol use. The authors hypothesized that the hypercapnic patients had depressed respiratory drives possibly secondary to the effects of alcohol. As effective treatment of OSA in patients with the overlap syndrome can result in a reduction of daytime $PCO_2$, nocturnal $CO_2$ retention secondary to apnea probably is contributory to the development of hypercapnia in overlap patients.

What are the implications of this combination of diseases (COPD + OSA)? The most obvious is that *both diseases need to be treated for optimal results.* Thus, the daytime gas exchange of the patient with OSA and mild COPD may improve when **bronchodilator therapy** is added to treatment of OSA (nasal CPAP therapy). In the patient with COPD and significant sleep apnea, treatment with oxygen alone may not adequately prevent nocturnal oxygen desaturation. In this group, low-flow oxygen also can result in significant nocturnal increases in $CO_2$. Studies suggest that oxygen alone does not improve right-sided heart failure if apnea is not adequately treated. Conversely, OSA patients with low $PO_2$ values when awake may need **oxygen plus nasal CPAP** to prevent nocturnal desaturation. When the upper airway obstruction of hypercapnic patients with the overlap syndrome is adequately treated, the daytime $PCO_2$ frequently improves.

When should a sleep study be ordered in a patient with known COPD? The major indication is a suspicion of sleep apnea (snoring, daytime sleepiness). Another is evaluation of a patient already using nocturnal oxygen who is not showing improvement in cor pulmonale. If resources are limited, a simple overnight pulse oximetry test may show the sawtooth pattern suggestive of sleep apnea. However, this approach can be more costly in the long run if a nasal CPAP titration is then required.

In the present patient, oximetry showed the sawtooth pattern of desaturation consistent with OSA. The worsening of $SaO_2$ at *A* is probably secondary to an episode of REM sleep (see figure). Note the low baseline $SaO_2$ and the persistence of decreased $SaO_2$ after each event. The patient underwent polysomnography while using his usual oxygen. An AHI of 50/hr was documented. Nasal CPAP was titrated, and apnea and hypopnea were abolished at 10 cm $H_2O$. Addition of oxygen at 2 L/min was needed to maintain $SaO_2$ above 90%. Treatment with a combination of nasal CPAP and oxygen was begun, and the patient's daytime sleepiness and pedal edema improved. After 1 month of nasal CPAP, the daytime $PCO_2$ had decreased to 45 mmHg.

## Clinical Pearls

1. A saw-tooth pattern on the $SaO_2$ trace in a patient with COPD suggests that OSA also is present.

2. If a COPD patient with only moderately severe airflow obstruction has daytime $CO_2$ retention, suspect the presence of the overlap syndrome.

3. In the overlap syndrome, adequate treatment of both COPD and OSA is required.

4. Supplemental oxygen therapy of nocturnal desaturation alone is not optimal treatment for most patients with COPD and significant OSA.

5. Nasal CPAP plus oxygen is probably the most effective therapy for patients with COPD and significant OSA who have a low $PO_2$ when awake.

# REFERENCES

1. Bradley TD, Rutherford R, Lue F, et al: Role of diffuse airway obstruction in the hypercapnia of obstructive sleep apnea. Am Rev Respir Dis 1986; 134:920–924.
2. Fletcher EC, Schaaf JW, Miller J, Fletcher JG: Long-term cardiopulmonary sequelae in patients with sleep apnea and chronic lung disease. Am Rev Respir Dis 1987; 135:525–533.
3. Chan CS, Grunstein RR, Bye PTP, et al: Obstructive sleep apnea with chronic airflow limitation: Comparison of hypercapnic and eucapnic patients. Am Rev Respir Dis 1989; 140:1274–1278.
4. Sampol G, Sagalés MT, Roca A, et al: Nasal continuous positive airway pressure with supplemental oxygen in coexistent sleep apnea-hypopnea syndrome and severe chronic obstructive pulmonary disease. Eur Respir J 1996; 9:111–116.

# PATIENT 65

## A 35-year-old woman with asthma and poor sleep at night

A 35-year-old woman had been treated for moderate-to-severe asthma since age 15. Her medications included sustained-action theophylline 450 mg qam and 300 mg at 6 PM, inhaled albuterol 2 puffs qid, inhaled flunisolide 4 puffs bid, and prednisone 20 mg po every other day. Attempts at weaning the prednisone to lower doses were associated with exacerbations. Over the last year, the patient had reported frequent awakenings with shortness of breath. In the morning she felt sleepy and somewhat wheezy. The patient's roommate reported loud snoring and gasping for air during the night.

**Physical Examination:** Height 5 feet 2 inches, weight 130 pounds. General: slightly "cushinoid" appearance. HEENT: edematous uvula and palate. Neck: 15-inch circumference. Chest: bilateral expiratory wheezes. Cardiac: normal. Extremities: no edema.

**Laboratory Findings:** Spirometry (3 PM): $FEV_1$ 1.8 L (63% of predicted), FVC 3.0 L (90% of predicted), $FEV_1/FVC$ 0.60. Theophylline level (12 noon): 12.0 μg/ml.

**Peak Flow Diary** (L/min)

|        | 6 AM | 10 PM | Awakenings[*] |       | 6 AM | 10 PM | Awakenings[*] |
|--------|------|-------|------------|-------|------|-------|------------|
| Day 1  | 200  | 300   | 3          | Day 4 | 225  | 325   | 4          |
| Day 2  | 225  | 325   | 2          | Day 5 | 180  | 300   | 3          |
| Day 3  | 225  | 300   | 3          | Day 6 | 200  | 300   | 3          |

[*] Awakenings are from the preceding night.

**Questions:** What is your diagnosis? What other evaluation do you suggest?

***Answers:*** Nocturnal asthma (documented diurnal variation in airflow). Consider a sleep study to rule out obstructive sleep apnea.

***Discussion:*** Nocturnal worsening of symptoms and sleep disturbance are significant problems for patients with asthma. In one study, up to 40% experienced symptoms every night. There is a normal **circadian variation in airway function**, with the highest airflow in the late afternoon (4 PM) and the lowest in the early morning (4 AM). This normal variation is exaggerated in patients with obstructive airway diseases: $FEV_1$ or peak flow can fall as much as 20–40% in the morning hours ("morning dippers"). The etiology of this variation is multifactorial and includes circadian changes in the amounts of circulating steroids and, possibly, inflammatory mediators in the lungs, as well as in cholinergic tone. Sleep also appears to have an adverse effect on asthma, independent of other factors. The easiest way to diagnose severe nocturnal worsening of asthma is to have the patient record peak flow measurements at bedtime and upon awakening.

Treatment of patients with nocturnal asthma should include **chronopharmacology**—the recognition that drug pharmacokinetics and effectiveness are influenced by circadian factors. For example, in dosing theophylline the goals should be to obtain the highest levels during the time of greatest airflow obstruction. Until recently, a particular limitation in the effectiveness of inhaled beta-agonists was their short half-life. When taken at bedtime, their power was weakest when it was needed the most (4 AM–6 AM). Salmeterol, a long-acting beta agonist, can be especially helpful in patients with nocturnal exacerbations of asthma. This inhaled medication may cause less central nervous system stimulation than sustained-action oral theophylline. However, a study comparing theophylline and salmeterol in nocturnal asthma found no difference in patient preference and no clinically meaningful differences in sleep quality. While asthmatics generally have a greater response to beta-agonists than anticholinergic medications, vagal tone is increased at night. Studies have shown an improvement in nocturnal peak flow after ipratropium bromide. A higher bedtime dose (4 puffs) may be needed for a more prolonged duration of action.

The circadian variation in inflammatory activity in the lung may have implications for the timing of steroid therapy. Some studies have suggested that the worsening of airflow is preceded by an influx of inflammatory cells into the lung. While not all studies have reproduced these findings, one study suggested that administration of prednisone at 3 PM was more effective than morning dosing in patients with nocturnal asthma. The usual morning timing of prednisone is thought to minimize adrenal suppression. However, no adrenal suppression was noted with the 3 PM dose. At present no clear consensus exists on whether a change in timing of steroid intake should be attempted.

Finally, asthmatic patients may have other sleep disorders. If obstructive sleep apnea (OSA) is present, adequate treatment may improve the control of asthma as well as symptoms of daytime sleepiness. The reasons that OSA may worsen asthma are at present unknown.

In the current case, the peak flow diary confirmed severe morning dipping. The theophylline dosing was changed to 450 mg at 10 PM and 300 mg qam to provide the highest levels when needed. The patient also was started on salmeterol, 2 puffs every 12 hours, with inhaled albuterol as needed between salmeterol doses. Morning peak flows improved to 300–325 L/min, and the patient reported a decrease in the number of prolonged awakenings to one or two per night. Despite these changes, complaints of falling asleep during the day persisted. A sleep study revealed an AHI of 30/hr. During the second half of the sleep study, a nasal CPAP titration documented elimination of snoring and apnea at 5.0 cm $H_2O$. Treatment with nasal CPAP resulted in improvement in symptoms of daytime sleepiness. In addition, the patient's asthma improved, and she eventually was weaned to a prednisone dose of 10 mg qod.

## Clinical Pearls

1. Consideration of chronobiology and chronopharmacology can assist in designing optimum treatment for nocturnal asthma.

2. The degree of diurnal variation in airflow can most easily be documented by peak flow measurements at bedtime and on awakening.

3. When OSA is present in asthmatic patients, adequate treatment of OSA may improve the asthma.

# REFERENCES

1. Chan CS, Woolcock AJ, Sullivan CE: Nocturnal asthma: Role of snoring and obstructive sleep apnea. Am Rev Respir Dis 1988; 137:1502–1504.
2. Beam WR, Weiner DE, Martin RJ: Timing of prednisone and alterations of airways inflammation in nocturnal asthma. Am Rev Respir Dis 1992; 146:1524–1530.
3. Martin RJ: Nocturnal asthma: Circadian rhythms and therapeutic interventions. Am Rev Respir Dis 1993; 147:525–528.
4. Selby C, Engleman HM, Fitzpatrick MF, et al: Inhaled salmeterol or oral theophylline in nocturnal asthma? Am J Respir Crit Care Med 1997; 155:104–108.

# PATIENT 66

## A 55-year-old man with daytime sleepiness

A 55-year-old man complained of daytime sleepiness of 2-year duration. His wife reported that he occasionally snored and was a "restless sleeper." There was no history of muscle weakness, orthopnea, pedal edema, or respiratory failure.

*Physical Examination:* Blood pressure 150/85 mmHg, pulse 80, temperature 37°C, respiratory rate 15. General: thin. HEENT: unremarkable. Neck: 15-inch circumference. Chest: clear to auscultation and percussion. Cardiac: normal. Extremities: no edema. Neurologic: normal.

*Sleep Study:* AHI 35/hr. No periodic limb movements in sleep noted.

*Figure:* Over 70% of the respiratory events (apneas and hypopneas) were similar to the one illustrated below.

*Question:* What is the cause of the patient's daytime sleepiness?

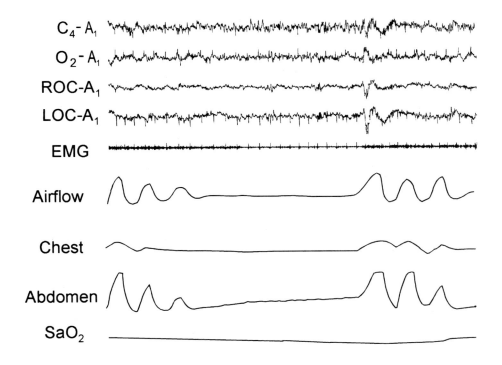

*Diagnosis:* Idiopathic central sleep apnea

*Discussion:* Central apnea is defined as a cessation in airflow of 10 seconds or longer that is associated with an absence of respiratory effort. A few central apneas are common in patients with obstructive sleep apnea (OSA). However, the diagnosis of the central sleep apnea (CSA) syndrome requires that the majority of apneic events be *central* in nature. The CSA syndrome affects a heterogeneous mix of patients that may be subdivided into a group with daytime hypoventilation and a group without hypoventilation. The **group with hypoventilation** includes patients with a defect in ventilatory control (primary alveolar hypoventilation) and patients with neuromuscular disorders. These patients usually have a history of bouts of respiratory failure and cor pulmonale. The **nonhypercapnic group** is composed of patients with Cheyne-Stokes breathing (usually secondary to congestive heart failure or neurologic disorders) and patients in whom no obvious cause for the CSA exists (idiopathic CSA).

**Cheyne-Stokes breathing** is a specific type of periodic breathing that is associated with a crescendo-decrescendo pattern of ventilation, with central apneas or hypopneas at the nadir (see figure below). Arousals tend to occur near the maximum point of ventilatory effort (sometime after apnea cessation) in Cheyne-Stokes breathing. In idiopathic central apnea, arousals tend to occur at apnea termination, and ventilatory drive returns abruptly. Most cases of Cheyne-Stokes breathing secondary to congestive heart failure also have a longer cycle time (longer ventilatory phase between apneas) and a long delay in the nadir in $SaO_2$ (long circulation time).

## Cheyne-Stokes Breathing

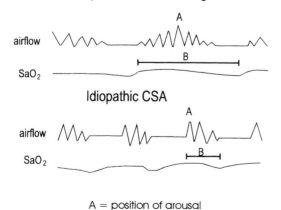

A = position of arousal

B = delay in saturation nadir

The presentation of idiopathic CSA is somewhat variable, including complaints of insomnia, daytime sleepiness, or choking during the night. In a recent series, the symptom of excessive daytime sleepiness was the major presenting complaint. Snoring may occur in idiopathic CSA, but is less prominent than in OSA. Patients with idiopathic CSA also tend to be thinner than those with OSA. CSA comprises less than 15% of patients with sleep apnea evaluated at most sleep centers. Of the patients with nonhypercapnic CSA, Cheyne-Stokes breathing is more common than idiopathic CSA. In one study, only 5% of over 300 patients with sleep apnea had idiopathic CSA.

Polysomnography in idiopathic CSA typically reveals frequent, isolated central apneas or runs of central apneas (one form of periodic breathing). A run of central apneas may follow arousal from a nonrespiratory stimulus. Central apneas during NREM sleep occur most commonly in stage 1 or 2 sleep. Central apnea is believed to occur because the $PCO_2$ level is below the apneic threshold (the lowest $PCO_2$ triggering ventilation during sleep). This is consistent with the findings that most patients with idiopathic CSA have relatively low $PCO_2$ values when awake and that central apneas usually follow periods of increased ventilation.

In a recent study, an increase in the baseline awake $PCO_2$—by either $CO_2$ administration or the addition of dead space—decreased the amount of central apnea. The periods of increased ventilation triggering central apneas often are associated with **arousal**. Arousal may trigger a transient increase in ventilation and a fall in $PCO_2$. This transient fall in $PCO_2$ is then associated with a central apnea as the patient returns to sleep. Thus, arousal may initiate or predispose to continuation of central apnea. In some patients with idiopathic CSA, central apnea occurs mainly in the supine position. Some investigators have hypothesized that reflexes triggered by upper airway collapse may inhibit respiration in these patients.

In the present patient, over 70% of the respiratory events were central apnea (see figure page 172). Note the absence of movement in the chest and abdominal tracings. The predominance of central apneas that were not of the Cheyne-Stokes type and the absence of symptoms or signs of congestive heart failure resulted in a diagnosis of idiopathic CSA. (See Patient 67 for a discussion of treatment for idiopathic CSA).

# Clinical Pearls

1. Patients with CSA are a heterogeneous group of patients with and without hypoventilation.

2. Idiopathic CSA occurs in nonhypercapnic patients without an obvious associated disease (neurologic disorder or congestive heart failure).

3. While many patients with idiopathic CSA complain of excessive daytime sleepiness and have a history of snoring, some complain primarily of insomnia (frequent awakenings).

## REFERENCES

1. Bradley TD, McNicholas WT, Rutherford R, et al: Clinical and physiologic heterogeneity of the central sleep apnea syndrome. Am Rev Respir Dis 1986; 134:217–221.
2. Dempsey JA, Skatrud JB: A sleep-induced apneic threshold and its consequences. Am Rev Respir Dis 1986; 133:1163–1170.
3. Xie A, Wong B, Phillipson EA, et al: Interaction of hyperventilation and arousal in pathogenesis of idiopathic central sleep apnea. Am J Respir Crit Care Med 1994; 150:489–495.
4. Xie A, Rankin F, Rutherford R, et al: Effects of inhaled $CO_2$ and added dead space on idiopathic central sleep apnea. Am Rev Respir Dis 1997; 82:918–926.

# PATIENT 67

## A 55-year-old man with central sleep apnea

A 55-year-old man with complaints of frequent awakenings and moderate daytime sleepiness was evaluated by polysomnography. He snored occasionally and his wife had noted some brief pauses in his breathing during the night. There was no history of leg jerks or symptoms of congestive heart failure. The patient's only medication was an angiotensin-converting enzyme inhibitor for hypertension.

*Physical Examination:*   Blood pressure 150/85 mmHg, pulse 80 and regular. HEENT: dependent palate. Cardiac: normal. Chest: clear, no rales. Extremities: no edema.

*Sleep Study:*   AHI 30/hr. Respiratory events: obstructive apnea 5%, mixed apnea 15%, central apnea 75%, hypopnea 5%.

*Figure:*   A sample tracing is shown below.

*Question:*   What treatment do you recommend?

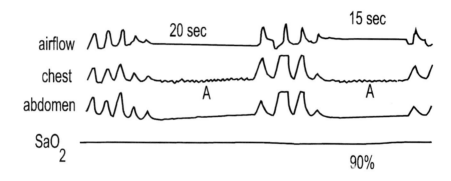

*Answer:* Nasal CPAP is effective treatment in some patients with idiopathic central sleep apnea.

*Discussion:* There is no uniform consensus about the best treatment for patients with idiopathic CSA (central sleep apnea). This group is heterogeneous, and treatment must be individualized. Because idiopathic CSA is relatively rare, no long-term studies of the effectiveness of any treatment have been published.

**Triazolam**, a benzodiazepine, reduced the frequency of idiopathic CSA in one study, probably by decreasing the number of arousals or the amount of hyperventilation associated with arousal. Obviously, sedatives are contraindicated in the hypercapnic forms of CSA. **Nasal CPAP** also has been reported to decrease central apnea in patients with idiopathic CSA. The mechanisms by which CPAP works are unknown. Two possibilities are that nasal CPAP slightly increases the sleeping $PCO_2$ or prevents upper airway reflexes from initiating apnea. The level of CPAP required to prevent central apnea may exceed the level necessary to prevent obstructive events.

Various respiratory stimulants have been tried as treatments for idiopathic CSA, with variable amounts of success. These include **acetazolamide** (Diamox), which is a carbonic anhydrase inhibitor, and **theophylline**. Acetazolamide induces a metabolic acidosis and reduces the pH even if the $PCO_2$ also decreases slightly. One study found modest success with a dose of 250 mg given 1 hour before bedtime: the AHI was reduced by about 50%, and symptoms improved, although sleep efficiency was not significantly better. Oxygen therapy also has been reported to decrease the amounts of nocturnal desaturation and central apnea in selected patients.

In the present patient, apnea was noted to be predominantly central. In the tracing, the small oscillations at *A* represent movement from cardiac contractions. The patient underwent a CPAP titration, and at 10 cm $H_2O$ the AHI was reduced to 8/hr. Treatment with nasal CPAP resulted in improvement of symptoms.

## Clinical Pearls

1. No consensus exists about the best treatment for idiopathic CSA. Treatment must be individualized.
2. Nasal CPAP may be effective in some patients with idiopathic CSA.
3. Alternative treatments include acetazolamide, hypnotics, and oxygen therapy.

## REFERENCES

1. Issa FG, Sullivan CE: Reversal of central sleep apnea using nasal CPAP. Chest 1986; 90:165–171.
2. Bonnet MH, Dexter JR, Arand DL: The effect of triazolam on arousal and respiration in central sleep apnea patients. Sleep 1990; 13:31–41.
3. DeBacker WA, Verbacken J, Willemen M et al: Central apnea index decreases after prolonged treatment with acetazolamide. Am J Resp Crit Care Med 1995; 151:87–91.
4. Franklin KA, Eriksoon P, Sahlin C, et al: Reversal of central sleep apnea with oxygen. Chest 1997; 111:163–169.

# PATIENT 68

## A 70-year-old man with daytime sleepiness and pedal edema

A 70-year-old man was evaluated for complaints of waking at night gasping for air and daytime sleepiness over several years. The patient's wife also reported that he snored while supine and occasionally stopped breathing. He was being treated for hypertension and occasional episodes of leg swelling.

*Physical Examination:* Blood pressure 130/80 mmHg, pulse 90, respiratory rate 15. General: no acute distress. Cardiac: $S_3$ gallop, PMI laterally displaced. Chest: rales at the lung bases. Extremities: 1+ pedal edema.

*Sleep Study:* AHI 52/hr. Respiratory events: obstructive apnea 0%, mixed apnea 75%, central apnea 15%, hypopnea 10%.

*Figure:* A mixed apnea characteristic of this patient is shown in the tracing below.

*Question:* Is this a typical case of obstructive sleep apnea?

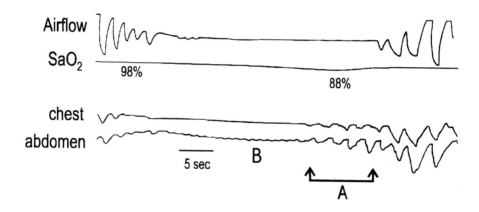

*Diagnosis:* Obstructive (mixed) sleep apnea with underlying Cheyne-Stokes breathing due to congestive heart failure

*Discussion:* Sleep-disordered breathing is common but often unrecognized in patients with congestive heart failure. At least **three forms of sleep apnea** exist in these patients: (1) Cheyne-Stokes breathing (CSB) with central apnea, (2) traditional obstructive sleep apnea (OSA), and (3) a combination of CSB and OSA, producing mixed and central apneas. Many clinicians fail to suspect sleep apnea because complaints of poor sleep are attributed to dyspnea secondary to congestive heart failure. Recognition of sleep-disordered breathing is important because treatment not only improves nocturnal oxygenation and sleep quality but may improve cardiac function.

Patients with CSB can mimic typical OSA presentation, with complaints of excessive daytime sleepiness and mixed apnea on polysomnography. The presence of CSB may be overlooked until treatment is attempted with nasal CPAP. Once the obstructive component is prevented, the repetitive central apneas of CSB are **unmasked**. Typical CSB is a crescendo-decrescendo pattern of ventilation with central apnea or hypopnea at the nadir in ventilatory effort. However, the return of ventilatory effort following central apnea is associated with upper airway closure in some patients. This causes an obstructive portion of apnea following the central part. In some patients, apnea is mixed in the supine position (predisposing to airway closure) and purely central (CSB pattern) in the lateral decubitus position.

Some differences between mixed apnea in the two disorders are notable. The mixed apnea of CSB tends to have a longer central than obstructive component. Also, in typical OSA a number of totally obstructive apneas usually are present. *When CSB is secondary to congestive heart failure, the nadir in arterial oxygen saturation is delayed* secondary to an increased circulation time. Finally, mixed apnea in patients with typical OSA resolves once upper airway obstruction is prevented. In contrast, patients with CSB have an underlying instability in ventilatory control that causes persistence of CSB. Although neurologic disease can cause CSB, congestive heart failure is by far the most common cause.

In the present case, the patient had mixed apnea with a long central component and a short obstructive portion (see figure, area *A*). The small, rapid deflections in the abdominal tracing represent cardiac contractions (*B*). The most interesting finding was the unusual position of the nadir (88%) in arterial oxygen saturation. At first glance the nadir appears to occur before, rather than after, apnea termination. However, the illustrated nadir is actually the consequence of the *preceding apnea* (not shown). The severity of congestive heart failure was unappreciated by the physicians taking care of the patient. A subsequent nuclear medicine study (multiple gated acquisition) revealed a left ventricular ejection fraction of 30%. (See Patients 69 and 70 for discussions on the treatment of CSB with and without an obstructive component).

# Clinical Pearls

1. Cheyne-Stokes breathing may present as a sleep apnea syndrome, with mixed and central apneas and daytime sleepiness.

2. A delay in the nadir of the arterial oxygen saturation is a clue that a long circulation time is present. This is evidence of significant cardiac dysfunction.

3. Sleep-disordered breathing in patients with congestive heart failure (obstructive sleep apnea, CSB, or a combination) frequently is unrecognized and may negatively impact patient outcome if not adequately treated.

## REFERENCES

1. Dowdell WT, Javaheri S, McGinnis W: Cheyne-Stokes respiration presenting as sleep apnea syndrome. Am Rev Respir Dis 1990; 141:871–879.
2. Javaheri S, Parker TJ, Wexler L, et al: Occult sleep-disordered breathing in stable congestive heart failure. Ann Intern Med 1995; 122:487–492.
3. Hanly PJ, Zuberi-Khokhar NS: Increased mortality associated with Cheyne-Stokes respiration in patients with congestive heart failure. Am J Resp Crit Care Med 1996; 153:272–276.

# PATIENT 69

## A 60-year-old man with severe congestive heart failure and daytime sleepiness

A 60-year-old man with known congestive heart failure (left ventricular ejection fraction 30%) was referred for complaints of daytime sleepiness. His wife denied hearing snoring but had noted her husband gasping for air and breathing irregularly during sleep. The patient also noted paroxysmal nocturnal dyspnea and had been admitted several times for exacerbations of congestive heart failure.

*Physical Examination:* Pulse 85 and regular, blood pressure 110/70 mmHg. HEENT: normal palate. Neck: no jugular venous distention, 15-inch circumference. Chest: bilateral rales. Cardiac: $S_3$ gallop, grade 2 holosystolic murmur at the apex. Extremities: 2+ pedal edema.

*Laboratory Findings:* Arterial oxygen saturation (room air): 94%.

*Sleep Study:* AHI 50/hr (70% central apneas, 30% hypopneas), arousal index 40/hr, desaturation index 30/hr ( < 85%).

*Figure:* This sample tracing of airflow shows multiple central apneas. Vertical arrows mark the timing of arousals.

*Question:* What is the diagnosis?

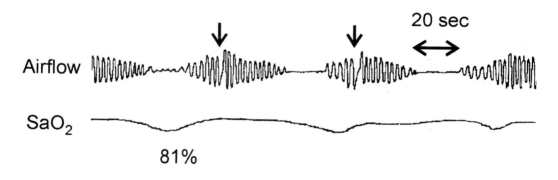

*Diagnosis*  Central apnea with Cheyne-Stokes breathing secondary to heart failure.

*Discussion:*  Cheyne-Stokes breathing (CSB) is defined as a crescendo-decrescendo pattern of breathing with central hypopnea or apnea at the nadir. CSB is caused by an instability in ventilatory control. The two most common causes of CSB are **neurologic disease** (cerebrovascular accidents) and **congestive heart failure** (CHF). The incidence of CSB in patients with severe CHF of any cause is as high as 40–50%. CSB often is unsuspected, as typical patients only exhibit it during sleep. The etiology of CSB in patients with CHF has been attributed to delayed feedback of changes in blood gases to the ventilatory controllers (**long circulation time**), thus producing an "overshoot" in ventilation. During sleep, when the $PCO_2$ drops below the apneic threshold, central apnea occurs. One would expect the CHF patients with CSB to have longer circulation times (as a consequence of worse cardiac function). However, when groups of CHF patients with and without CSB were compared, the main difference was *not* the degree of cardiac dysfunction, but the slightly lower daytime $PCO_2$ levels in CSB patients.

CSB may be associated with frequent arousal from sleep and daytime sleepiness. Unfortunately, clinicians typically assume that these symptoms are secondary to dyspnea associated with CHF. Interestingly, the arousals associated with CSB tend to occur at the *zenith* of ventilatory effort, rather than at apnea termination. Significant arterial oxygen desaturation is common in CSB patients, despite a normal daytime $SaO_2$. Neither oxygen desaturation nor repetitive activation of the sympathetic nervous system is beneficial to patients already suffering from cardiac dysfunction. It is not surprising that the presence of CSB in patients with CHF signals a worse prognosis.

The optimal treatment of CSB associated with CHF is not yet known. Certainly treatment starts with optimization of cardiac function. Other treatments for CSB associated with CHF include **oxygen therapy**, **nasal CPAP**, and **theophylline**. Oxygen improves CSB-associated desaturation, reduces the amount of CSB, and improves sleep quality. Theophylline also lowers the amount of CSB; however, treatment may not reduce the number of arousals. One concern is the possibility of inducing arrhythmias with this medication. Nasal CPAP can acutely reduce the amount of CSB by improving oxygenation and inducing a modest increase in the sleeping $PCO_2$. In some patients, nasal CPAP acutely improves the $SaO_2$ and reduces arousals without eliminating CSB (see Patient 70). Even if CSB cannot be eliminated during CPAP titration, several studies have shown that chronic treatment with empirically determined levels of 10–12 cm $H_2O$ can improve cardiac function and ultimately the amount of CSB. A period of "desensitization" to CPAP may be required. Other studies are in progress to determine which of these treatments is best and if any improve long-term survival in this patient population.

The present patient was treated with ongoing nasal CPAP at 10–12 cm $H_2O$. He reported improved sleep quality and over the next several weeks noted a dramatic decrease in pedal edema although his medications were unchanged.

## Clinical Pearls

1. The CSB type of central apnea is common and often unsuspected in patients with significant CHF.

2. CSB can present with symptoms of daytime sleepiness and disturbed sleep.

3. Adequate treatment of CSB associated with CHF can improve sleep, cardiac function, and perhaps even the long-term prognosis of these patients.

## REFERENCES

1. Hanly PJ, Millar TW, Steljes DG, et al: The effect of oxygen on respiration and sleep in patients with congestive heart failure. Ann Int Med 1989; 111:777–782.
2. Takasaki Y, Orr D, Popkin J, et al: Effect of nasal continuous positive airway pressure on sleep apnea in congestive heart failure. Am Rev Respir Dis 1989; 140:1578–1584.
3. Naughton M, Bernard D, Tam A, et al: Role of hyperventilation in the pathogenesis of central sleep apnea in patients with congestive heart failure. Am Rev Respir Dis 1993; 148:330–338.
4. Jahavheri S, Parker TJ, Wexler L, et al: Effect of theophylline on sleep-disordered breathing in heart failure. N Engl J Med 1996; 335:562–567.

# PATIENT 70

## A 60-year-old man with obstructive sleep apnea
## and numerous central apneas on CPAP

A 60-year-old man with a diagnosis of obstructive sleep apnea (OSA) was referred from another sleep laboratory for a nasal CPAP titration. His previous sleep study showed an AHI of 60/hr.

### Sleep Study

| | | | | | | |
|---|---|---|---|---|---|---|
| CPAP (cm H$_2$O) | 0 | 5 | 7.5 | 10 | 12 | 15 |
| NREM (min) | 120 | 60 | 60 | 60 | 20 | 30 |
| AHI (/hr) | 55 | 50 | 50 | 40 | 35 | 30 |
| % obstructive apnea | 0 | 0 | 0 | 0 | 0 | 0 |
| % mixed apnea | 100 | 50 | 0 | 0 | 0 | 0 |
| % central apnea | 0 | 0 | 0 | **100** | **100** | **100** |
| % hypopnea | 0 | 50 | 100 | 0 | 0 | 0 |
| Desaturations < 85% | 40 | 30 | 10 | 0 | 0 | 0 |
| Arousal index (/hr) | 40 | 35 | 20 | 10 | 10 | 10 |

*Figure*:   A tracing of a central apnea at a CPAP level of 12 cm H2O is shown below.

*Question:*   What is causing the central apnea?

### Nasal CPAP 12 cm H$_2$O

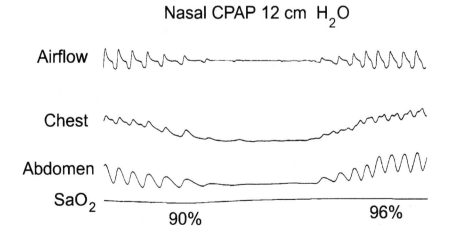

181

**Diagnosis:**   Cheyne-Stokes breathing presenting as obstructive sleep apnea (mixed apnea)

**Discussion:**   When patients with OSA (mixed apnea) and underlying Cheyne-Stokes breathing (CSB) are treated with nasal CPAP, the CSB tends to be unmasked. CPAP abolishes the obstructive component of mixed apnea by preventing upper airway obstruction. However, unlike typical cases of mixed apnea, the central component persists secondary to underlying CSB. The sudden appearance of **repetitive central apnea** during a CPAP titration may be a surprise if the underlying CSB was not appreciated on the diagnostic study. Note that central apneas also may appear during upward titration of CPAP if high levels of pressure trigger arousal and hyperventilation (followed by central apnea on return to sleep). However, these central apneas will not be of the Cheyne-Stokes type.

The first goal of CPAP titration in these patients is to prevent upper airway obstruction. As discussed in the previous case, further upward titration of CPAP usually does not abolish CSB, but may reduce desaturation and arousal. Acute reduction of CSB may be secondary to increases in $PCO_2$ or a reduction in the severity of desaturation. When no level of CPAP abolishes CSB, one approach is to treat with pressure at **10–12.5 cm $H_2O$** (or a higher level if needed to prevent upper airway obstruction). Several studies have shown that treatment during sleep with this level of nasal CPAP in patients with congestive heart failure produces long-term improvements in cardiac function—by improving oxygenation, decreasing afterload, and decreasing sympathetic stimulation from frequent arousals. Improvements in cardiac function should eventually improve the amount of CSB. However, note that one study of similar patients showed no improvement in symptoms of cardiac function when nasal CPAP at a level of 7.5 cm $H_2O$ was compared with placebo. This result emphasizes that treatment must be individualized and monitored carefully. Long-term effects of CPAP may depend on the preload status of the patient.

In the present case, the tabular summary of the CPAP trial shows a conversion of the apnea type from mixed apnea to hypopnea and finally to central apnea as the level of CPAP was increased. Further upward titration did not eliminate the central apneas. Detailed examination of the central apnea showed a crescendo-decrescendo pattern of breathing with central apneas or hypopneas at the nadir, consistent with CSB. The time from end apnea to saturation nadir was increased in this patient (long circulation time). Although no level of CPAP eliminated the central apneas, the number of arousals was decreased and oxygenation was much improved. The present patient was prescribed nasal CPAP at a level of 12 cm $H_2O$, resulting in improved symptoms of both daytime sleepiness and congestive heart failure.

## Clinical Pearls

1. CPAP therapy may uncover CSB in patients with congestive heart failure once the obstructive component has been eliminated.

2. CSB (central apnea) usually persists despite upward titration of CPAP.

3. The goals of CPAP therapy in patients with both upper airway obstruction and CSB secondary to heart failure are to prevent airway obstruction, improve oxygenation, and provide a pressure sufficient to improve cardiac function (10–12 cm $H_2O$ in most patients).

## REFERENCES

1. Takasaki Y, Orr D, Popkin J, et al: Effect of nasal continuous positive airway pressure on sleep apnea in congestive heart failure. Am Rev Respir Dis 1989; 140:1578–1584.
2. Dowdell WT, Javaheri S, McGinnis W: Cheyne-Stokes respiration presenting as sleep apnea syndrome. Am Rev Respir Dis 1990; 141:871–879.
3. Bradley TD, Holloway RM, McLaughlin PR, et al: Cardiac output response to continuous positive airway pressure in congestive heart failure. Am Rev Respir Dis 1992; 145:377–382.
4. Davies RJO, Harrington KJ, Ormerod OJM, et al: Nasal continuous positive airway pressure in chronic heart failure with sleep disordered breathing. Am Rev Respir Dis 1993; 147:630–634.

# PATIENT 71

## A 75-year-old man with a history of polio

A 75-year-old man was seen for complaints of daytime somnolence and pedal edema. At age 30 he had a severe case of poliomyelitis with weakness in the arms and legs. After partial recovery, he enjoyed good health until the last few years. About 2 years ago, unexplained pedal edema began to occur. An arterial blood gas test (room air) at that time revealed: pH 7.36, $PCO_2$ 50 mmHg, $pO_2$ 65 mmHg, $HCO_3$ 25 mmol/L. The patient was started on nocturnal oxygen, at 2 L/min by nasal cannula at night, and his pedal edema improved. No sleep study was performed at that time. The patient's wife reported that he rarely snored or gasped for air at night. Over the last few months, the patient had become increasingly somnolent during the day, and his ankles began to swell.

***Physical Examination:*** Vital signs: unremarkable. HEENT: edentulous, otherwise normal. Chest: clear to ausculation and percussion. Cardiac: no murmurs. Abdomen: normal. Extremities: 2+ pedal edema. Neurologic: mild-to-moderate symmetric reduction in strength in the arms and legs; gag reflex intact.

***Laboratory Findings:*** ABG (room air): pH 7.34, $PCO_2$ 60 mmHg, $PO_2$ 55 mmHg, $HCO_3$ 27 mmol/L.

***Question:*** What evaluation and treatment would you suggest?

*Answer:* Sleep study with titration of bilevel positive airway pressure.

*Discussion:* Patients with a distant history of poliomyelitis may experience a worsening of the muscle weakness later in life (post-polio syndrome). Respiratory muscle weakness can result in hypoventilation during the day, with a worsening during sleep. The associated desaturation during sleep may result in findings consistent with cor pulmonale. During NREM sleep, periods of central apnea, hypopnea, obstructive apnea, or regular breathing with hypoventilation may occur. During REM sleep, more profound arterial oxygen desaturation usually is noted. Transcutaneous $PCO_2$ monitoring reveals an increase in $PCO_2$ during NREM sleep and a further increase during REM sleep.

The treatment of this syndrome must be individualized. Milder cases may respond to oxygen administration. As hypoventilation worsens, some degree of ventilatory support, such as bilevel pressure via nasal mask, is indicated. The level of expiratory positive airway pressure (EPAP) is titrated to maintain upper airway patency. The level of inspiratory positive airway pressure (IPAP) is adjusted to provide a level of pressure support (pressure support = IPAP – EPAP). The level of pressure support is adjusted until the spontaneous tidal volume is in a normal range (400–500 cc). Oxygen can be added if desaturation persists despite pressure support of ventilation.

Negative-pressure ventilation via body wrap or cuirass also has been used successfully in some patients. One potential problem is the development of upper airway obstruction because upper airway muscle activity is not coordinated with the negative-pressure breaths.

If patients do not improve adequately with the aforementioned approaches, the next step is positive-pressure, volume-cycled ventilation via nasal mask. Mouth leaks may require chin straps or a full face mask. In very severe cases, tracheostomy and volume ventilation can be employed. Even then, many patients may only require ventilatory support at night. Nocturnal ventilation can improve the daytime $PCO_2$ by preventing hypoxic depression of ventilatory drive and resting the respiratory muscles.

In the present patient, a sleep study revealed desaturation to 80% without discrete hypopneas during NREM sleep. During REM sleep, central apneas and arterial oxygen desaturation to 50% were noted. During the second part of the night, bilevel pressure was titrated to a level of 15/5 cm $H_2O$, and oxygen at 2 L/min was added to prevent desaturation. Using this approach, nocturnal desaturation was prevented. After 1 week of treatment the patient felt more awake, and his daytime $PCO_2$ decreased to 50 mmHg. He was followed carefully so that the amount of pressure support could be increased or volume-cycled ventilation via mask instituted if a progressive rise in $PCO_2$ was noted.

## Clinical Pearls

1. Respiratory failure can develop many years after the initial infection in patients with a history of poliomyelitis.

2. Patients with neuromuscular disorders may experience severe nocturnal hypoventilation (with or without obstructive or central sleep apnea) and symptoms of cor pulmonale and daytime sleepiness.

3. Nocturnal ventilatory assistance with bilevel pressure or volume-cycled ventilation via nasal or full face mask can prevent nocturnal hypoventilation and allow many patients to function during the day without ventilatory support.

## REFERENCES
1. Bach JR, Alba MS: Management of chronic alveolar hypoventilation by nasal ventilation. Chest 1990; 97:52–57.
2. Steljes DG, Kryger MH, Kirk BW, Millar TW: Sleep in postpolio syndrome. Chest 1990; 98:133–140.
3. Claman DM, Piper AM, Sanders MH, et al: Nocturnal noninvasive positive pressure ventilatory assistance. Chest 1996; 110:1581–1588.

# PATIENT 72

## A 40-year-old man who kicks in his sleep

A 40-year-old man was referred for daytime sleepiness of 2-year duration. His wife reported that he snored occasionally and sometimes "kicked" during sleep. There was no history of recent weight gain, cataplexy, sleep paralysis, or hypnagogic hallucinations. The patient remembered awakening several times each night but never noticed any discomfort at those times. The patient denied any unusual sensations in his legs at bedtime.

***Physical Examination:*** Normal.

***Sleep Study:*** Total sleep time 360 minutes. AHI 10/hr.

***Figure:*** There were 250 events similar to the two identified (*A* and *B*) in the tracing below. Sixty percent of these events were associated with arousal.

***Question:*** What is your diagnosis?

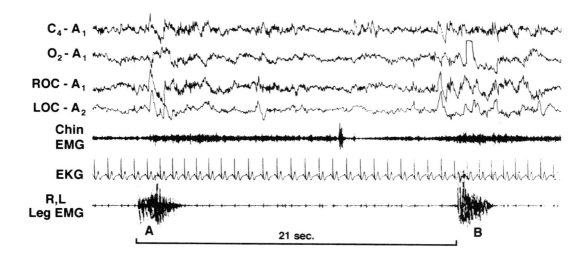

*Diagnosis:* Periodic leg movement in sleep.

*Discussion:* The syndrome of periodic leg (or limb) movement (PLM), also known as nocturnal myoclonus, consists of stereotypic periodic leg (arm) movements during sleep that may or may not be associated with arousals. When enough arousals occur, sleep is fragmented, and daytime sleepiness results. While PLM is the etiology in about 10–12% of patients seen in sleep centers for insomnia complaints, only 2–3% of patients presenting with excessive daytime sleepiness are found to have PLM as the major cause of their sleepiness. Probably a much higher percentage of elderly patients have PLM but no symptoms.

The cause of the PLM syndrome is unknown, but conditions associated with PLM include withdrawal of anticonvulsants, barbiturates, and other hypnotics; the use of tricyclic antidepressants; and renal failure. Patients with excessive daytime sleepiness due to PLM may or may not remember the awakenings during the night, but almost never remember the leg movements. The movements usually consist of dorsiflexion of the foot at the ankle, extension of the big toe, and partial flexion of the knee and hip. This differs from hypnic jerks (sleep starts) in which the entire body jerks at sleep onset. A small portion of the patients have the restless leg syndrome (RLS), which involves a creeping sensation in the legs associated with a desire to move them. These sensations commonly occur at bedtime. It is important to question patients about these sensations because if a patient has RLS, he or she frequently also has PLM. (See Patient 74 for more information on RLS.)

The diagnosis of the PLM syndrome requires monitoring of leg EMG. Surface electrodes usually are placed over the anterior tibialis muscle (lateral calf). Movements may occur in one or both legs; therefore, monitoring of *both* legs is suggested. This dual monitoring can be performed using a single polygraph channel.

A leg movement is considered part of a PLM sequence if it belongs to a group of four or more leg movements separated by more than 5 and less than 90 seconds (most separations are 20–40 seconds). Leg movements resulting from arousals due to respiratory disturbances usually are not counted as PLMs. Simultaneous movements in both legs are counted as one movement. Some labs tabulate all leg movements (including those during wake and associated with respiratory events); others count only leg movements in a sequence during sleep.

Not all leg movements are associated with arousals, and a significant number of arousals following PLMs must be documented to identify PLM as the cause of excessive sleepiness or insomnia. The PLM index is computed by dividing the total number of PLMs by the total sleep time in hours (movements / hour of sleep). The PLM-arousal index is the total number of PLMs *associated with arousal* divided by the total sleep time in hours. A PLM index > 5 is considered abnormal, 5–24 mild, 25–49 moderate, and ≥ 50 severe. However, the true impact of the disorder is more accurately assessed by looking at the PLM-arousal index. Severe insomnia or excessive daytime sleepiness usually is associated with a PLM-arousal index > 25/hr. In many patients, PLMs are almost completely restricted to NREM sleep. However, PLMs in REM sleep can occur.

In the present patient, 400 PLMs occurred as part of a sequence and were not associated with respiratory events. The PLM index was 400 movements / 6 hours of sleep = 66.7/hr. The PLM-arousal index was 40/hr. The patient was diagnosed with the PLM syndrome and was treated with carbidopa/levodopa 25 mg/100 mg at bedtime. He reported a decrease in daytime sleepiness. (See Patient 73 for a discussion of treatment of PLM.)

# Clinical Pearls

1. PLM can cause insomnia and/or excessive daytime sleepiness.
2. Patients with the restless leg syndrome almost always have PLM. In contrast, only a small portion of patients with PLM have the restless leg syndrome.
3. Patients usually do not remember PLMs, but bedmates may report movement.
4. The PLM-arousal index reflects the impact of PLM on sleep quality. Significant symptoms are usually associated with a PLM arousal index > 25/hr.

## REFERENCES

1. Coleman RM: Periodic movements in sleep (nocturnal myoclonus) and restless legs syndrome. *In* Guilleminault C (ed): Sleeping and Waking Disorders: Indications and Techniques. Boston, Butterworths, 1982, pp 265–295.
2. American Sleep Disorders Association: International Classification of Sleep Disorders: Diagnostic and Coding Manual. Lawrence, KS, Allen Press, 1990, pp 65–71.
3. The Atlas Task Force of the American Sleep Disorders Association: Recording and scoring leg movements. Sleep 1993; 16:749–759.

# PATIENT 73

## A 50-year-old man groggy in the morning after treatment
## for periodic leg movements

A 50-year-old man who complained of excessive daytime sleepiness was diagnosed as having periodic limb movement (PLM) in sleep on a previous study. That evaluation showed a PLM index of 50/hr and a PLM-arousal index (number of PLMs per hour associated with arousal) of 30/hr. He was treated with clonazepam starting at 0.5 mg qhs and increasing to 1 mg at bedtime. He reported improved sleep but grogginess in the morning. A repeat polysomnogram was ordered (results below).

### Sleep Study*

| | | Sleep Stages | % SPT |
|---|---|---|---|
| Time in bed | 480 min (378–468) | | |
| Total sleep time | 350 min (340–439 | Stage Wake | 18 (2–7) |
| Sleep period time (SPT) | 425 min (361–453) | Stage 1 | 13 (4–12) |
| Sleep latency | 10 min (1–22) | Stage 2 | 49 (51–72) |
| REM latency | 80 min (65–104) | Stages 3 and 4 | 5 (0–13) |
| Arousal index | 15/hr | Stage REM | 15 (17–25) |
| AHI | 8/hr (<5) | | |
| PLM index | 55/hr | | |
| PLM-arousal index | 10/hr | | |

*On clonazepam

( ) = normal values for age, PLM = periodic leg movement

*Question:* Why is there no reduction in the PLM index with treatment?

*Answer:* Clonazapam reduces the number of PLM-related arousals, but generally does not change the frequency of leg movements.

*Discussion:* The traditional treatment for symptomatic PLM in sleep is the benzodiazepine clonazepam (Klonopin). The drug typically is started at 0.5 mg at bedtime and titrated upward to 1.5–2 mg if necessary. Clonazepam's efficacy is primarily due to a **decrease in the arousals** associated with the leg movements. Most studies have documented no decrease in the number of leg movements.

Although clonazepam is relatively free of side effects, morning somnolence is a common complaint. This side effect can be minimized by starting a low dose (allowing tolerance to develop) and taking the medication earlier in the evening (about 1 hour before bedtime). Patients should be cautioned about drinking alcohol, driving, or performing any potentially dangerous activity while under the influence of the medication.

The overall efficacy of clonazepam is only mild-to-moderate. Other benzodiazepines with shorter half-lives, such as temazepam (Restoril) or triazolam (Halcion) also have been used for treatment of the PLM syndrome. It is important to remember that benzodiazepines can worsen obstructive sleep apnea and should not be used in patients with hypoventilation.

An alternative to the benzodiazepines is the carbidopa/levodopa (25/100 mg) combination. This drug does appear to **decrease the amount of leg movements**. The usual starting dose is one-half pill at bedtime, which can be increased in half-tablet increments every 3 days until symptoms are controlled (maximum dose is four pills). Initial side effects such as nausea are minimized by a slow upward titration. This medication is short-acting, and a single dose generally suppresses PLM only during the first half of the night. If the patient awakens and has difficulty falling asleep or maintaining sleep, an additional dose of one-half to two tablets may be taken. To avoid repeat dosing during the night, an equivalent dose of a continuous preparation of carbidopa/levodopa (Sinemet CR) may be taken at bedtime (one 25/100 mg Sinemet CR at bedtime versus one-half pill of the usual 25/100 mg preparation at bedtime and one-half at 3 AM.)

Unfortunately, up to 80% of patients with restless leg syndrome (RLS) and 30% with PLM but no RLS eventually experience some augmentation of symptoms. Augmentation is less likely at lower doses. Should augmentation occur, it may respond to higher doses, but the problem commonly returns. Some patients using the short-acting medication also may experience restlessness or paresthesia in the morning. Moreover, a concern to all physicians prescribing levodopa is the possibility of tardive dyskinesia (involuntary movements), a side effect seen in patients with Parkinson's disease who are treated with levodopa at higher doses. This side effect has not been a problem in patients with PLM taking lower doses. Therefore, a prescription for the lowest effective dose is the prudent course.

In the present patient, the second sleep study showed a reduction in PLM-associated arousals without a change in the frequency of PLMs. This is typical of clonazepam treatment, as is morning grogginess. The patient tried taking clonazepam 1 hour before bedtime, but still had morning symptoms. He was switched to carbidopa/levodopa 25/100 mg starting with one-half pill at bedtime, to be repeated if necessary. On one pill at bedtime (repeated if necessary), the patient noted good sleep and control of his daytime sleepiness.

## Clinical Pearls

1. Treatment of PLM with clonazepam improves sleep quality (reduces arousals), but often does not reduce the frequency of leg movements.

2. Early morning somnolence, a common side effect of clonazepam, may limit the usefulness of this medication.

3. Carbidopa/levodopa appears to reduce the number of PLMs and improve sleep quality. Many clinicians consider this medication the drug of choice for treating PLM.

## REFERENCES

1. Mitler, MM, Browman CP, Menn SJ, et al: Nocturnal myoclonus: treatment efficacy of clonazepam and temazepam. Sleep 1986; 9:385–392.
2. Peled R, Lavie P: Double-blind evaluation of clonazepam on periodic leg movements in sleep. J Neurol Neurosurg Psych 1987; 50:1679–1681.
3. Doghramji K, Browman CP, Gaddy JR, et al: Triazolam diminishes daytime sleepiness and sleep fragmentation in patients with periodic leg movements in sleep. J Clin Psychopharmacol 1991; 11:284–290.
4. Becker PM, Jamieson AO, Brown WD: Dopaminergic agents in restless leg syndrome and periodic leg movements of sleep: Response and complications of extended treatment in 49 cases. Sleep 1993; 16:713–716.

# PATIENT 74

## A 56-year-old man with crawling sensations in his legs at bedtime

A 56-year-old patient reported an inability to fall asleep at night secondary to a crawling sensation in both legs. These unpleasant sensations frequently started an hour before bedtime when he was seated or recumbent in bed. The discomfort usually was relieved by moving his legs or walking, but it returned as soon as he became inactive. After great difficulty falling asleep, the patient experienced frequent and prolonged awakenings during the night. His wife reported that he kicked and jerked during sleep, but did not snore. Because of these problems, the patient was quite fatigued. An evaluation by the patient's primary care physician revealed no evidence of anemia, iron or folate deficiency, or renal failure.

***Physical Examination:*** Neurologic: intact position and vibration sense; sensation to pin and touch normal; deep tendon reflexes normal and symmetric.

***Laboratory Finding:*** Hct 40%.

***Questions:*** What is the diagnosis? Should a sleep study be ordered?

***Diagnosis:*** Restless leg syndrome. A sleep study is not needed unless other sleep pathology is suspected.

***Discussion:*** The restless leg syndrome (RLS) consists of paresthesia in the legs, usually described as crawling or creeping, that occurs during wakefulness exclusively while the patient is at rest (inactive) in the seated or recumbent position. Walking or moving brings quick relief, but the sensations return once the patient is inactive. Sometimes a sensation of pain also is present. Most patients with RLS have periodic leg movement (PLM) during sleep. Because of this fact, a sleep study is not needed in someone with unequivocal symptoms of RLS when no other sleep pathology (e.g., sleep apnea) is suspected. In contrast, only a small fraction of all patients with PLM have RLS. Thus, the absence of a history of RLS does not diminish the possibility that PLM is present during sleep.

RLS symptoms make sleep onset difficult, and associated PLM causes frequent awakenings. Thus, patients with RLS usually complain of insomnia (difficulty initiating and maintaining sleep) and/or excessive daytime sleepiness. The differential diagnosis of RLS includes paresthesia due to neuropathy. This paresthesia is constant, usually not relieved by moving or walking, and sometimes worsens at night. Unlike peripheral neuropathy, the neurologic examination and nerve conduction/EMG studies usually are normal in RLS. Neuroleptic akathisia (motor restlessness in which patients feel compelled to move their extremities) can be eliminated from the differential because there is no history of prior neuroleptic use. Akathisia movements also are not associated with dysesthesia (crawling sensations) characteristic of RLS symptoms.

The etiology of RLS is unknown. The condition has been associated with iron deficiency (less commonly, folate or B12 deficiency), vascular insufficiency, uremic neuropathy, and caffeine abuse. Some of the described associations are based on relatively few anecdotal reports. When sleep monitoring is performed in patients with RLS, there are quasiperiodic movements of the legs during wakefulness, and the sleep latency is prolonged. After sleep onset, PLM usually is noted.

Treatment of RLS includes many of the agents used for treatment of PLM. One important principle is to administer the agents early enough so that an effect is present at bedtime. Many clinicians consider dopamine agents to be the first line of treatment in RLS, with some reporting efficacy in over 90% of patients. Carbidopa/levodopa (25/100 mg) has been the most frequently used agent. However, this short-acting preparation may lead to a rebound in symptoms (and PLM) in the second half of the night. The dose usually is repeated if the patient awakens in the middle of the night. One approach is to start with one-half pill of the 25/100 mg preparation 20–30 minutes before bedtime (with a repeat if needed during the night). The dose can be increased by one-half pill every few days if there are no side effects (e.g., nausea) until symptoms are controlled. The usual maximum dose is two to four pills per night. An alternative to repeat dosing during the night is Sinemet CR, a continuous release form of carbidopa/levodopa.

Unfortunately, use of these medications sometimes results in morning symptoms of RLS and often increases symptoms. This augmentation is manifested as spread of the crawling sensations to the arms as well as the legs and/or symptoms occurring throughout the day. Symptom augmentation usually responds to discontinuation of the medication. Augmentation is less likely at lower doses. If the side effects of carbidopa/levodopa are intolerable, dopamine agonists, opiates, or benzodiazepines can be tried. (See Patient 75 for a discussion of these treatment options.)

In the present patient, clear-cut symptoms of RLS were present, so a sleep study was not ordered. The patient was started on carbidopa/levodopa 25/100 mg at one-half pill 90 minutes before bedtime, with a repeat during the night if needed. The dose was gradually increased to one pill, and the RLS symptoms were reasonably controlled on most nights.

## Clinical Pearls

1. Diagnosis of RLS usually can be made by history and physical examination.
2. Iron-deficiency anemia should be excluded in patients with RLS.
3. Most patients with RLS have PLM during sleep.

## REFERENCES

1. Monteplaisir J, Lapierre O, Warnes H, et al: The treatment of the restless leg syndrome with or without periodic leg movements in sleep. Sleep 1992; 15:391–395.
2. Earley CJ, Allen RP: Pergolide and carbidopa/levodopa treatment of restless leg syndrome and periodic leg movements in sleep in a consecutive series of patients. Sleep 1996; 19:801–810.

# PATIENT 75

**A 72-year-old man with worsening symptoms during treatment for restless legs**

A 72-year-old man was diagnosed as having the restless leg syndrome (RLS) on the basis of a history of crawling sensation in both legs. These unpleasant sensations frequently started 30 minutes before bedtime when he was seated or recumbent in bed. The discomfort usually was relieved by moving his legs or walking, but the sensations returned once he became inactive. The patient was started on one-half pill of carbidopa/levodopa 25/100 mg, and the dose was slowly increased to two pills 90 minutes before bedtime. This treatment resulted in good control of his symptoms. However, he began to notice RLS symptoms in the early evening that involved his arms as well as his legs.

*Physical Examination:* Unremarkable. Neurologic: no involuntary movements, normal muscle tone, sensation intact.

*Question:* What treatment do you recommend?

***Answer:*** Discontinue carbidopa/levodopa and try a dopamine agonist.

***Discussion:*** Treatment of RLS with carbidopa/levodopa eventually results in some augmentation of symptoms in up to 80% of patients with RLS and in 30% of patients with PLM and no RLS. The **rebound effect** describes increased symptoms in the early morning and is secondary to the relative short duration of the medication. The **augmentation effect** describes: (1) earlier onset of the usual bedtime symptoms (early evening or late afternoon), (2) increased severity of symptoms, and (3) spread of symptoms to the arms. Augmentation is less likely at lower doses. It may temporarily improve with an increase in dosage, but the symptoms eventually occur again. Augmentation usually responds to discontinuing the medication and switching to another agent.

If the side effects of carbidopa/levodopa are intolerable, then other **dopamine agonists**, such as bromocriptine and pergolide (Permax), can be tried. Of these, pergolide has a longer duration of efficacy (10–12 hours versus 5–6 hours) and is less expensive. Pergolide is started at .05 mg (one tablet) 2 hours before bedtime (or one-half tablet with dinner and one-half before bed). The dose may be increased every 3–4 days up to a maximum daily dose of 1 mg. Nausea is the most common side effect.

**Opiates** are more often used for RLS than PLM, and they can be very effective in some patients. Two problems are the potential for abuse and the development of tolerance. Some clinicians combine opiates and dopamine agents so that a lower dose of each agent is effective, resulting in fewer side effects. Another approach is to use different medications on alternate weeks. Carbamazepine (Tegretol) also has been reported to be beneficial in RLS. This medication has been used for symptoms of peripheral neuropathy, and an occasional patient with RLS also has symptoms consistent with this disorder.

**Benzodiazepines** were once the main type of medication used for RLS. Due to their sedative effects, patients are less bothered by sensations of RLS during wakefulness and when asleep are less likely to arouse from PLM. Clonazepam (Klonopin) was the traditional agent, but it frequently is associated with daytime drowsiness. This side effect can be minimized by starting with a low dose (0.5 mg) and taking the medication earlier in the evening. The usual effective dose is 1–2 mg. Other benzodiazepines with shorter half-lives, such as tempazepam (Restoril), may avoid the problem of daytime sleepiness.

In the present patient, carbidopa/levodopa was discontinued, and the early evening symptoms as well as the spread to his arms gradually ceased. The patient was begun on pergolide .05 mg, one-half tablet with dinner and one-half before bed. He initially experienced mild nausea, but this diminished with time. On a dose of one tablet with dinner and one at bedtime, the patient noted reasonable control of his bedtime symptoms on most nights.

# Clinical Pearls

1. Augmentation of RLS symptoms can occur while on treatment with levodopa/carbidopa, but usually responds to a discontinuation of medication.

2. Augmentation is more likely in patients with RLS than with PLM only. The lowest effective dose of carbidopa/levodopa should be used to decrease the risk of augmentation.

3. Alternative effective treatments for RLS include other dopamine agonists (e.g., pergolide and bromocriptine), opiates, and benzodiazepines.

4. Treatment of RLS must be individualized. Prescribing different medications on alternate weeks or using lower doses of two medications in combined therapy can minimize side effects and avoid tolerance and augmentation.

## REFERENCES

1. Monteplaisir J, Lapierre O, Warnes H, et al: The treatment of the restless leg syndrome with or without periodic leg movements in sleep. Sleep 1992; 15:391–395.
2. Walters AS, Wagner ML, Hening WA, et al: Successful treatment of the idiopathic restless leg syndrome in a randomized double-blind trial of oxycodone versus placebo. Sleep 1993; 16:327–332.
3. Allen RP, Earley CJ: Augmentation of the restless leg syndrome with carbidopa/levodopa. Sleep 1996; 19:205–213.
4. Earley CJ, Allen RP: Pergolide and carbidopa/levodopa treatment of restless leg syndrome and periodic leg movements in sleep in a consecutive series of patients. Sleep 1996; 19:801–810.

# PATIENT 76

## A 58-year-old man with sleep apnea and leg jerks during sleep

A 58-year-old man was diagnosed as having severe obstructive sleep apnea (OSA) on an initial study. He then underwent a nasal CPAP titration, after which he remarked that he had had the "best night of sleep in years." However, there was a drastic change in his PLM index on CPAP.

***Physical Examination:*** Vital signs: normal. HEENT: large tongue, dependent palate. Neck: 16-inch circumference. Chest: clear. Cardiac: normal. Extremities: no edema. Neurologic: sensation in extremities intact.

### Sleep Study

|  | Diagnostic | CPAP Titration (12 cm $H_2O$) |
|---|---|---|
| AHI | 66/hr | 10/hr |
| PLM index | 10/hr | 60/hr |
| PLM-arousal index | 5/hr | 10/hr |
| Arousal index | 50/hr | 15/hr |

All indices are the number of events per hour of sleep.

***Question:*** What is your diagnosis?

*Diagnosis:* Periodic leg movements associated with nasal CPAP treatment of OSA.

*Discussion:* A significant increase in periodic leg movement (PLM) has been reported in patients with OSA following the initiation of nasal CPAP. The etiology of this change is unknown, but several possibilities have been suggested. One is that the severe fragmentation of sleep by apnea (pre-CPAP) did not allow manifestation of the PLM, and treatment with CPAP **unmasked the PLM** by allowing continuous sleep. Another is that the **rebound in sleep** following initial CPAP treatment results in less spontaneous patient movement, and the stasis or pressure on the nerves due to immobility leads to PLM. Many patients spend more time supine when treated with CPAP than in the untreated state. Whatever the etiology, the clinician must decide whether to treat the PLM or follow the patient's symptoms after nasal CPAP therapy is initiated.

In some patients on nasal CPAP, the large increase in PLM is **transient**. In others, the PLM-arousal index is low, and the impact on sleep is **insignificant**. In such cases, observation is adequate, and if symptoms of daytime sleepiness resolve, no additional treatment is necessary. However, if daytime sleepiness persists or returns after treatment of OSA is initiated, PLM could be one cause of treatment failure. Note that the mere presence of PLM should not exclude consideration of other causes of persistent daytime sleepiness, such as poor compli-

ance, inadequate sleep, and narcolepsy (which often coexists with PLM). The patient's bed partner should be questioned about the frequency of body movements while the patient is on nasal CPAP. Repeat sleep monitoring to determine the PLM-arousal index (with the patient on nasal CPAP) may be needed for clarification and to document that the level of CPAP is adequate.

Special treatment consideration is necessary in patients with PLM and significant OSA. Benzodiazepines, a common treatment for PLM, have the potential to worsen sleep apnea. The risk probably is small if the patient is on an adequate amount of nasal CPAP. However, the effect of benzodiazepines on the efficacy of nasal CPAP has not been specifically studied. In addition, there is always the possibility that the medication will be taken on nights when CPAP is not used. An alternative treatment for PLM, such as levodopa/carbidopa, may be a better choice in this situation. Certainly, benzodiazepines are *absolutely contraindicated* in patients with hypoventilation.

In the present case, the PLM-arousal index was modest, and the patient noted a marked improvement in daytime sleepiness almost immediately. Good control of his symptoms persisted on nasal CPAP therapy, and no treatment for the PLM was initiated.

## Clinical Pearls

1. A large increase in PLM can follow initiation of nasal CPAP therapy in patients with OSA.

2. In many patients with OSA and PLM, treatment of the OSA alone can result in a complete resolution of symptoms. PLM treatment may not be needed.

3. When adequate treatment of OSA (nasal CPAP) fails to abolish symptoms of daytime sleepiness, PLM may be one cause of persistent sleepiness.

4. Benzodiazepines can worsen OSA. This fact should be considered in choosing a treatment for PLM in patients with sleep apnea.

## REFERENCES

1. Fry JM, Diphillip MA, Pressman MR: Periodic leg movements in sleep following treatment of obstructive sleep apnea with nasal CPAP. Chest 1989; 96:89–91.
2. Berry RB, Kouchi K, Bower J, et al: Effect of triazolam in obstructive sleep apnea. Am J Resp Crit Care Med 1995; 151:450–454.
3. Guilleminault C, Phillip P: Tiredness and somnolence despite initial treatment of obstructive sleep apnea syndrome. Sleep 1996; 19:S117–S122.

# PATIENT 77

## A 30-year-old man with daytime sleepiness and episodes of weakness

A 30-year-old man was evaluated for excessive daytime sleepiness of 5-year duration. There was no history of snoring or observed apnea. The patient recalled feeling weak in the knees when he laughed or was embarrassed. The patient's wife reported that sometimes he kicked the covers at night. Rarely, the patient felt he could not move for awhile as he was falling asleep at night.

***Physical Examination:*** Normal.

***Sleep Study***

| | | Sleep Stages | % SPT |
|---|---|---|---|
| Time in bed | 480 min (414–455) | | |
| Total sleep time | 350 min (400–443) | Stage Wake | 18 (0–3) |
| Sleep period time (SPT) | 425 min (405–451) | Stage 1 | 13 (2–9) |
| Sleep efficiency | .73 (.95–.99) | Stage 2 | 49 (50–64) |
| Sleep latency | 10 min (2–10 min) | Stages 3 and 4 | 5 (7–18) |
| REM latency | 2.5 min (70–100) | Stage REM | 15 (20–27) |
| Arousal index | 20/hr | | |
| AHI | 3/hr (< 5) | PLM index | 30/hr |
| | | PLM-arousal index | 15/hr |

( ) = normal values for age, PLM = periodic leg movement

***Question:*** What is the likely diagnosis?

*Diagnosis* Narcolepsy.

*Discussion:* Narcolepsy is a disorder of unknown etiology that causes excessive daytime sleepiness and usually is associated with cataplexy as well as other phenomena linked to REM sleep. A relatively young age of onset (10–30 years old) is typical; in 70–80% of cases, symptoms start before age 25. Interestingly, 5% of cases start after age 50. The history of **cataplexy** (episodes of weakness preceded by high emotion such as lauger, surprise, or embarrassment) is strong evidence for narcolepsy. This symptom is the only member of the classic tetrad of narcoleptic symptoms (sleep attacks, cataplexy, hypnogogic hallucinations, and sleep paralysis) that is pathognomonic for a narcolepsy. The entire tetrad is present in only 10–15% of patients.

**Sleep paralysis** is characterized by an inability to move while still awake at sleep onset (hypnagogic) or, less commonly, on awakening (hypnopompic). This symptom can occur in normal individuals, especially after periods of sleep deprivation. **Hypnagogic hallucinations** are vivid sensory images occurring while awake at sleep onset (hypnopompic just after awakening). **Sleep attacks** are sudden periods of irresistable daytime sleepiness. While this is a classic symptom of narcolepsy, many patients complain of sleepiness throughout the day. Sleep attacks also can be a symptom of other disorders, such as sleep apnea. Daytime naps are said to be more refreshing in narcolepsy than OSA. However, not all studies have documented this difference. The onset of sleep attacks may precede cataplexy by several years (rarely, by as many as 40 years) making the diagnosis of narcolepsy more difficult. Even when present, episodes of cataplexy may be uncommon and subtle, so that obtaining an unequivocal history of cataplexy is not a simple task.

Polysomnography usually reveals sleep fragmentation and PLM. A brief REM latency (time from sleep onset to the first REM sleep) of 10–15 minutes or less (termed sleep-onset REM), is the characteristic finding, although it is not always present (about 40–50% of the time). Again, this symptom can occur with other disorders, such as sleep apnea, depression, withdrawal of REM-suppressing medication, and prior REM deprivation of any cause. The laboratory diagnosis of narcolepsy depends on a nocturnal polysomnogram to rule out other causes of daytime sleepiness (e.g., sleep apnea, PLM in sleep) and the multiple sleep latency test (MSLT) performed on the following day. (See Patient 78 for a detailed discussion of the use of the MSLT in the diagnosis of narcolepsy.) The MSLT documents and quantifies daytime sleepiness (short sleep latency) and provides more opportunities to detect a short REM latency. In cases of unequivocal cataplexy, polysomnography and an MSLT are used to rule out other coexistent sleep disorders and provide objective confirmation of the diagnosis. However, an MSLT showing a short sleep latency but fewer than two REM periods does not rule out narcolepsy in such a situation.

In the current case, the patient noted a young age of onset and had symptoms consistent with cataplexy and sleep paralysis. The sleep study showed a short REM latency, a low sleep efficiency, reduced slow wave sleep, and PLM in sleep. PLM is not uncommon in narcoleptics and can disturb sleep enough to contribute to the symptoms of daytime sleepiness. However, PLM does not typically result in a short REM latency. In the present patient, a PLM arousal index of 20/hr, while disturbing sleep, is unlikely to be responsible for the severe symptoms. All of these findings are highly suggestive of narcolepsy.

## Clinical Pearls

1. A very short REM latency should always suggest the possibility of narcolepsy. Other conditions that can cause a short REM latency must be ruled out.

2. Cataplexy is the only pathognomonic symptom of narcolepsy. Unfortunately, sleep attacks may precede symptoms of cataplexy by several (rarely, many) years.

3. PLM in sleep can occur in patients with narcolepsy. However, the PLM syndrome usually is not associated with a short REM latency.

4. Absence of a short REM latency during a nocturnal polysomnogram does not rule out narcolepsy. An MSLT following nocturnal polysomnography should be ordered if narcolepsy is suspected.

## REFERENCES

1. Van den Hood J, Kraemer H, Guilleminault C, et al: Disorders of excessive daytime sleepiness. Sleep 1981; 4:23–38.
2. Mosko SS, Shampain DS, Sassin JF: Nocturnal REM latency and sleep disturbance in narcolepsy. Sleep 1984; 7:115–125.
3. Gelb M, Guilleminault C, Kraemer H, et al: Stability of cataplexy over several months. Sleep 1994; 17:265–273.
4. Guilleminault C: Narcolepsy syndrome. *In* Kryger MH, Roth T, Dement WC (eds): Principles and Practice of Sleep Medicine. Philadelphia, WB Saunders, 1994, pp 549–561.

# PATIENT 78

**A 23-year-old man with daytime sleepiness but no symptoms of cataplexy**

A 23-year-old man complained of severe attacks of daytime sleepiness present for at least 2 years. If the patient was able to take a nap, he usually awoke feeling refreshed. There was no history of cataplexy or hypnagogic hallucinations, and the patient denied snoring. However, he did remember a few episodes of sleep paralysis during which he was aware of having awakened but could not move for a few minutes. The patient provided a sleep log (diary) documenting at least 7 hours of sleep each night. A sleep study and multiple sleep latency test (MSLT) were ordered.

***Physical Examination:*** Normal.

***Sleep Study***

| | | Sleep Stages | % SPT |
|---|---|---|---|
| Time in bed | 440 min (430–454) | | |
| Total sleep time | 390 min (405–434) | Stage Wake | 8 (0–1) |
| Sleep period time (SPT) | 425 min (410–439) | Stage 1 | 13 (3–6) |
| Sleep efficiency | .88 (.91–.99) | Stage 2 | 49 (40–51) |
| Sleep latency | 10 min (3–26 min) | Stages 3 and 4 | 15 (16–26) |
| REM latency | 40 min (78–99) | Stage REM | 15 (22–34) |
| Arousal index | 20/hr | | |
| | | AHI | 0/hr ($<$ 5) |
| | | PLM index | 0/hr |

( ) = normal values for age, PLM = periodic leg movement

| MSLT | Sleep Latency (min) | REM Latency (min) |
|---|---|---|
| Nap 1 | 3.5 | 5 |
| Nap 2 | 2.0 | 3 |
| Nap 3 | 3.5 | None |
| Nap 4 | 1.0 | 3 |
| Nap 5 | 4.0 | None |
| mean | 2.8 (min) | 3 of 5 naps with REM |

***Question:*** What is the cause of the patient's daytime sleepiness?

***Diagnosis:*** Narcolepsy on the basis of the MSLT.

***Discussion:*** The MSLT can help support the diagnosis of narcolepsy, but the characteristic findings are neither absolutely sensitive nor specific for this disorder. The findings must be analyzed with the results of the previous nocturnal polysomnogram, the clinical history, and the patient's recent medication and sleep history in mind. The usual MSLT criteria for narcolepsy include a mean sleep latency < 5 minutes, documenting severe daytime sleepiness, and REM sleep present in two or more of five naps. However, narcoleptic subjects occasionally have REM onsets and a slightly longer mean sleep latency (5–10 minutes). Only about 60–80% of patients with classic narcolepsy (excessive daytime sleepiness plus cataplexy) have a positive MSLT on any one day. Therefore, unfortunately, a negative MSLT does not rule out the possibility of narcolepsy. In such cases, a history of unequivocal cataplexy still allows the diagnosis of narcolepsy.

In cases where the polysomnogram does not suggest another cause for daytime sleepiness, and the MSLT documents a short sleep latency but insufficient REM periods, there are three major possibilities: narcolepsy, idiopathic hypersomnolence, and upper airway resistance syndrome. This scenario assumes that insufficient sleep (during the sleep study or in the prior week) or acute withdrawal of stimulants is not responsible for the short sleep latency on the MSLT.

Conversely, a MSLT meeting criteria for narcolepsy is not specific for this diagnosis. REM onsets are seen in other sleep pathology, such as obstructive sleep apnea. This is why the preceding nocturnal polysomonography is absolutely essential to rule out sleep apnea or sleep disturbance (decreased REM sleep) that may alter the REM latency. A sleep diary should reveal if recent sleep deprivation caused a false positive MSLT. A drug history (and often a urine drug screen) helps clarify if medication or medication withdrawal altered the MSLT results. All drugs affecting sleepiness or REM sleep should be withdrawn for 2–3 weeks before testing, if possible.

In the present case, the patient reported sleep attacks and sleep paralysis, but neither of these symptoms is specific for narcolepsy. The sleep study showed a slightly shortened REM latency, but not as short as is typical in narcolepsy. Neither sleep apnea nor PLM was recorded, and the amount of sleep (and REM sleep) was adequate. Thus, the sleep study did not indicate a reason for daytime sleepiness or REM onsets. The MSLT met criteria for narcolepsy, as the patient exhibited severe sleepiness (sleep latency < 5 minutes) and three of five naps included REM sleep. The sleep log and medication history showed no reasons to suspect another cause for these findings. Thus, a diagnosis of narcolepsy was well-supported, despite an absence of cataplexy (which may not be present for several years following the onset of sleep attacks). Some have suggested that narcolepsy should be subdivided into a classic syndrome with cataplexy and a syndrome without cataplexy (excessive daytime sleepiness and positive MSLT). However, at the present time both are treated in the same manner.

## Clinical Pearls

1. MSLT testing can help support a diagnosis of narcolepsy. However, a negative test does not eliminate the possibility that narcolepsy is present.

2. A positive MSLT is not specific for narcolepsy and must be interpreted in light of information from the prior nocturnal polysomnogram, a medication history, and the recent pattern and amount of sleep.

3. The MSLT criteria for narcolepsy are a mean sleep latency < 5 minutes and REM sleep present in two or more of five naps.

REFERENCES

1. American Sleep Disorders Association: The clinical use of the multiple sleep latency test. Sleep 1992; 15:268–276.
2. Bassetti C, Aldrich MS: Narcolepsy. Neurol Clin 1996; 14:545–569.
3. Aldrich MS, Chervin RD, Malow BA: Value of the multiple sleep latency test for the diagnosis of narcolepsy. Sleep 1997; 20:620–629.

# PATIENT 79

**A 25-year-old man with narcolepsy who is still sleepy on medication**

A 25-year-old man was diagnosed with narcolepsy on the basis of symptoms of excessive daytime sleepiness and cataplexy. A polysomnogram revealed no apnea or periodic leg movement (PLM) in sleep. A multiple sleep latency test showed a mean sleep latency of 3 minutes and REM sleep in two of five naps. The patient was started on methylphenidate (Ritalin) 10 mg tid, but still had severe daytime sleepiness in the early afternoon. The patient filled out a sleep diary which showed that some nights he only slept for 6 hours due to late bedtimes. He also admitted to taking an additional pill at night to allow him to study into the late-night hours.

*Physical Examination:*   Normal.

*Question:*   What treatment would you recommend?

.

*Answer:* Longer sleep time, improved sleep hygiene, and increased medication—especially before the most sleepy periods of the day.

*Discussion:* The treatment of narcolepsy can be divided into **treatment of daytime sleepiness** and **treatment of cataplexy/hypnagogic hallucinations**. The treatment of daytime sleepiness begins with evaluation of the polysomnogram to determine if arousals from PLM or sleep apnea could be worsening daytime sleepiness. Next, sleep hygiene and the amount of sleep must be optimized. Regular bedtime and an adequate sleep period are essential. Any sleep disturbance magnifies symptoms of narcolepsy. Those patients who find a short nap restorative may benefit from regularly scheduled naps during the day.

A number of stimulant medications are available to treat the daytime sleepiness of narcolepsy, including indirect sympathomimetics, which increase the synaptic availability of norepinepherine and dopamine (see table). Adequate control of daytime sleepiness can be attained in about 60–80% of patients. **Methamphetamine, dextroamphetamine**, and **methylphenidate** appear to be the more efficacious medications. Methylphenidate is less expensive, has a shorter half-life, and is the preferred agent for moderate-to-severe narcolepsy. However, milder cases often can be treated with pemoline or mazindol, which have the advantage of not being schedule II medications.

There are several potential problems with the use of stimulant medications. First, tolerance may develop, requiring escalating doses and leading to ineffectiveness at the highest dose. In some patients effectiveness can be restored by a "drug holiday"—no medications for several days. Unfortunately, severe sleepiness may occur during that time. Second, the medications can increase blood pressure, although this effect is not usual in normotensive patients. Third, side effects of stimulants include nervousness, irritability, headache, and insomnia. Thus, *they should not be taken near bedtime*, especially methamphetamine and dextroamphetamine, both of which have a relatively long half-life. Fourth, attacks of paranoia or hallucinations have been reported with amphetamines, but major psychiatric side effects are rare in the absence of underlying psychiatric disorders. In addition, pemoline has been reported to cause hepatotoxicity.

The peak action of dextroamphetamine, methamphetamine, and methylphenidate is 1–3 hours from ingestion, so the medications should be taken at least 1 hour before the time of desired effectiveness. If a sleep attack has begun before medication is taken, then a nap may be the best treatment in some patients.

**Modafinil**, a new treatment for narcolepsy, is not yet available in the United States. It differs from the other agents in that it is an alpha-1 agonist with relatively few side effects (headache, dry mouth), and it has a low potential for substance abuse. Unlike the indirect sympathomimetics, withdrawal of modafinil does not result in a rebound of REM and slow wave sleep. The usual dose is 50 mg bid (maximum of 400 mg daily).

In the present case, the dose of methylphenidate was changed to 10 mg every morning, 20 mg before lunch, and 10 mg at 4 PM, with improvement in early afternoon symptoms. As an alternative, on nonworking days the patient was encouraged to take an early-afternoon nap. He also was encouraged to get 7–8 hours of sleep each night and to avoid any stimulant medication after supper.

# Clinical Pearls

1. With proper dose titration, stimulant medication can control symptoms of daytime sleepiness in 60–80% of narcoleptic patients.

2. Good sleep hygiene, regular sleep habits, and scheduled naps also can help control symptoms of sleepiness.

3. It is essential to plan dosing according to the time profile of symptoms and to avoid medication-induced insomnia or sleep disturbance.

4. If patients fail to respond to treatment, the coexistence of other sleep disorders such as PLM or obstructive sleep apnea should be suspected.

## Stimulant Medications

| Drug | Brand Name | Dose | Maximum Dose (daily) | Half-Life | Selected Side-Effects |
|------|-----------|------|----------------------|-----------|----------------------|
| Pemoline | Cylert | 18.75–37.5 mg qd (18.75, 37.5 mg tabs) | 150 mg | 12 hrs (adults) | Hepatitis |
| Mazindol | Mazanor Sanorex | 1–2 mg bid (1, 2 mg tabs) | 8 mg | 8–15 hrs | Gastrointestinal disorders |
| Methylphenidate* | Ritalin | 5–10 mg bid or tid (5, 10, 20 mg tabs) | 100 mg | 2–4 hrs | Nervousness, tremulousness, headache |
| Dextroamphetamine* | Dexedrine Dextrostat and others | 5 mg qd to bid (5, 10 mg tabs) | 60 mg | 10–30 hrs | Nervousness, tremulousness, headache |
| Methamphetamine* | Desoxyn | 5 mg qd (5, 10 mg tabs) | 60 mg | 12–34 hrs | Nervousness, tremulousness, headache |

* = schedule II medication

## REFERENCES

1. Billiard M, Besset A, Montplaisir J, et al: Modafinil: A double-blind multicentric study. Sleep 1994; 17(8 Suppl):S107–S112.
2. Mitler M, Aldrich MS, Koob GF, et al: ASDA standards of practice: Narcolepsy and its treatment with stimulants. Sleep 1994; 17:352–371.
3. Bassetti C, Aldrich MS: Narcolepsy.  Neurol Clin 1996; 14:545–569.
4. U.S. Modafinil in  Narcolepsy Study Group: Randomized trial of modafinil for the treatment of pathological somnolence in narcolepsy. Ann Neurol 1998; 43:88–97.

# PATIENT 80

## A 25-year-old man with frequent episodes of cataplexy

A 25-year-old man who was diagnosed with narcolepsy experienced almost daily episodes of cataplexy that commonly were associated with laughter or surprise. At these times, the patient felt weakness in his legs; a few times he almost fell to the ground. The episodes varied in frequency, but were increased after periods of irregular sleep.

In addition to cataplexy, the patient also was troubled with hypnagogic hallucinations, which consisted of seeing a stranger in the room as he was falling asleep. While he realized the imagery was not real, the patient sometimes felt quite anxious about the episodes.

He was treated with protriptyline and later imipramine (two tricyclic antidepressants), with decreases in the frequency of the episodes of cataplexy and hypnagogic hallucinations. However, at doses that controlled his cataplexy, he found both medications intolerable secondary to side effects (especially dry mouth). When he abruptly stopped the medicines, he noted a significant increase in the episodes of cataplexy.

***Physical Examination:*** Normal.

***Question:*** What treatment would you recommend?

*Answer:*    A trial of fluoxetine.

*Discussion:*    Cataplexy is the only manifestation of narcolepsy that is virtually pathognomonic for this disorder. This symptom is characterized by sudden bilateral loss of muscle tone at moments of emotion (e.g., surprise, laughter, anger, embarrassment). The severity varies from minor facial drooping with eye closure, slurred speech, and a sagging jaw to loss of postural muscle tone and falling. The loss of muscle tone is not always instantaneous; it may progress over a few minutes. Duration of a cataplectic episode usually is about 1 minute, but it can last up to 20 minutes in the rare patient.

During cataplexy, consciousness is preserved. However, the patient can enter a period of sleep and dream during the attacks or can have hallucinations. The frequency of cataplectic episodes varies widely between patients with narcolepsy. In general, patients with the most severe cataplectic episodes tend to have them frequently, and they are very disturbing. In some patients, cataplexy is infrequent and requires no treatment. Cataplexy typically is treated more successfully than daytime sleepiness.

Hypnagogic hallucinations are images occurring while the patient is still awake at sleep onset or on awakening (hypnopompic). They usually are visual, but may include or feature exclusively other senses, such as smell and hearing. Images may be simple or complex and bizarre. Patients typically know the hallucinations are not real, but are still quite frightened. The most common hypnagogic hallucination is a stranger or animal in the room.

The usual treatment for cataplexy is low doses of tricyclic antidepressants. **Protriptyline** (5–30 mg daily) is a nonsedative medication, but it is commonly associated with anticholinergic side effects. Urinary retention is a typical side effect in older patients. **Imipramine** (Tofranil) is another commonly used medication (25–200 mg daily) Successful treatment also has been reported with **fluoxetine** (Prozac), a selective serotonin reuptake inhibitor (20–80 mg daily). However, fluoxetine can cause sleep disturbance, thereby worsening daytime sleepiness. All of these medications tend to suppress REM sleep. Recently, **carbamazepine** (Tegretol) was reported to decrease cataplexy in a patient who did not respond to the traditional medications. In that study, a dose of 200 mg twice daily was effective.

Abrupt withdrawal of medications used to treat cataplexy can result in an exacerbation of this symptom. A form of continuous cataplectic attacks (status cataplecticus) has been reported after abrupt cessation of treatment. The use of alpha-1 adrenergic blockers (e.g., prazosin) also has been reported to worsen cataplexy. Therefore, these medications should be avoided in patients with narcolepsy. The medications used to treat cataplexy also suppress hypnagogic hallucinations and sleep paralysis; however, treatment of these two symptoms usually is not required.

In the current patient, treatment was begun with fluoxetine 20 mg daily. On this medication the frequency of cataplexy was significantly reduced. The patient tolerated the medication well and was satisfied with the treatment.

# Clinical Pearls

1. Specific treatment for cataplexy may not be required in all patients with narcolepsy.

2. An increase in the frequency of cataplectic episodes can occur after withdrawal of medications treating this symptom or after initiation of treatment of other disorders with alpha-1 adrenergic receptor antagonists (e.g., prazosin).

3. While the traditional treatment of cataplexy has been tricyclic antidepressants, fluoxetine (a selective serotonin reuptake inhibitor) also has proven effective.

4. Carbamazepine can be efficacious when cataplexy does not respond to more conventional treatments.

## REFERENCES
1. Aldrich M, Rogers AE: Exacerbation of human cataplexy by prazosin. Sleep 1989; 12:254–256.
2. Frey J, Darbonne C: Fluoxetine suppresses human cataplexy. Neurology 1994; 44:707–709.
3. Guilleminault C, Gelb M: Clinical aspects and features of cataplexy. Adv Neurol 1995; 67:65–77.
4. Vaughn BV, D'Cruz OF: Carbamazepine as a treatment for cataplexy. Sleep 1996; 19:101–103.

# PATIENT 81

## A 35-year-old man with sleep apnea and a short REM latency

A 35-year-old man complained of severe sleepiness of 5-year duration. His wife reported that he snored heavily and had severe attacks of sleepiness in social situations and even at meals. However, she was unable to comment on the existence of periods of apnea because she slept in a separate bedroom. The patient had recently been fired for falling asleep on the job. He denied sleep paralysis but reported feeling "funny" when angry. The sensation was more like being dizzy than weak. A multiple sleep latency test (MSLT) performed without nocturnal polysomnography at another hospital showed a mean sleep latency of 4 minutes (severe sleepiness) and two of five naps with REM sleep. The patient was diagnosed with narcolepsy, but treatment with stimulants was ineffective.

### Sleep Study

| | | Sleep Stages | % SPT |
|---|---|---|---|
| Time in bed | 480 min (414–455) | | |
| Total sleep time | 350 min (400–443) | Stage Wake | 18 (0–3) |
| Sleep period time | 425 min (405–451) | Stage 1 | 13 (2–9) |
| Sleep latency | 10 min (2–20 min) | Stage 2 | 49 (50–64) |
| REM latency | 5 min (70–100) | Stages 3 and 4 | 5 (7–18) |
| Arousal index | 65/hr | Stage REM | 10 (20–27) |
| | | AHI | 80/hr (< 5) |
| | | PLM index | 0/hr |

( )= normal values for age, PLM = periodic leg movement

*Questions:*   What is your diagnosis? Should another MSLT be performed immediately?

***Diagnosis:*** Obstructive sleep apnea. An MSLT would not be useful until after the sleep apnea is adequately treated.

***Discussion:*** Obstructive sleep apnea (OSA) can be associated with both a short sleep latency and two or more REM periods. Thus, these MSLT findings cannot be used to support a diagnosis of narcolepsy in patients with significant sleep apnea. The usual approach is to *first treat the sleep apnea* and then repeat the MSLT if clinically indicated.

For example, treatment is begun with nasal CPAP. If daytime sleepiness completely resolves, then narcolepsy probably is not present. If some degree of sleepiness persists or there is a history of **cataplexy**, then further evaluation is indicated. After several weeks of treatment, another sleep study (on nasal CPAP) confirms adequate treatment and REM sleep, and a subsequent MSLT (also on CPAP) determines the severity of residual sleepiness as well as the presence of REM periods. A diagnosis of narcolepsy is supported when there is evidence of persistent, **severe sleepiness** (sleep latency < 5 minutes) and two of five naps with REM sleep—assuming that the nocturnal sleep study showed reasonable sleep quality (and no evidence of REM or slow wave sleep rebound). No further evaluation is needed when the MSLT is normal. However, if the MSLT shows **significant sleepiness** (sleep latency < 10 minutes) and no REM periods, then several possibilities must be considered, including: poor compliance with nasal CPAP, inadequate CPAP pressure, idiopathic hypersomnia, periodic leg movements, insufficient sleep, and narcolepsy. Remember, failure on an MSLT to show two or more REM periods in five naps does not rule out narcolepsy. When cataplexy is present, narcolepsy is likely.

In the present patient, the polysomnogram revealed severe OSA and sleep fragmentation (high arousal index) with reduced amounts of slow wave and REM sleep. In addition, the REM latency was very short. These findings suggested narcolepsy. While there was no history of unequivocal cataplexy, daytime sleepiness can be present for several years before the onset of cataplexy. The patient underwent a nasal CPAP titration, and on 12 cm $H_2O$ the AHI was reduced to 5/hr. A large rebound in slow wave and REM sleep was noted. Treatment was begun with nasal CPAP, resulting in a complete resolution of symptoms: this fact alone made narcolepsy unlikely. However, because of the past diagnosis and the equivocal history of cataplexy, a repeat sleep study and MSLT (both on CPAP) were performed several weeks later. The nocturnal study showed a normal REM latency and adequate treatment of OSA. The MSLT showed a sleep latency of 12 minutes and an absence of REM sleep. These findings demonstrated that coexistent narcolepsy was unlikely.

# Clinical Pearls

1. When significant sleep apnea is present on a nocturnal sleep study, testing for narcolepsy (MSLT) should be delayed until after the sleep apnea is adequately treated.

2. REM deprivation associated with OSA can result in both a short nocturnal REM latency and two REM periods during MSLT testing.

3. A nocturnal study documenting effective treatment of OSA (and a normal amount of REM sleep) coupled with a subsequent MSLT (on treatment) satisfying the diagnostic criteria for narcolepsy supports this additional diagnosis in a patient with OSA.

4. An MSLT without preceding nocturnal polysomnography can be misleading and is rarely indicated.

## REFERENCES

1. Walsh JK, Smitson SS, Kramer M: Sleep-onset REM sleep: Comparison of narcoleptic and sleep apnea patients. Clin Electroencephalogr 1982; 13:57–60.
2. American Sleep Disorders Association: The clinical use of the multiple sleep latency test. Sleep 1992; 15:268–276.

# PATIENT 82

## A 40-year-old man with sleep apnea and persistent daytime sleepiness

A 40-year-old African-American man with excessive daytime sleepiness since age 20 was diagnosed as having obstructive sleep apnea (AHI 80/hr) at another hospital. Nasal CPAP at 12 cm $H_2O$ reduced the AHI to 3/hr. The patient was started on treatment, and he noted some improvement in his symptoms. However, significant daytime sleepiness persisted despite using CPAP for at least 6 hours a night. There was no history of cataplexy or sleep paralysis. Narcolepsy was considered but the patient was HLA-DR15 (a subtype of HLA-DR2) negative. He was referred for another opinion.

*Physical Examination:*  HEENT: dependent palate. Neck: 17-inch circumference. Chest: clear. Cardiac: normal. Extremities: no edema.

*Sleep Study*   (on nasal CPAP 12 cm $H_2O$)

| | | Sleep Stages | % SPT |
|---|---|---|---|
| Time in bed | 450 min (390–468) | | |
| Total sleep time | 395.5 min (343–436) | Stage Awake | 8 (1–12) |
| Sleep period time (SPT) | 430 min (378–452 | Stage 1 | 10 (5–11) |
| WASO | 34.5 min | Stage 2 | 52 (44–66) |
| Sleep efficiency | .88 (.85–.97) | Stages 3 and 4 | 10 (2–15) |
| Sleep latency | 10 min (2–18) | Stage REM | 20 (19–27) |
| REM latency | 15 min (55–78) | | |
| | | AHI (< 5/hr) | 3/hr |
| | | PLM index | 10/hr |

( ) = normal values for age, AHI = apnea + hypopnea index, PLM = periodic limb movement

*MSLT:*   On nasal CPAP 12 cm $H_2O$: mean sleep latency 4 minutes; three of five naps with REM sleep.

*Question:*   What is causing the persistent sleepiness?

***Diagnosis:*** Narcolepsy.

***Discussion:*** A combination of narcolepsy and obstructive sleep apnea (OSA) is not uncommon. Adequate treatment of both disorders is required for control of daytime sleepiness. If cataplexy is *unequivocal*, a diagnosis of narcolepsy can be made in patients with OSA on clinical grounds. However, cataplexy makes a delayed appearance in many patients with narcolepsy—sometimes years after sleep attacks begin. The MSLT is used to support the diagnosis of narcolepsy in these patients with OSA and suspected narcolepsy without cataplexy.

The first step in all of these cases is successful **treatment of the OSA**. Then a repeat sleep study (on treatment) is followed by an MSLT (also on treatment). The sleep study documents adequate treatment (and adequate sleep) and the MSLT provides objective evidence of continued daytime sleepiness (sleep latency < 5 min) and the presence of two or more REM periods. The differential of a patient with OSA still sleepy on CPAP includes: poor compliance, inadequate CPAP pressure, narcolepsy, periodic limb movements in sleep, idiopathic hypersomnia, insufficient sleep, and depression.

**HLA haplotyping** has been used in evaluation of suspected narcolepsy since early studies showed that most Caucasian patients with narcolepsy (with cataplexy) were HLA-DR2 positive. Obviously, many patients without narcolepsy are HLA-DR2 positive, so the main utility of haplotyping is excluding the diagnosis in HLA-DR2 negative patients. Subsequent studies have found that DR15 (a subtype of HLA-DR2) and DQ6 (a subtype of HLA-DQ1) are present in 95–100% of Caucasian and Japanese patients with narcolepsy, and DQ6 also is present in 95% of narcoleptic African-American patients. However, 40% of the latter are DR15 negative. Therefore, **DQ6** appears to be the best marker across all races, but the utility of genetic testing is limited by the fact that 1–5% of all patients with narcolepsy are negative for both DR2 and DQ6. Patients with narcolepsy without cataplexy are more likely to be DQ6 negative. Of note, there appear to be factors other than genetic that determine the appearance of the syndrome. Cases of monozygotic twins have been reported where only one twin developed narcolepsy.

In the present patient, a negative DR15 test did not rule out narcolepsy—the patient was, in fact, DQ6 positive. The early age of onset of symptoms was consistent with narcolepsy. The sleep study on CPAP showed excellent treatment of his sleep apnea and sleep of fairly good quality (no evidence of REM rebound). The MSLT documented both severe daytime sleepiness and REM periods in three of five naps. The absence of other reasons to explain these MSLT findings makes narcolepsy highly likely. The patient was treated with methylphenidate 10 mg tid, with improvement in his symptoms of daytime sleepiness.

# Clinical Pearls

1. While most narcolepsy patients are DQ6 positive (all races), a negative result does not rule out narcolepsy.

2. When daytime sleepiness persists on nasal CPAP, consider the possibility of other sleep disorders as well as poor compliance or inadequate pressure.

3. An MSLT can provide objective evidence of persistent sleepiness on nasal CPAP and help support a diagnosis of narcolepsy.

REFERENCES
1. Mignot E, Lin X, Arrigoni J, et al: DQB1*0602 and DQA1*0101 are better markers than DR2 for narcolepsy in Caucasians and African-Americans. Sleep 1994; 17:60–67.
2. Bassetti C, Aldrich MS: Narcolepsy. Neurol Clin, 1996; 14:545–569.

# PATIENT 83

## A 65-year-old woman with excessive daytime sleepiness and a short REM latency

A 65-year-old woman complained of fatigue and sleepiness of 8-month duration. There was no history of snoring. The patient lived by herself; her husband had died 5 years previously. She denied feeling depressed. Her only medication was clonidine for hypertension (started about 8 months previously). Her normal bedtime was 9 PM and normal waketime was 5 AM. There was no history of head trauma or cataplexy (loss of muscle tone during periods of high emotion).

The patient reported to the sleep technician that her primary care physician had switched her from clonidine to another medicine a few days prior to her sleep test appointment, and she "already felt much less sleepy."

***Physical Examination:***   Normal for age.

***Sleep Study:***   (Lights out 11 PM, Lights on 6:30 AM)

| | | Sleep Stages | % SPT |
|---|---|---|---|
| Time in bed (TIB) | 450 min (420–511) | | |
| Total sleep time (TST) | 360 min (349–446) | Stage Wake | 10 (0–17) |
| Sleep period time (SPT) | 400 min (397–492) | Stage 1 | 13 (4–12) |
| Sleep latency | 5 min (3–30 min) | Stage 2 | 54 (46–63) |
| REM latency | 40 min (69–111) | Stages 3 and 4 | 5 (0–14) |
| Sleep efficiency | .80 (.78–.96) | Stage REM | 18 (17–25) |
| Arousal index | 15/hr | | |
| | | AHI | 0/hr (< 5) |
| | | PLM index | 0/hr |

( ) = normal values for age

***Question:***   Why is the REM latency decreased?

*Answer:* Short nocturnal REM latency secondary to delay of bedtime or withdrawal of clonidine.

*Discussion:* The normal REM latency (time from the beginning of sleep onset until the beginning of REM sleep) normally is around 70–120 minutes and may decrease slightly with **age**. Both sleep and nonsleep factors are influential. REM sleep normally follows NREM sleep. REM propensity tracks the circadian nadir in body temperature. A short nocturnal REM latency is seen in several conditions, including narcolepsy (usually $< 20$ minutes), depression (usually 20–50 minutes), obstructive sleep apnea, withdrawal from REM-suppressing medication, and REM deprivation or fragmentation from any cause. Rarely, circadian factors (e.g., later than normal bedtime) can abbreviate REM latency. A very short REM latency (10–15 minutes), known as sleep-onset REM, is most characteristic of narcolepsy.

In the present case, the sleep study results are fairly normal except for the low sleep efficiency and the modestly shortened REM latency. The time from lights out to final awakening (sleep latency + SPT) was 405 minutes, and the patient was awake for the remaining 45 minutes of the monitoring period. Thus, the sleep efficiency (TST *100 / TIB) is low due to the early final awakening. The patient's **usual waketime** is 5 AM, which partly accounts for the early awakening.

There are many causes of a short REM latency that are associated with daytime sleepiness. While the nocturnal REM latency in narcolepsy usually is $< 20$ minutes, mildly decreased or normal values also can occur in this disorder. However, the late age of onset in this patient makes narcolepsy unlikely. The nocturnal sleep study showed no sleep apnea. Early-morning awakening and a modestly shortened REM latency are seen with depression. However, many older patients have early bedtimes and awakening times; they are "phase-advanced" relative to typical societal habits. In addition, the improvement in sleepiness after discontinuing the clonidine makes depression unlikely. Note that the lights out time of the sleep study was much later than the patient's **normal bedtime**—it was even later than her normal REM onset time of around 10:30 PM. By delaying sleep onset until 11 PM, the likelihood of a short REM latency was increased.

Another possible cause of the short REM latency is **withdrawal of clonidine**. This medication can cause daytime sleepiness and tends to increase the REM latency. Clonidine withdrawal has not been reported to definitely shorten the REM latency, but it is a possibility.

When seen in clinic to discuss the sleep study results, the present patient declared herself "cured and back to her old self." No further sleep studies or evaluations were ordered.

# Clinical Pearls

1. To avoid possible circadian effects on the REM and sleep latency, bedtime in the sleep lab should mimic the patient's normal schedule.

2. Medications always should be considered in evaluating daytime sleepiness, especially in older patients.

3. Clonidine, an antihypertensive, has been associated with daytime somnolence.

## REFERENCES

1. Czeisler CA, Zimmerman JC, Rhonda JM, et al: Timing of REM sleep is coupled to the circadian rhythm of body temperature in man. Sleep 1980; 2:329–346.
2. Nicholson AN, Pascoe PA: Presynaptic alpha-2-adrenoreceptor function and sleep in man: Studies with clonidine and diazoxan. Neuropharmacology 1991; 30:367–372.
3. American Sleep Disorders Association: The clinical use of the multiple sleep latency test. Sleep 1992; 15:268–276.

# PATIENT 84

## A 35-year-old man requesting stimulant medication

A 35-year-old man was evaluated for complaints of excessive daytime sleepiness of 6-year duration. He had been diagnosed with idiopathic hypersomnia by another physician and had been receiving stimulant medications for more than 2 years. After having recently moved, he sought medical attention for medication refills. For the previous 2 months he had not taken stimulant medications, and at work he drank large amounts of coffee to combat sleepiness. His usual bedtime was 11:00 PM, and he awoke at 4:30 AM by alarm. The early awake time was necessary because of a lengthy commute to work. On the weekends, he slept to 9:00 AM and felt somewhat less sleepy.

The patient denied a history of cataplexy, hypnagogic hallucinations, sleep paralysis, head trauma, or depression. There was no history of snoring. His previous evaluations included a normal nocturnal polysomnogram, and an MSLT showed a short sleep latency (8 minutes) with no episodes of REM sleep. The patient was asked to keep a sleep log and to obtain at least 7 hours of sleep nightly before a repeat polysomnogram and MSLT.

***Physical Examination:*** Normal.
***Laboratory Findings:*** Normal thyroid function.
***Sleep Study***

| Time in bed | 440 min (414–455) | | Sleep Stages | % SPT |
|---|---|---|---|---|
| Total sleep time | 417 min (400–443) | | Stage Wake | 3 (0–3) |
| Sleep period time (SPT) | 430 min (405–451) | | Stage 1 | 13 (2–9) |
| Sleep efficiency | .95 (.95–.99) | | Stage 2 | 49 (50–64) |
| Sleep latency | 10 min (2–10 min) | | Stages 3 and 4 | 15 (7–18) |
| REM latency | 110 min (70–100) | | Stage REM | 20 (20–27) |
| Arousal index | 10/hr | | | |
| AHI | 2/hr (< 5) | | PLM index | 0/hr |
| | | | PLM-arousal index | 0/hr |

AHI = apnea + hypopnea index, PLM = periodic leg movement, ( ) = normal values for age

***MSLT:*** Mean sleep latency 13 minutes, no REM periods in five naps.

***Question:*** What is your diagnosis?

***Diagnosis:*** Insufficient sleep syndrome.

***Discussion:*** In the insufficient sleep syndrome, an inadequate amount of time is allotted for sleep by the patient due to personal or societal (work) schedules. The amount of sleep required for normal function varies considerably between individuals, with a population mean around 7.5 hours. This sleep need is genetically determined. When less sleep is obtained, a sleep debt accumulates. Commonly, such patients sleep considerably more on weekends. A study of patients with the insufficient sleep syndrome found that this disparity between the amount of sleep obtained on weekday nights and on weekends was an important clinical clue. These patients had normal-to-high sleep efficiencies during nocturnal sleep testing, with greater total sleep times than reported for a typical night, and they showed moderate reductions in sleep latency without REM periods on MSLT.

One study in normal subjects found that a reduction of the time in bed from 8 to 6 hours reduced the mean sleep latency from approximately 12.5 to 8.5 minutes. Thus, a mild reduction in nocturnal sleep can increase daytime sleepiness, although usually not to a severe degree (i.e., sleep latency < 5 minutes). Remember, though, that any reduction in nocturnal sleep magnifies the sleepiness associated with other sleep disorders, such as narcolepsy or sleep apnea.

The present patient's normal duration of sleep was, at most, 5.5 hours. Thus, the possibility of insufficient sleep was considered. This short sleep time would make interpretation of an MSLT difficult, which is why the patient was asked to sleep for at least 7 hours and keep a sleep log prior to testing. The nocturnal polysomnogram documented fairly normal sleep. The MSLT revealed a sleep latency in the "grey" zone: traditionally, a sleep latency > 15 minutes is considered normal, < 10 minutes abnormal, and 10–15 minutes could be either (mild sleepiness). Certainly a sleep latency of 13 minutes is inconsistent with the severe symptoms reported by this patient.

When confronted with the results of his testing, the patient admitted that he thinks "sleep is a waste of time" and that he always tries to function on as little sleep as possible. Although he could not remember his sleep habits before the previous sleep testing, he believed he had allotted the usual short amount of time. While not entirely happy with the decision not to prescribe stimulants, the patient did understand that the test proved he would be less sleepy during the day if he had more nocturnal sleep.

# Clinical Pearls

1. Proper interpretation of the MSLT depends on the patient having an adequate amount of sleep (ideally 7–7.5 hours a night) for at least one week before testing.

2. An accurate sleep log is an essential part of the evaluation of daytime sleepiness. It also is helpful in interpreting the results of both the nocturnal sleep study and the MSLT.

3. A modest shortening of nocturnal sleep (to about 6 hours) can shorten the mean sleep latency on the MSLT to < 10 minutes.

4. The insufficient sleep syndrome should be considered in the differential of excessive daytime sleepiness.

## REFERENCES

1. Roehrs T, Zorick F. Sicklesteel J, et al: Excessive daytime sleepiness associated with insufficient sleep. Sleep 1983; 6:319–325.
2. American Sleep Disorders Association: The clinical use of the multiple sleep latency test. Sleep 1992; 15:268–276.
3. Rosenthal L, Roehrs TA, Rosen A, et al: Level of sleepiness and total sleep time following various time in bed conditions. Sleep 1993; 16:226–232.
4. Aldrich MS: The clinical spectrum of narcolepsy and idiopathic hypersomnia. Neurology 1996; 46:383–401.

# PATIENT 85

## A 64-year-old man with daytime sleepiness since age 21

A 64-year-old man was evaluated for the complaint of excessive daytime sleepiness present since age 21. He sometimes fell asleep while driving and in social situations. He denied a history of cataplexy, sleep paralysis, or hypnagogic hallucinations. There was a history of mild snoring. The patient retired nightly around 9:30 PM and reported falling asleep in less than 30 minutes. He usually arose at 6:30 AM (awakened by alarm clock). The patient commonly slept for up to 9 hours on the weekend, with no reduction in his symptoms of sleepiness. There was no history of head trauma nor symptoms to suggest depression.

*Physical Examination:* Vital signs: normal. General: thin, in no distress. HEENT: normal. Chest: clear to auscultation and percussion. Cardiac: normal. Abdomen: normal. Extremities: normal. Neurologic: normal.

### Sleep Study

| | | Sleep Stages | % SPT |
|---|---|---|---|
| Time in bed | 435 min (414–489) | | |
| Total sleep time | 360 min (363–452) | Stage Wake | 12 (2–14) |
| Sleep period time (SPT) | 410 min (404–479) | Stage 1 | 14 (6–14) |
| Sleep efficiency | .83 (.83–.97) | Stage 2 | 49 (48–66) |
| Sleep latency | 4.5 min (1–15 min) | Stages 3 and 4 | 7 (0–8) |
| REM latency | 177 min (65–103) | Stage REM | 18 (20–27) |
| Arousal index | 10/hr | | |
| | | AHI | 0/hr (< 5) |
| | | PLM index | 0/hr |

( ) = normal values for age, AHI = apnea + hypopnea index, PLM = periodic leg movement

*MSLT:* Mean sleep latency 4.8 minutes, no REM sleep in five naps.

*Question:* What is the most likely cause of the patient's daytime sleepiness?

*Diagnosis:*   Idiopathic hypersomnia.

*Discussion:*   The diagnosis of idiopathic hypersomnia (IHS) is made by documenting excessive daytime sleepiness despite adequate sleep and excluding other disorders that cause daytime sleepiness, such as narcolepsy. Patients with IHS may complain of persistent daytime drowsiness or discrete sleep attacks. IHS, like narcolepsy, usually begins in adolescence or the early twenties. The syndrome accounts for 5–10% of patients seen in sleep clinics with complaints of excessive daytime sleepiness. The sleep period may be long (> 8 hours). Some patients are able to wake normally; others report difficulty waking and/or disorientation at awakening ("sleep drunkenness"). Unlike narcolepsy, naps are not refreshing. A minority of patients have associated symptoms suggesting problems with the autonomic nervous system, including headache, syncope, orthostatic hypotension, and peripheral vascular complaints (Raynaud-type symptoms).

The polysomnography of IHS patients shows a **normal or increased quantity of sleep**. Sleep quality usually is normal, and the amount of slow wave sleep may be increased. The REM latency is not decreased. The sleep latency usually is < 10 minutes. In contrast, the sleep of narcoleptics typically is shortened or fragmented, and the REM latency may be very short (< 20 minutes). The multiple sleep latency test (MSLT) in patients with IHS documents excessive daytime sleepiness (sleep latency < 10 minutes) while showing no REM sleep episode (rarely, one) in five naps. Some have suggested that 24-hour sleep recording may be useful in patients with IHS. Common results are long nocturnal sleep and long daytime naps, with 10–12 hrs of total sleep. Some patients with IHS report hypnagogic hallucinations and sleep paralysis. Thus, eliciting such symptoms does not necessarily differentiate IHS from narcolepsy.

Before the diagnosis of IHS can be made with confidence, medical and psychiatric causes of excessive sleepiness should be excluded. **Chronic low-grade depression** may be difficult to eliminate as a possibility. A moderately reduced nocturnal REM latency (< 60 minutes) might be a clue that depression is present. Sleepiness also can be a symptom of progressive **hydrocephalus**. Recent onset, worsening of symptoms, or impairment of cognitive functioning suggests a need for neurologic evaluation and computed axial tomography or other studies to rule out this possibility. **Posttraumatic hypersomnia** is a syndrome in which symptoms and findings of hypersomnia develop 6–18 months after head trauma. **Sedative/hypnotic abuse** is another possible cause of daytime sleepiness. Urine or blood tests can screen for use of these agents. The insufficient sleep syndrome and the upper airway resistance syndrome also should be excluded.

The treatment of patients with IHS involves the same stimulant medications as used in narcolepsy, but patients with IHS do not always respond. Patients also are instructed to avoid reductions in sleep time or irregular sleep/wake schedules.

The present patient snored lightly but aroused rarely, making the upper airway resistance syndrome unlikely. There was no history of depression or head trauma. The MSLT documented severe sleepiness (sleep latency < 5 min) despite fairly normal sleep. The MSLT was not consistent with narcolepsy, and there was no history of cataplexy. However, neither of these facts absolutely excludes narcolepsy. Therefore, the diagnosis of IHS always is made with some uncertainty.

## Clinical Pearls

1. The diagnosis of idiopathic hypersomnia depends on exclusion of other disorders causing excessive daytime sleepiness, including sleep apnea (and the upper airway resistance syndrome), period limb movements in sleep, narcolepsy, affective disorders, stimulant withdrawal, and insufficient sleep.

2. History of recent head trauma suggests the posttraumatic hypersomnia syndrome.

3. When polysomnography fails to explain the recent onset of hypersomnia in an older patient, exclude neurologic disease (e.g., brain tumors, hydrocephalus), medical illness, medication side effects, and depression.

## REFERENCES

1. Guilleminault C, van den Hoed J, Miles L: Posttraumatic excessive daytime sleepiness. Neurology 1983; 33:1584–1589.
2. Baker TL, Guilleminault C, Nino-Murcia G, Dement WC: Comparative polysomnographic study of narcolepsy and idiopathic central nervous system hypersomnia. Sleep 1986; 9:232–242, 1986.
3. Aldrich MS: The clinical spectrum of narcolepsy and idiopathic hypersomnia. Neurology 1996; 46:383–401.
4. Billiard M: Idiopathic hypersomnia. Neurol Clin 1996; 14:573–582.

# PATIENT 86

## A 55-year-old man with violent dreams

A 55-year-old man complained of violent movements during sleep, present for the previous 14 months. The movements tended to occur during the last half of the night and varied from simply moving his arms to hitting his wife. On some occasions, the patient got up from the bed. When awakened he was not confused, but only rarely remembered dream content. During some of the episodes, the patient also screamed or talked about harming someone. The episodes seemed to be worse after periods of interrupted sleep or a change in sleep schedule. There was no history of head trauma or change in intellectual functioning, motor strength, sensation, or coordination. There was no history of sleepwalking (somnambulism) during childhood.

***Physical Examination:*** Normal.
***Sleep Study:*** Normal.

***Question:*** What diagnosis most likely explains the patient's problem?

*Diagnosis:* Rapid eye movement behavior disorder.

*Discussion:* The REM behavior disorder (RBD) is characterized by a **loss of the normal muscle hypotonia** associated with REM sleep; thus, dreams can be "acted out." Limb and body movements often are violent (e.g., hitting a wall, kicking) and may be associated with emotionally charged utterances. The movements can be related to dream content ("kicking an attacker"), but the patient may not remember associated dream material when awakened during an episode. *Serious injury to the patient or the bed partner can result* from these episodes, which typically occur one to four times a week. The median age of onset is about 50 years, and a milder prodrome of sleeptalking, simple limb-jerking, or vividly violent dreams may precede the full blown syndrome. Because the episodes occur during REM sleep, they are most common during the early morning hours (the second half of the night).

The differential diagnosis of abnormal movement and behavior arising from sleep includes sleep-related seizure activity, periodic limb movements in sleep, sleepwalking, night terrors, nocturnal panic attacks, nightmares, and the posttraumatic stress disorder. In contrast to RBD, sleepwalking (and variants) classically occurs during slow wave sleep (stages 3 and 4) and, hence, is most common in the early portion of the night. Unlike RBD, most adults with sleepwalking had episodes during childhood. When patients are awakened during sleepwalking or night terror episodes, they are quite confused and tend to have no memory of dream content. If content is remembered, usually it is not as complex as a typical dream. However, note that recent studies of sleepwalking and night terrors in adults have shown that episodes can begin in stage 2 sleep and during the second part of the night.

The separation between sleepwalking/night terrors and RBD is not absolute—some patients have violent behavioral episodes occurring in both NREM and REM sleep (mixed disorder). However, while both nightmares and the posttraumatic stress syndrome can be associated with violent or terrifying dream content and arousal from sleep, complex body movements are uncommon. Additionally, nocturnal seizure activity usually occurs in NREM sleep, and behaviors typically are more stereotyped and less complex than in RBD. A few patients with abnormal EEG activity and complex and violent behavior have been described. These patients responded to antiseizure medication.

In animal experiments, lesions in the pons can result in body movements during REM sleep. Thus, degeneration of the brain stem is believed to be one possible cause of RBD in humans. However, even with extensive evaluation, about 60% of cases are idiopathic. Others are associated with multiple sclerosis, subarachnoid hemorrhage, dementia, ischemic cerebrovascular disease, and brain stem neoplasm. In one study, almost 40% of patients with idiopathic RBD later developed Parkinson's syndrome. An acute form of RBD can occur after withdrawal from REM suppressants, such as ethanol. Drug-induced cases also have been reported, with the use of tricyclic antidepressants or selective serotonin reuptake inhibitors (e.g., fluoxetine).

Polysomnography may or may not reveal an episode, as most patients do not have nightly attacks. Some sleep centers routinely perform at least three serial sleep studies. Simultaneous video and sleep recording (including both leg and arm EMG) is recommended. An episode is evidenced by bursts of limb movement or persistent augmented muscle tone during REM sleep. At first glance the episode may appear as stage Wake (eye movements and elevated chin EMG). Clues to the fact that abnormal REM sleep is present include phasic EMG bursts in the limbs and alterations in airflow associated with bursts of eye movements. The heart rate also may remain constant despite the sudden appearance of increased EMG tone (as opposed to an awakening). Detailed neurologic evaluation of patients suspected of having RBD is indicated and should include MRI of the brain, a full clinical EEG, and a thorough neurologic examination.

Successful treatment of RBD has been achieved with **clonazepam** 0.5–2 mg in approximately 90% of patients. Clonazepam dramatically reduces episode frequency. However, occasional breakthrough attacks can occur, and **environmental precautions** (e.g., bedmate sleeping in a separate bed, closed windows and doors) are essential.

The present patient responded well to clonazepam, and his episodes of violent movement during sleep became infrequent, occurring only once every 1–2 months. The patient's wife began sleeping in another room.

# Clinical Pearls

1. Episodes of violent limb or body movements during sleep suggest the REM behavior disorder.

2. A detailed neurologic examination is essential to rule out an associated neurologic problem.

3. Polysomnography with video recording can help confirm the diagnosis. If seizures are suspected, a full clinical EEG montage should be monitored.

4. Treatment with clonazepam usually is successful, although breakthrough episodes can occur. Environmental precautions are essential.

## REFERENCES

1. Schenck CH, Bundlie SR, Patterson AL, et al: Rapid eye movement sleep behavior disorder: A treatable parasomnia affecting older males. JAMA 1987; 257:1786–1789.
2. Schenck CH, Mahowald MW: A polysomnographic, neurologic, psychiatric and clinical outcome report on 70 consecutive cases with REM sleep behavior disorder: Sustained clonazepam efficacy in 89.5% of 57 treated patients. Clev Clin J Med 1990; 57(Suppl); 10–24.
3. Schenck CH, Bundlie SR, Mahowald MW: Delayed emergence of a parkinsonian disorder in 38% of 29 older men initially diagnosed with idiopathic rapid eye movement sleep disorder. Neurology 1996; 46:388–393.

# PATIENT 87

## A 25-year-old woman walking in her sleep

A 25-year-old woman was referred for evaluation of sleepwalking. She had a history of sleepwalking beginning at age 10, at which time she had about five episodes a month. These gradually decreased until they were uncommon (one or two a year) from age 13 on. However, recently the episodes had been occurring weekly. During this time she had been sleeping poorly because of stress related to college. She sometimes got as little as 3 hours of sleep because of studying for examinations. The patient sought evaluation because she had read that persistence of sleepwalking into adulthood implied psychiatric problems. She denied symptoms of depression and anxiety and did not abuse alcohol or stimulant medications.

*Physical Examination:*   Normal.

*Figure:*   The tracings below occurred when the patient was noted to sit up in bed and pick at the sheets. When the technician entered the room and tried to talk to the patient, she did not respond.

*Question:*   Should the patient be referred for psychiatric evaluation?

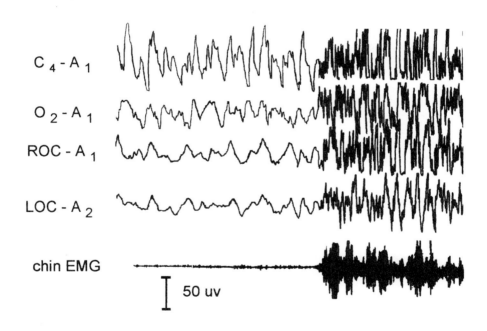

*Answer:* No. Sleepwalking in adults is not always associated with psychopathology. Referral is indicated only if the history suggests an emotional problem.

*Discussion:* Sleepwalking (somnambulism) is defined as a series of complex behaviors that are initiated during **slow wave sleep** and result in ambulation during sleep. Activity can vary from simply sitting up in bed to walking. Patients usually are difficult to awaken during these episodes, and if awakened, are confused. Talking during sleep (somniloquy) can occur simultaneously. In children, sleepwalking usually occurs during the first third of the night, when slow wave sleep is present. However, recent studies in adults have recorded episodes beginning in **stage 2 NREM sleep** and frequently in the second half of the night. Episodes in children are rarely violent, and movements often are slow, but *episodes in adults can be frenzied and violent*. Sleepwalking may be terminated by the patient returning to bed or by the patient simply lying down and continuing sleep out of bed. Typically, there is total amnesia for the episodes.

Sleepwalking can occur as soon as children can walk, but peaks between the ages of 4 and 8. The onset of sleepwalking can occur in adulthood; however, most adult sleepwalkers had episodes during childhood. Sleepwalking usually disappears in adolescence. Fever, sleep deprivation, and certain medications (e.g., phenothiazines, tricyclic antidepressants, lithium) can precipitate the events. Sleepwalking during slow wave sleep rebound has been reported in a patient with obstructive sleep apnea (OSA).

While it was once thought that persistence of sleepwalking into adulthood was a manifestation of underlying psychopathology, several studies have found that at least **50% of adult sleepwalkers have no psychopathology**. Sleepwalking is considered a disorder of arousal. Because there is some overlap with night terrors, some refer to the syndrome as sleepwalking/night terrors. Although polysomnography rarely is performed to evaluate cases of sleepwalking, the classic finding is a sudden arousal occurring in slow wave sleep. During the prolonged arousal, there usually is tachycardia and persistence of slow wave EEG activity—despite the presence of high-frequency EEG activity and an increase in EMG amplitude. Evaluation of parasomnias in the sleep laboratory is best performed with simultaneous video recording to document body movements. Sleep monitoring is indicated when sleepwalking has resulted in bodily injury or has failed to respond to simple measures.

The differential diagnosis of sleepwalking includes the REM behavior disorder, seizure disorders (such as temporal lobe seizures), and dissociative states. The walking associated with the REM behavior disorder occurs during REM sleep usually in the later part of the night. When awakened, subjects generally are not confused and may relate a dream in which they were moving. Patients with nocturnal seizures also may have seizures during wakefulness. However, if seizure activity only occurs during sleep, this diagnosis is more difficult. Diagnosis of temporal lobe seizures may not be possible with conventional scalp electrodes.

In one study of 100 adults referred for evaluation of sleep-related injury, 54 had night terrors/sleepwalking, 36 had the REM behavior disorder, and two had nocturnal seizures. Interestingly, 33% of the group with sleepwalking had an age of onset after age 16, and 70% had episodes arising from both stages 1 and 2 as well as slow wave sleep. The sleepwalking behaviors were variable in duration and intensity. Psychological evaluation identified 50% with psychiatric disorders (e.g., depression, substance abuse, dysthymia). However, 50% of the group had no identifiable psychopathology.

The main complications of sleepwalking are social embarrassment and danger of self-injury. Reports of violent behavior (homicide) have been reported. The treatment of sleepwalking includes environmental precautions (e.g., closed doors and windows, sleeping on the first level, avoidance of precipitating causes such as sleep deprivation), and reassurance. If the episodes seem to require medication, then benzodiazepines or tricyclic antidepressants may be tried. Clonazepam 0.5–2 mg qhs or temazepam 30 mg qhs are commonly prescribed. Medications should be given early enough before bedtime so that sleepwalking in the first slow wave cycle is prevented. Selective serotonin reuptake inhibitors also have been reported to work.

In the present case, the irregular sleep schedule and sleep deprivation were the most likely causes of the return of sleepwalking. The sample sleep tracing shows evidence of arousal from slow wave sleep. Note that some slow wave activity still is present, despite the large amount of high-frequency EEG activity. As the history did not suggest psychopathology, referral for psychological evaluation was not deemed necessary. The patient was instructed to keep a regular sleep schedule and to take environmental precautions. She was reassured that the return of her sleepwalking did not necessarily imply that she had emotional problems. After she began following instructions, the sleepwalking episodes decreased to less than one every 2–3 months.

# Clinical Pearls

1. Not all adults with sleepwalking had episodes as children.

2. Sleepwalking classically occurs during slow wave sleep. In some adults, onset can occur in stage 2 sleep and in the second half of the night.

3. The persistence of sleepwalking into adulthood does *not* necessarily imply underlying psychopathology.

4. Prior sleep deprivation with resulting slow wave sleep rebound (as with nasal CPAP treatment for OSA) can trigger episodes of sleepwalking.

## REFERENCES

1. Schenck CH, Milner DM, Hurwitz TD, et al: A polysomnographic and clinical report of sleep related injury in 100 adult patients. Am J Psych 1989; 146:1166–1172.
2. Kavey NB, Whyte J, Resor SA, et al: Somnabulism in adults. Neurology 1990; 40:749–752.
3. Millman RF, Kipp GJ, Carskadon MA: Sleepwalking precipitated by treatment of sleep apnea with nasal CPAP. Chest 1991; 99:750–751.
4. Mahowald MW, Schenck CH: NREM sleep parasomnias. Neurol Clin 1996; 14:675–696.

# PATIENT 88

## A 20-year-old man with severe "nightmares"

A 20-year-old man was evaluated for complaints of awakening with screaming and severe sweating once or twice a week, usually before 3 AM in the morning. According to his roommate, the patient was diaphoretic and difficult to communicate with during these episodes. Total amnesia for the events was reported. The patient admitted that he had severe nightmares as a child, but that they were infrequent until recently. The events typically occurred after he had missed his normal amount of sleep the night before because of social events or studying for tests.

*Physical Examination:* Normal.

*Question:* How should these "nightmares" be treated?

*Diagnosis:* Night terrors (pavor nocturnus).

*Discussion:* Night terrors, also called sleep terrors or pavor nocturnus, consist of sudden arousal, usually from **stage 3 or 4 sleep**, accompanied by a scream or cry and manifestations of severe fear (behavioral and autonomic). The affected individual typically is confused, diaphoretic, and tachycardic, and he or she frequently sits up in bed. It is difficult or impossible to communicate with a person having a night terror, and **total amnesia** for the event is usual. Night terrors typically occur in prepubertal children (up to 3%) and subside by adolescence; they are uncommon in adults. Some studies have suggested that the presence of night terrors in adulthood indicates psychopathology. However, other authorities disagree with this conclusion.

Patients may sleepwalk during episodes of night terrors. Thus, many consider sleepwalking and night terrors to be one syndrome with a spectrum of manifestations. Both are considered **disorders of arousal**. In adults, night terrors/sleep walking can occur out of stage 2 NREM sleep and during the second part of the night. Stress, febrile illness, sleep deprivation, and heavy caffeine intake have been identified as inciting agents for night terrors. Slow wave sleep rebound, such as occurs with nasal CPAP treatment of OSA, also has been associated with episodes of night terrors.

The differential diagnosis of night terrors includes nightmares, nocturnal seizure activity, the REM behavior disorder (RBD), and the posttraumatic stress syndrome. Nightmares (dream anxiety attacks) and RBD occur within REM sleep and are more common in the second part of the night. RBD usually does not begin until after age 40. Differentiation from partial complex seizures is difficult without complete EEG monitoring. Seizures tend to be more stereotypic and may occur during the day. Patients with nightmares, the posttraumatic stress syndrome, and RBD typically *can* relate complex dream mentation that promoted the event.

Polysomnography usually is not required to evaluate night terrors unless the episodes are frequent, violent, or have the potential to result in self-injury. When polysomnography is performed, inclusion of video monitoring (synchronized if possible) is ideal. If seizures are suspected, then a complete clinical EEG montage is needed. When a night terror is captured, it appears as a sudden arousal from slow wave sleep. The EMG amplitude is greatly increased, and alpha waves are present; however, persistent slow wave activity also is noted.

If the episodes of night terrors are infrequent, treatment beyond simple environmental precautions is unnecessary. Several medications, including benzodiazepines, tricyclic antidepressants, and selective serotonin reuptake inhibitors, have been used with some success. Avoidance of inciting agents is recommended.

In the present case, the patient seemed well-adjusted emotionally. He was told that irregular sleep patterns were probably responsible for the reappearance of the episodes. As he wanted to avoid medication at all costs, the patient diligently maintained good sleep habits and reported only one minor episode every 2–3 months.

## Clinical Pearls

1. Night terrors usually occur from slow wave sleep and are more common in the first part of the night in children. In adults, night terrors can occur from stage 2 sleep and in the second half of the night.

2. The persistence of night terrors into adulthood or onset in adulthood is not necessarily evidence that psychopathology is present.

3. Unlike nightmares and RBD, patients with night terrors cannot relate dream mentation associated with the event.

REFERENCES

1. Guilleminault C, Moscovithc A, et al: Forensic sleep medicine: Nocturnal wanderings and violence. Sleep 1995; 18:740–748.
2. Crisp AH: The sleepwalking/night terrors syndrome in adults. Postgrad Med J 1996; 72:599–604.
3. Mahowald MW, Schenck CH: NREM sleep parasomnias. Neurol Clin 1996; 14:675–696.

# PATIENT 89

## A 55-year-old man with unusual movements during sleep

A 55-year-old man was evaluated for arm movements and confusion during sleep. The episodes, which occurred once or twice weekly, had begun 1 year previously. During an episode the patient did not get out of bed, but was unresponsive. Afterwards, he was groggy. There was no history of daytime sleepiness or insomnia. The patient had no recall of the events in the morning.

*Physical Examination:*   Unremarkable.

*Sleep Study:*   No overt body movements or PLM were noted.

*Figure:*   The following was noted on a tracing when the patient had just fallen asleep.

*Question:*   What is causing the body movements during sleep?

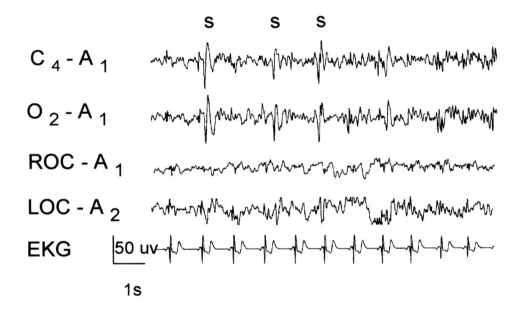

**Diagnosis:** Seizure activity.

**Discussion:** Seizure disorders are part of the differential diagnosis of "nocturnal spells"—episodes of abnormal motor activity during sleep. Depending on the type of patients studied, as many as 45% of seizures occur exclusively or mainly during sleep. The peak incidence of nocturnal seizures is 2 hours after bedtime and between 4 and 5 AM. Daytime seizures are most prevalent in the first hour after awakening. In general, all manifestations of nocturnal seizure disorders are much more common in NREM than REM sleep. Prior sleep deprivation activates seizures; therefore, patients often undergo clinical EEG monitoring in a sleep-deprived state to increase the likelihood of recording seizure activity.

Seizure activity comprises interictal and ictal phases (see table). Interictal refers to transient focal or generalized discharges between seizure events. Ictal discharge refers to the event itself, which, depending on the type of seizure, may be manifested by partial motor activity (limb jerking and twitching), a generalized tonic-clonic seizure (GTC), myoclonic jerking, an absence seizure (brief period of unresponsiveness), or complex motor behavior. When these symptoms occur during sleep, they may not be recognized. Seizures are classified as partial (focal) onset, arising from a localized area of the brain (with or without subsequent generalization), and generalized onset, arising from both hemispheres.

Primary generalized epilepsies include idiopathic GTC seizures, absence seizures (petit mal), and juvenile myoclonic seizures. **Absence seizures** are manifested as a blank stare during which the patient is unresponsive. The characteristic waking EEG pattern is a 3-second spike and wave. **Juvenile myoclonic epilepsy** is a genetically determined condition involving myoclonic jerks in the arms shortly after awakening. These disorders sometimes are called *awakening epilepsies* because they commonly occur when the patient is in a drowsy state upon awakening from sleep. Patients with both absence and juvenile myoclonic disorders also can have GTC seizures. GTC seizures associated with these disorders usually occur on awakening.

Focal seizure disorders are sometimes called *sleeping epilepsies* because they frequently are associated with interictal discharges or seizure activity in NREM sleep. They may be manifested by focal motor activity, impairment of consciousness (during wakefulness), and automatisms (partial complex). Overnight EEG recording is especially useful in diagnosing these disorders, which often are mislabeled as other sleep-related conditions (e.g., PLM, sleepwalking). **Temporal lobe seizures** begin focally and impair consciousness. Staring, orofacial or limb automatisms, and head and body movements frequently occur. Temporal lobe seizures are more common in NREM sleep but also occur at the transition from NREM to REM sleep. **Frontal lobe seizures** are brief and are associated with kicking, thrashing, vocalization, and minimal postictal confusion. Seizures arising from the supplemental motor area involve thrashing with maintenance of consciousness and often are misdiagnosed as psychogenic seizures. Partial seizures with complex automatisms have been described in a few patients; unusual sleepwalking episodes, vocalization, and violent behavior were noted. These patients responded to antiseizure medications.

Diagnosis of nocturnal seizures requires a full EEG montage and, ideally, simultaneous synchronized video recording. Temporal lobe epilepsy is especially difficult to document and often requires internal electrodes. Sometimes a diagnosis is elusive, and an empiric trial of antiseizure medications is needed. In routine clinical EEG monitoring, the paper speed is faster (30 mm/sec) and the EEG amplitude is less sensitive than in sleep monitoring. Therefore, on routine sleep monitoring interictal activity appears sharper and often with a higher amplitude. Unlike usual sleep patterns, interictal activity often manifests as repetitive occurrences of nearly identical patterns. If a computerized system is used to record sleep, the tracing can be reviewed at a simulated clinical EEG paper speed (30 mm/sec). The differential of nocturnal seizures includes bruxism, PLM, night terrors, sleepwalking, and the REM behavior disorder. General motor activity arising from seizures is simpler and more stereotypic than motor activity associated with sleepwalking, night terrors, and the REM behavior disorder.

In the present case, a routine sleep study was initially performed (see figure). This showed no PLM, but frequent spike and wave complexes (*S*) occurred during NREM sleep. Note that the activity does not coincide with the EKG complexes. The complexes were not the usual vertex sharp waves, which are upgoing and sporadic. The patient was referred to a neurologist, and a full clinical EEG confirmed the presence of interictal activity in the right temporal area. The patient was treated with carbamazepine, with resolution of the episodes. An MRI of the brain showed increased size of the temporal horn of the right lateral ventricle, as well as scarring. The patient had a history of head trauma during an automobile accident 10 years earlier, and the seizure activity and MRI findings were thought to be posttraumatic.

**Typical Seizure Occurrence**

| Seizure Type | Interictal Discharge | | Ictal Discharge | | |
|---|---|---|---|---|---|
| | NREM | REM | NREM | REM | After NREM* |
| Primary generalized | Common | Rare | Rare | Rare | Common |
| Focal | Common | Rare | Common | Rare | Possible |

*After awakening from NREM sleep

# Clinical Pearls

1. Seizures are part of the differential diagnosis of abnormal motor behavior occurring during sleep.

2. Optimal diagnosis of nocturnal seizures requires a full EEG montage, with simultaneous video recording if possible.

3. Episodes of repetitive, high-amplitude, sharp EEG activity during a routine sleep study could represent interictal seizure activity.

## REFERENCES

1. Guilleminault C, Moscovithc A, et al: Forensic sleep medicine: Nocturnal wanderings and violence. Sleep 1995; 18:740–748.
2. Malow BA: Sleep and epilepsy. Neurol Clin 1996;14:765–789.
3. Shouse MN, Martins da Silva A, Sammaritano M: Circadian rhythm, sleep, and epilepsy. J Clin Neurophysiol 1996; 13:32–50.

## Evaluation of Insomnia

Insomnia is a broad term denoting unsatisfactory sleep. It includes difficulty initiating sleep (sleep-onset insomnia), difficulty maintaining sleep (sleep-maintenance insomnia), early morning awakening (short sleep period), and nonrestorative sleep. Most causes of insomnia are associated with problems both initiating and maintaining sleep. Some, like the delayed sleep-phase syndrome, are associated mainly with sleep-onset insomnia. The causes of insomnia are many and diverse, complicating the evaluation of patients with this complaint (see table).

### Common Causes of Insomnia

| Primary Insomnia | Secondary Insomnia* |
|---|---|
| Psychophysiological | Sleep disorders (sleep apnea, PLM) |
|   Acute (adjustment sleep disorder) | Psychiatric disorder (depression, panic attacks) |
|   Chronic | Drugs (nicotine, ethanol, caffeine) |
| Idiopathic | Medical conditions/medications |
| Sleep state misperception |   Fibromyalgia and chronic pain syndromes |
| |   COPD and other respiratory disorders |
| |   Medications for illness (theophylline, |
| |     beta blockers) |
| | Circadian disorders |
| |   Delayed sleep-phase syndrome |
| |   Advanced sleep-phase syndrome |
| |   Shift work or jet lag syndrome |
| | Inadequate sleep hygiene |
| | Environmental sleep disorder |

\* "Secondary" means another disorder can be diagnosed.
PLM = periodic leg movement, COPD = chronic obstructive pulmonary disease

An exhaustive **history** and collection of a **sleep diary** are the key elements in making a diagnosis. Obtaining a good history from a patient with insomnia can be difficult because of the many factors to be addressed (see table below).

### Insomnia History

| | |
|---|---|
| Nature and duration of problem | Effects of a new sleep environment (vacations) |
| Sleep habits | Medication/beverage history |
|   Time in bed, lights out, sleep onset, waketime | Symptoms of depression |
|   Bedroom environment | History of leg jerks, restless leg syndrome, |
|   Timing and duration of naps |   snoring, apnea |
|   Changes on weekends | |

Rather than relying on the patient's memory, a sleep log (diary) is an essential tool in the evaluation of insomnia. Most sleep centers have patients complete such a diary for 2 weeks prior to the initial evaluation. There are many types of sleep diaries. The example below shows sleep behavior Monday night through Tuesday morning (see figure). The patient got into bed at 10 PM (↓) but did not try to fall asleep until 11 PM (X). The first sleep did not occur until around 1 AM and lasted until 3 AM (←→). A prolonged awakening between 3 and 5 AM was noted. Another episode of sleep occurred from 5 to 7 AM. The patient got out of bed at 8 AM (↑).

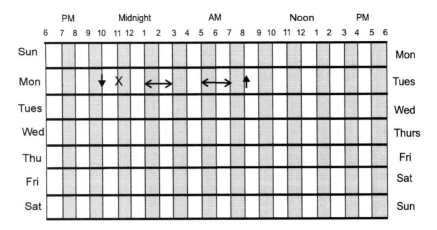

Polysomnography has a minor role in evaluation of most types of insomnia. Conditions with specific polysomnographic findings are sleep apnea, periodic leg movement (PLM), and alpha-delta sleep. Although excessive daytime sleepiness usually is the major complaint of patients with **obstructive sleep apnea,** a few patients complain of insomnia. Complaints of insomnia are more prominent in central sleep apnea. **Periodic limb movement** in sleep may result in complaints of both insomnia and excessive sleepiness, but a complaint of insomnia is more common. **Alpha-delta sleep** is a polysomnographic finding of alpha intrusion into slow wave sleep. It has many causes, such as fibromyalgia (see Patient 96). In most cases of insomnia, polysomnography is not indicated unless sleep apnea or PLM is suspected. However, if the disorder is severe or does not respond to empiric treatment, then a sleep study may be warranted.

For cases of insomnia in which polysomnography is obtained, the study tends to simply confirm patient complaints of a prolonged sleep latency ($> 30$ minutes), frequent prolonged awakenings, frequent arousals, reduction in total sleep time, reduced sleep efficiency, and decreased amount of slow wave and REM sleep. A short REM latency or early morning awakening suggests the diagnosis of depression. In **sleep misperception,** a fairly normal night of sleep is recorded, but the patient believes that good sleep was not obtained. In **psychophysiologic insomnia,** both the sleep study and the patient confirm a good night of sleep, suggesting that the home sleep environment is either suboptimal or has become a stimulus for anxiety regarding sleep.

## REFERENCES

1. Buysse DJ, Reynolds CF: Insomnia. *In* Thorpy MJ (ed): Handbook of Sleep Disorders. New York, Marcel Dekker, 1990, pp 375–433.
2. Kupfer DJ, Reynolds CF: Management of insomnia. N Engl J Med 1997; 336:341–346.

# PATIENT 90

## A 30-year-old woman having difficulty falling asleep

A 30-year-old woman was referred for complaints of an inability to sleep (insomnia). This problem had been severe for more than 5 years. The patient usually retired at 10 PM each night, but did not fall asleep until 1 AM. Three to four awakenings occurred each night, with the final awakening at 6:30 AM (spontaneous). After each, the patient required at least 30 minutes to fall asleep. Self-medication with over-the-counter sleeping pills and alcohol sometimes was effective. The only good night of sleep occurred when the patient went on vacations.

The sleep environment was reported to be quiet and dark. The patient did keep a lighted clock at bedside. During the day, fatigue but not definite sleepiness was noted. No naps were taken. There were no symptoms of depression and no history of marital conflicts. The patient's husband reported that his wife did not snore, kick, or jerk during sleep.

**Physical Examination:**   General: thin and nervous. Otherwise unremarkable.

**Sleep Study**

| | | Sleep Stages | % SPT |
|---|---|---|---|
| Time in bed (monitoring time) | 460 min (425–462) | | |
| Total sleep time | 411 min (394–457) | Stage Wake | 5 (0–6) |
| Sleep period time (SPT) | 432.5 min (414–453) | Stage 1 | 11.8 (3–6) |
| Wake after sleep onset | 21.5 min | Stage 2 | 45 (46–62) |
| Sleep efficiency | .89 (.90–1.0) | Stages 3 and 4 | 18 (7–21) |
| Sleep latency | 20 min (0–19) | Stage REM | 20.2 (21–31) |
| REM latency | 85 min (69–88) | | |
| | | AHI | 0/hr |
| | | PLM index | 0/hr |

( ) = normal values for age, AHI = apnea + hypopnea index, PLM = periodic limb movement

**Question:**   Why is the sleep study relatively normal?

*Diagnosis:* Psychophysiologic insomnia.

*Discussion:* Psychophysiologic insomnia is defined as a disorder of somatized tension and learned sleep-preventing associations. In most sleep disorder centers, up to 15% of insomniacs receive a diagnosis of psychophysiologic insomnia. These individuals tend to react to stress with increased tension, and there is a marked overconcern and frustration with an inability to sleep. The bedroom and lights-out time become stimuli for increased tension and anxiety. The insomnia usually is fairly fixed, although it may vary in severity. A precipitating event may have caused the problem's onset, but it now has taken on a life of its own. Patients with this disorder frequently have a history of being "light sleepers" for many years. Inadequate sleep hygiene also may be present, but even after correction the problem persists. This diagnosis is not made if the patient can be classified as having an anxiety disorder, obsessive-compulsive neurosis, or major depression.

The diagnosis of **adjustment sleep disorder** (transient psychophysiologic insomnia) is made if the insomnia is transient (usually less than 6 months) and clearly follows an acute stress or conflict. In this case the sleep problems are a change from the patient's norm. **Environmental sleep disorder** is the diagnosis when insomnia is clearly secondary to problems with the sleep environment, such as noise, bed-partner disturbance, or the necessity of remaining vigilant (e.g., sick children).

Polysomnography is of limited utility in evaluating most cases of insomnia; therefore, it is not routinely recommended and often is not reimbursed by health insurance plans. The results usually corroborate the patient's complaints (long sleep latency, low sleep efficiency, frequent arousals, prolonged awakenings) and seldom reveal a specific reason for the sleep disturbance. However, identification of periodic limb movement (PLM) in sleep, a shortened REM latency (possible depression), or, rarely, central or obstructive sleep apnea can provide clues to the cause of the insomnia.

When polysomnography is performed to evaluate insomnia, the results may be amazingly normal. In such a case, if the patient believes it was a poor night of sleep, then the diagnosis is **sleep state misperception.** In this disorder, patients do not seem to recognize that they were asleep. Conversely, if the patient recognizes that sleep was fairly normal and, in fact, expected a good night of sleep, then either the home sleep environment is suboptimal or it has become a conditioned stimulus for sleep difficulty. This phenomenon is called the **reverse first-night effect,** as normal subjects tend to sleep poorly in a novel environment (sleep lab).

In the current case, the patient complained of both sleep-onset and sleep-maintenance insomnia. There was no historical information to suggest sleep apnea, PLM, or depression. A sleep study was performed at the patient's insistence. The study showed a near normal night of sleep in the sleep laboratory and an absence of evidence for other etiologies, making psychophysiologic insomnia the most likely disorder. The patient was treated with improved sleep hygiene and stimulus control therapy (see Patient 91). Treatment resulted in better sleep latency and sleep continuity.

# Clinical Pearls

1. Diagnosis of the cause of insomnia usually is made on the basis of a careful history and review of a patient sleep diary (log).

2. Polysomnography generally is not indicated in evaluation of insomnia. Two exceptions are when there is a suspicion of PLM in sleep or sleep apnea and when the insomnia is severe and does not respond to empiric therapy.

3. A better-than-normal night of sleep in the sleep laboratory (a reverse first-night effect) suggests that the home sleep environment is suboptimal or has become a conditioned stimulus for sleep difficulty.

4. In psychophysiologic insomnia, sleeping in a novel location may temporarily improve insomnia.

## REFERENCES
1. Reynolds CF, Taska LS, Sewitch DE, et al: Persistent psychophysiological insomnia: Preliminary diagnostic criteria and EEG sleep data. Am J Psych 1984; 141:804–805.
2. American Sleep Disorders Association: The International Classification of Sleep Disorders: Diagnostic and Coding Manual. Lawrence, Kansas, Allen Press, 1990, pp 28–32.
3. Reite M, Buysse D, Reynolds C, Mendelson W: The use of polysomnography in the evaluation of insomnia. Sleep 1995; 18:58–70.
4. Standards of Practice Committee of the American Sleep Disorders Association: Practice parameters of the use of polysomnography in evaluation of insomnia. Sleep 1995; 18:55–57.

# PATIENT 91

## A 30-year-old woman with insomnia

A 30-year-old woman with complaints of insomnia was diagnosed with psychophysiologic insomnia after an evaluation that included a polysomnogram. She admitted that she was a tense person and had problems relaxing. When she had problems falling asleep, she became very anxious: "I look at the clock and am upset that the night is almost over and I haven't fallen asleep." The patient denied drinking coffee, but admitted that she drank wine at bedtime to help her fall asleep. She reported being less tense about falling asleep on the weekends because she could sleep later the next day. Interestingly, the patient reported sleeping better on vacations than in her own bedroom. There was no history of snoring or leg movements during sleep.

*Sleep Diary*

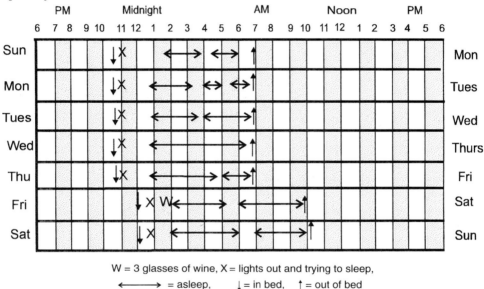

W = 3 glasses of wine, X = lights out and trying to sleep,
⟵⟶ = asleep,  ↓ = in bed,  ↑ = out of bed

*Question:* What treatment options, other than medication, would you recommend?

*Answer:*    Good sleep hygiene, stimulus control therapy, relaxation therapy.

*Discussion:*    The treatment of insomnia must be individualized. The mainstay of any treatment is to optimize sleep hygiene by educating patients about habits that interfere with good sleep. Good sleep hygiene includes maintaining a favorable sleep environment (e.g., quiet, dark, comfortable), keeping a regular sleep routine (constant bedtime and waketime), avoiding stimulants such as **caffeine** and other medications that interrupt sleep (e.g., ethanol), and avoiding long naps. Note that caffeine can impair sleep up to 10 hours later, and some patients are quite sensitive to just a tiny amount. Therefore, patients with insomnia should be questioned carefully about their caffeine intake, including colas and tea. **Ethanol** frequently is used to help promote sleep onset; however, ethanol intake near bedtime can cause awakenings and fragmented sleep later in the night, even at low doses.

Behavioral techniques, although widely recommended as treatment for insomnia, are applied less commonly than the pharmacologic approach. One reason is that they are time-intensive for both clinician and patient. Readily available educational materials and instruction by knowledgeable ancillary personnel may reduce clinician involvement and make these techniques more cost-effective. Relaxation therapy is a commonly used behavioral treatment. Many patients with insomnia report physiologic (tension) and cognitive/emotional (racing thoughts and worrying) arousal at bedtime. **Progressive muscle relaxation** (Jacobson) consists of first tensing then relaxing each muscle group in a systematic way. Patients receive instruction in this technique and then practice twice daily, with the last session at bedtime. **Biofeedback treatment** uses feedback from EMG monitoring of a muscle, such as the frontalis muscle, to teach the patient how to relax. Patients with cognitive arousal at bedtime may benefit from **meditation** or guided-imagery techniques (refocusing on a pleasant mental target). For some patients, regular **exercise** may improve sleep. Exercise should not be within 2 hours of bedtime as it raises the body temperature, making sleep onset more difficult.

A second behavioral option is **stimulus control therapy**. This treatment recognizes that insomniacs typically associate the bedroom with difficulty falling asleep: they become anxious as they stay in bed and "watch the clock," and over several nights the bedroom itself becomes a stimulus for anxiety and insomnia. This association explains why some patients with insomnia sleep better in a new setting. Stimulus control therapy seeks to create a conditioned association between the bedroom and sleep. Activities in the bedroom are restricted to sleep and sex. Patient do not get in bed unless sleepy and do not remain in bed unless drowsy or asleep. If they fail to fall asleep in a reasonable time, they are instructed to get out of bed until they feel sleepy. Regular bedtime and waketime as well as avoidance of naps are part of the instructions.

A third option is called **sleep restriction therapy.** The clinician looks at the sleep diary and estimates the time spent in bed and the time asleep. The patient is then asked to restrict the time in bed to match the previous time spent asleep. This induces mild sleep deprivation and increases sleep efficiency. As the efficiency is improved the time allowed in bed is slowly increased.

The present patient, when questioned in detail, reported consumption of at least ten caffeine-containing carbonated beverages a day. Her sleep diary shows a lights-out time of 11 PM during the week and a long sleep latency. The patient typically was in bed an hour before lights out, and she sometimes read work-related materials during this time. On the weekends, bedtime was delayed and ethanol was consumed, resulting in a shorter sleep latency. One or two awakenings most nights were recorded. The history of sleeping better on vacation suggested that the patient had an association between her bedroom and problems falling asleep.

Treatment included instructions to switch to noncaffeinated drinks and avoid ethanol near bedtime. The patient removed the clock from her bedroom and went to bed just before lights out. If unable to fall asleep within a reasonable time, she got out of bed and read (recreational reading) until she felt sleepy, and then she returned to bed. If she awakened during the night and was unable to return to sleep, she again got out of bed until sleepy (stimulus control). In addition, the patient was given tapes instructing her in relaxation techniques. She practiced relaxation rather than engaging in work-related activities near bedtime. Initially, despite this combined approach, the patient still had some difficulty falling asleep. However, within a few weeks she reported falling asleep within 20 minutes on most nights and having fewer awakenings.

230

# Clinical Pearls

1. Every patient with insomnia must be questioned in detail about sleep habits and intake of beverages that can disturb sleep.

2. Treatment of insomnia always should begin with establishment of good sleep hygiene.

3. Relaxation therapy may be especially helpful in patients with emotional or physical tension at bedtime.

4. Stimulus control treatment can break the association between the bedroom and poor sleep.

## REFERENCES

1. Bootzin RR, Nicassio PM: Behavioral treatments for insomnia. *In* Hersen M, Eisler RM, Miller PM (eds): Progress in Behavior Modification. New York, Academic Press, 1978, p 6.
2. Buysse DJ, Reynolds CF: Insomnia. *In* Thorpy MJ (ed): Handbook of Sleep Disorders. New York, Marcel Dekker, 1990, pp 375–433.
3. Morin CM, Culbert JP, Schwartz SM: Nonpharmacologic interventions for insomnia: A meta-analysis of treatment efficacy. Am J Psych 1994; 151:1172–1180.
4. Stepanski EJ: Behavior therapy for insomnia. *In* Kryger M, Roth T, Dement W (eds): Principles and Practice of Sleep Medicine. Philadelphia, WB Saunders 1994, pp 535–541.

# PATIENT 92

**A 40-year-old man with difficulty falling asleep after the death of his brother**

A 40-year-old man who previously had no sleep problems developed difficulty falling asleep and staying asleep after the death of his brother 3 months previously. He had tried improvement in sleep hygiene and did not remain in bed unless sleepy. However, he was still unable to sleep for at least 1 hour after retiring at his normal bedtime. He had seen a psychiatrist who had started him on amitriptyline, but this made the patient very groggy the next day. The patient's primary care physician had given him triazolam, which enabled him to fall asleep quickly, but he sometimes felt very anxious in the mornings. The patient's wife noted that his legs jerked on occasion when he was asleep.

### Sleep Study

| | | Sleep Stages | % SPT |
|---|---|---|---|
| Time in bed (TIB) | 440 min (390–468) | | |
| Total sleep time (TST) | 314 min (343–436) | Stage Wake | 15 (1–12) |
| Sleep period time (SPT) | 370 min (378–452) | Stage 1 | 20 (5–11) |
| Wake after sleep onset | 55.5 min | Stage 2 | 45 (44–66) |
| Sleep efficiency | .71 (.90–1.0) | Stages 3 and 4 | 5 (2–15) |
| Sleep latency | 50 min (2–18) | Stage REM | 15 (19–27) |
| REM latency | 85 min (55–78) | | |
| | | AHI | 3/hr |
| | | PLM index | 5/hr |

( ) = normal values for age, AHI = apnea + hypopnea index, PLM = periodic limb movement

**Question:** What is your diagnosis? Which hypnotic would you suggest for this patient?

***Diagnosis:*** Adjustment sleep disorder. An intermediate-duration benzodiazepine is a reasonable treatment option.

***Discussion:*** Adjustment sleep disorder (transient psychophysiologic insomnia) is defined as insomnia related to an **acute stress, conflict, or environmental change**. Rather than a true disorder, it is a normal reaction to one of life's many stresses. The course usually is brief, lasting only days: an acute state is less than one week; subacute is up to 3 months. However, insomnia can become chronic (duration longer than 3 months) following a precipitating event. It then might be classified as psychophysiologic insomnia if *the initial stressor is no longer present or a major concern.* An example of the adjustment sleep disorder is the difficulty many people have in sleeping in a novel environment, such as a sleep lab. This is called the first-night effect and usually is rather mild.

**Benzodiazepines** are the most widely used hypnotic medications (see table on next page). They are relatively safe and well-tolerated. Generally, it is safer to start with a low dose and increase gradually. The lowest dose should be used in older patients who are susceptible to side effects. Agents with a long half-life tend to cause daytime grogginess (flurazepam), but they can be useful in anxious patients. Benzodiazepines with a short half-life may cause rebound irritability (triazolam). All benzodiazepines tend to increase the amount of stage 2 sleep (increased sleep spindles) and cause mild decreases in slow wave and REM sleep. When ceasing treatment it is wise to slowly decrease the dose, weaning the patient to minimize any rebound effects secondary to withdrawal.

A new nonbenzodiazepine agent, zolpidem, was introduced recently. Unlike a benzodiazepine, this agent does not decrease the amount of slow wave sleep. However, zolpidem gives little warning of impending sleep and is relatively expensive. Additionally, behavior in some elderly patients is altered by this medication. The usual dose is 10 mg at bedtime (5 mg in older or small patients).

**Tricyclic antidepressants** are another class of agents that sometimes are used as hypnotics. They are especially beneficial in cases of insomnia associated with depression. Typically, tricyclic medications with sedating properties such as doxepin (Sinequan) or amitriptyline (Elavil) are prescribed. Trazadone, a sedating nontricyclic antidepressant, also is used as a hypnotic when depression is present. The tricyclic antidepressants have anticholinergic and cardiovascular side effects (e.g., widened QRS, arrhythmias). Of the tricyclics, doxepin is thought to have a relatively safe cardiovascular profile. However, trazadone and all tricyclic antidepressants can cause profound orthostatic hypotension in some patients. Trazadone also can cause intractable priapism, and patients should be cautioned to stop the medication immediately if this occurs.

The following **guidelines for hypnotic use** are suggested:

1. Limit to a course of 4 weeks if possible (unless treating depression with an antidepressant)
2. Use the lowest effective dose
3. Use a low dose in elderly patients
4. Monitor for side effects
5. Avoid abrupt discontinuation of the medication (wean off over several days).

In the present patient, the absence of prior sleep problems and the obvious association with the recent death of a family member makes adjustment sleep disorder the likely diagnosis. The need for a sleep study in this case is debatable; it was ordered because of the history of leg kicks. However, the study showed no evidence of significant leg movement. It did document a long sleep latency ($> 30$ minutes) and a low sleep efficiency consistent with the patient's complaints. The amount of slow wave and REM sleep also was reduced. The patient was treated with temazepam 30 mg qhs and **bereavement counseling.** On this therapy his sleep improved, and he was weaned off the temazepam after 3 weeks.

## Commonly Prescribed Benzodiazepines

| | Dose* | Half-life | Comments |
|---|---|---|---|
| Flurazepam (Dalmane) | 15, 30 mg | Long | Daytime drowsiness common<br>Rarely used today |
| Clonazepam (Klonopin)** | 0.5–2 mg | Long | Used for PLM, REM behavior disorder<br>Can cause morning drowsiness |
| Temazepam (Restoril) | 15, 30 mg | Intermediate | |
| Estazolam (ProSom) | 1–2 mg | Intermediate | Can cause agranulocytosis |
| Triazolam (Halcion) | 0.125, 0.25 mg | Short | Rebound insomnia may occur |
| Zolpidem (Ambien) | 5, 10 mg | Short | A nonbenzodiazepine |

*Use lower dose in elderly  **Not FDA-approved as a hypnotic

PLM = periodic leg movement

# Clinical Pearls

1. The "first-night effect" refers to the insomnia many people experience when sleeping in a novel environment.

2. Adjustment sleep disorder follows an obvious life event and usually is transient.

3. The selection of hypnotics depends on the desired duration of action, the patient's age, and the presence or absence of depression. The lowest dose should be used in older patients.

4. When hypnotics are prescribed for treatment of insomnia, the goal should be a limited course with a taper of medication to minimize rebound insomnia.

## REFERENCES

1. Agnew H, Webb W, Williams RL: The first-night effect: An EEG study of sleep. Psychophysiology 1966; 7:263–266.
2. Buysee DJ, Reynolds CF: Insomnia. In Thorpy MJ (ed): Handbook of Sleep Disorders. New York, Marcel Dekker, 1990, pp 375–433.
3. Kupfer DJ, Reynolds CF: Management of insomnia. N Engl J Med 1997; 336:341–346.

# PATIENT 93

## A 40-year-old woman complaining of difficulty falling asleep

A 40-year-old woman had been having trouble falling asleep for more than 10 years. She typically went to bed around 11 PM, did not fall asleep until 2–3 AM and awakened to the alarm clock at 6 AM. Thus, she obtained only 4 hours of sleep per night during the work week and felt tired throughout the day. On the weekends, she slept until 10–11 AM and awoke feeling refreshed. The patient rarely took naps during the day. There was no history of depression or recent stressful life events. The patient avoided caffeine intake completely. Because she rarely felt sleepy at 11 PM, she sometimes took either a drink of ethanol or an over-the-counter sleeping medication, both of which were only moderately successful at inducing sleep. Sleeping pills left her feeling groggy in the morning.

***Physical Examination:*** Normal

***Sleep Diary***

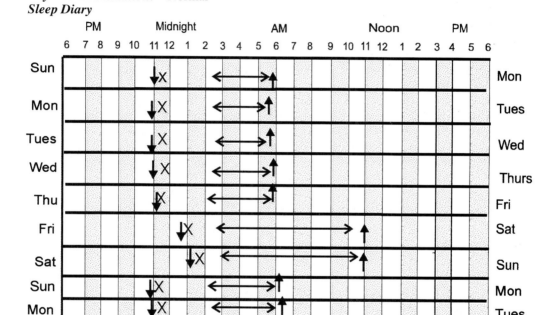

X = lights out and trying to sleep,
⟵⟶ = asleep,  ↓ = in bed,  ↑ = out of bed

***Question:*** What is the reason for this patient's difficulty falling asleep?

*Diagnosis:*   Delayed sleep-phase syndrome.

*Discussion:* The delayed sleep-phase syndrome (DSPS) is classified as a **circadian rhythm sleep disorder.** "Circadian" means related to the daily time period (*circa,* about; *dian,* day). The physiology of many human processes, including body temperature and sleep onset, is related to the daily 24-hour clock. In DSPS, the timing of sleep onset is delayed relative to clock time. Attempts to start sleep by getting into bed at the usual time are unsuccessful at inducing sleep. Sleep-onset time tends to be regular, but delayed (2–6 AM). There usually is no problem maintaining sleep, and when sleep is undisturbed, the sleep period is of normal length. However, waking at a typical clock time to fulfill social obligations results in a short duration of sleep.

The duration of DSPS varies from months to decades. Adolescence is the most common age of onset; onset after age 30 is rare. True DSPS must be differentiated from sleep-onset insomnia in individuals who delay sleep for social reasons and then experience difficulty falling asleep when they sporadically try to go to bed earlier. These individuals have a transient sleep-wake cycle disorder caused by a self-enforced phase shift. When they maintain a regular bedtime and waketime for several days, they quickly adjust to this schedule. Patients with bipolar affective disorder in the mania phase also may have sleep-onset insomnia. The sleep period is short in these patients, but they have no difficulty arising at a conventional time. The non–24-hour sleep-wake syndrome is characterized by a progressive, incremental phase delay in sleep onset and waketimes.

Treatment of DSPS often is difficult. While hypnotics may be temporarily successful at inducing sleep at normal clock times, daytime grogginess typically results. **Chronotherapy** is the traditional therapy for this disorder. This therapy is based on the fact that it is easier to phase delay (delay the time of sleep onset) than phase advance. Bedtime is progressively delayed by several hours on successive days. The sleep period is allowed to run its course with later and later waketimes. Thus, the sleep period moves around the clock until sleep onset occurs at normal societal times. However, this therapy requires that the patient be free from societal constraints (e.g., job, child care) for the duration of the treatment, and the bedroom must be dark and quiet. Obviously, many patients are unable to commit to chronotherapy.

Recently, **bright light** has been shown to shift the phase of the internal clock if applied at appropriate times. Therapy with bright light in the early morning (end of dark phase) may help phase advance patients with DSPS. The source must be either bright outdoor light or indoor artificial light of > 2500 lux for 30 minutes to 2 hours, beginning soon after waking in the morning (6–8 AM). The result is patient sleepiness earlier in the evening (phase advance). In some patients, the bright light can be discontinued. However, maintaining a fixed bedtime and waketime is essential. Staying up late for any reason tends to reshift the internal clock. Bright light should be avoided near bedtime, as it can induce a phase delay. Commercial bright light units are available for use in the winter months.

Another potential treatment of DSPS is the ingestion of **melatonin** in the evening. This hormone is manufactured in the pineal gland during the dark phase. When given at the end of the day, it can induce a phase advance (opposite timing from bright light). In supraphysiologic doses (greater than 0.5 mg), it also may have direct, mild, sleep-inducing effects (this is controversial). In one study, 5 mg was given at 2200 hours (5 hours before usual sleep-onset time) for 4 weeks. A mean advance of 72 minutes in sleep-onset time was noted. There are no clinical trials showing long-term efficacy and safety. In general, the phase-shifting effects of melatonin are weaker than bright light.

In the current case, the sleep diary shows that the patient had mainly sleep-onset insomnia. Once asleep, there was little difficulty maintaining sleep. Due to societal constraints, the waketime was set at 6 AM. Thus, a delayed sleep onset resulted in a reduced total sleep time. The patient underwent a regimen of fixed waketimes (6 AM) on all days and avoided naps. She was advised to walk or jog for an hour in bright morning light during the summer, and use bright, artificial light in the winter. This approach improved her ability to fall asleep, and sleep onset occurred by 12–12:30 on most nights.

# Clinical Pearls

1. Insomnia primarily of the sleep-onset type suggests the possibility of the delayed sleep-phase syndrome.

2. A sleep log is helpful in documenting a pattern of delayed sleep onset but relatively normal sleep maintenance.

3. Chronotherapy (progressive phase delay) is the traditional treatment for this problem.

4. Bright light therapy in the morning is an important new treatment for this disorder.

## REFERENCES

1. Czeisler CA, Richardson GS, Coleman RM, et al: Chronotherapy: Resetting the circadian clocks of patients with delayed sleep phase insomnia. Sleep 1981; 4:1–21.
2. Weitzman ED, Czeisler CA, Coleman RM, et al: Delayed sleep-phase syndrome: A chronobiological disorder with sleep-onset insomnia. Arch Gen Psych 1981; 38:737–746.
3. Rosenthal NE, Joseph-Vanderpool JR, Levendosky AA, et al: Phase-shifting effects of bright morning light as treatment for delayed sleep-phase syndrome. Sleep 1990; 13:354–361.
4. Dahlitz M, Alvarez B, Vignau J: Delayed sleep-phase syndrome response to melatonin. Lancet 1991; 337:112–104.

# PATIENT 94

## A 70-year-old man with early morning awakening

A 70-year-old man was seen for complaints of early morning awakening. This problem had worsened since his retirement 5 years ago. His typical bedtime was 9 PM; he fell asleep within 5 minutes, and staying up later was difficult for him. During the night, the patient awakened twice with nocturia, usually at midnight and 2 AM, but returned quickly to sleep. He then awoke spontaneously between 4 and 5 AM and typically was unable to fall back asleep, but remained in bed until 6:30 AM. The patient's futile efforts to return to sleep caused him considerably distress. During the day, the patient was able to stay awake without difficulty. He normally took a 1–1½ hour nap at 1 PM. He denied feeling sad or depressed. He had many hobbies and a good relationship with his wife. The patient took a diuretic for hypertension and denied taking any hypnotic medication.

***Physical Examination:*** Normal.

***Sleep Diary***

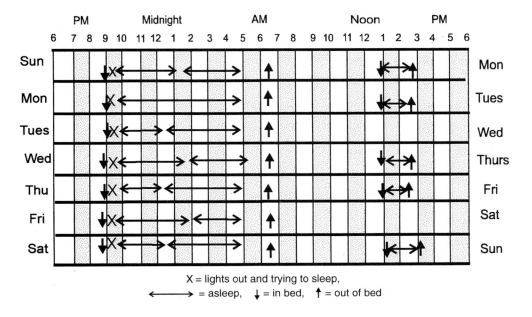

X = lights out and trying to sleep,
⟵⟶ = asleep, ↓ = in bed, ↑ = out of bed

*Question:* What is causing this patient's early awakening time?

*Diagnosis:*  Advanced sleep-phase syndrome.

*Discussion:*  The advanced sleep-phase syndrome (ASPS) is characterized by an **early sleep onset** (6–9 PM) and an **early waketime** (3–4 AM) relative to clock time. There usually is no difficulty initiating sleep or maintaining sleep until early spontaneous awakening. Delaying bedtime past 9 PM is difficult. While some patients complain of an inability to maintain wakefulness for evening social functions, the main presenting complaint is early morning awakening. The early awakening produces anxiety in patients who feel they are not getting a full night of sleep. However, as long as the total amount and quality of sleep is adequate, the early morning awakening causes no physiologic problems.

ASPS is exacerbated by naps during the day (reduce total nocturnal sleep need) and early morning walks in the sunshine—both of which are common habits of many elderly patients. The exposure to bright light in the early morning hours results in a phase advance. In contrast, exposure to bright light near bedtime results in a **phase delay** and is a possible treatment for this syndrome. Typical indoor light is not strong enough to reset the circadian phase; therefore, outside daylight or special indoor lighting ($> 2500$ lux) is required. Avoiding naps and enforcing a delayed bedtime, perhaps by engaging in physical activity in a brightly lit setting, may help. In addition, education can reduce the anxiety and frustration.

Severe forms of ASPS (intractable sleepiness before 8 PM) are rare. A tendency for mild phase advancement is common in elderly persons and may be one cause of sleep maintenance problems in these patients. In one study, bright light in the evening induced a phase delay in the nadir of body temperature and improved sleep maintenance. However, this treatment may not be practical on a long-term basis.

**Depression** is the other major cause of early morning awakening. The symptoms of depression in older patients (e.g., loss of appetite, weight loss) should be carefully elicited. Evaluation of a patient with suspected ASPS should include a daily sleep log to document the pattern of sleep. A sleep study might help reveal depression: an early REM latency is suggestive, but this finding is not specific for depression. Otherwise, a sleep study probably is not useful, unless sleep apnea or periodic leg movement is suspected.

The present patient complained mainly of an early waketime. Daily sleep was reported to be approximately 7 hours at night plus a 1-1½ hour daytime nap. Thus, total sleep time was adequate. Symptoms of depression can be subtle in elderly patients. However, the patient denied any symptoms of depression and reported an active lifestyle. The most likely diagnosis was a mild form of ASPS. The patient was instructed to avoid naps and take his daily walk in the evening. These changes enabled him to delay his sleep onset to 10 PM and sleep until 5–5:30 AM. Upon awakening, the patient got out of bed and worked on one of his hobbies until breakfast time. He seemed satisfied with his new schedule.

## Clinical Pearls

1. A mild form of ASPS is common in elderly patients; severe forms are rare.
2. An early waketime is the main complaint in ASPS.
3. Exposure to bright light (outside sunshine) in the early morning advances the sleep phase and should be avoided in patients with ASPS.
4. The main differential of ASPS (early morning awakening) is depression.

## REFERENCES

1. American Sleep Disorders Association: International Classification of Sleep Disorders: Diagnostic and Coding Manual. Lawrence, Kansas, Allen Press, 1990, pp 133–136.
2. Campbell SS, Dawson D, Anderson MW: Alleviation of sleep-maintenance insomnia with timed exposure to bright light. J Am Geriatr Soc 1993; 41:829–836.
3. Ando K, Kripke DP, Ancoli-Israel S: Estimated prevalence of delayed and advanced sleep-phase syndrome. Sleep Research 1995; 14:509.

# PATIENT 95

## A 44-year-old man with jet lag

A 44-year-old business executive was referred for complaints of increasing difficulty adjusting to business trips from the West to the East Coast. He found it extremely difficulty to fall asleep at an East Coast bedtime and wake up for his early morning business appointments. If he did make it to the meetings, he was drowsy and found it hard to stay awake. These problems had seemed to worsen over the last 3 years. His normal bedtime was 11 PM and normal waketime was 6 AM. At home he awakened refreshed and had no problems with daytime sleepiness. There was no history of snoring. The patient had tried triazolam for the first night on the East Coast—he was able to fall asleep and sleep better, but still had problems maintaining alertness in the morning.

***Physical Examination:*** Normal.

***Question:*** What treatments would you advise?

*Answer:*    Phase advancing with early-morning, bright light exposure.

*Discussion:*    Time zone change ( jet lag) syndrome describes the condition arising from **asynchrony** between a patient's internal circadian pacemaker and external clock time secondary to rapid travel across several time zones. Symptoms include problems with sleep onset or maintenance and/or decreased alertness and performance in the new time zone. Traveling eastward is the more difficult direction, as patients find it easier to phase delay than phase advance. For example, West to East Coast travel results in a patient retiring at a clock time of 11 PM but an **internal circadian time** of 8 PM. Sleep onset is delayed, and sleep is easily disturbed. At 7 AM clock time, the circadian time is 4 AM, and the patient finds it difficult to awaken and achieve normal alertness. It appears that adjusting to jet lag is more difficult with increasing age.

Propensity for sleep and wakefulness, cognitive function, hormonal secretion, and many other physiologic functions cycle regularly across each day. These circadian ("about a day") rhythms are generated by an internal pacemaker in the suprachiasmic nucleus (SCN) of the hypothalamus. The major afferents to the SCN are retinal neurons whose axons leave the optic chiasm and synapse on SCN cells (retinohypothalamic pathway). The afferents transmit nonvisual light information. The main role of the SCN is to synchronize bodily functions with the environmental light-dark cycle. **Light** is the most potent stimulus for shifting the phase of the circadian cycle. The amplitude and direction of the phase shifts vary with timing of the stimulus (phase response curve). Light exposure in the early-evening-to-bedtime period shifts the internal rhythm to an earlier time (phase delay) decreasing the propensity to sleep. Light exposure in the early morning causes a phase advance. While the largest phase shifts are induced by very bright light (outdoor sunlight), regular indoor illumination also can have a small effect. Indoor sources of bright light (> 2500 lux) have been used clinically to effectively shift the circadian clock.

**Melatonin**, a hormone secreted by the pineal gland only during darkness, appears to play a role in synchronizing the SCN to the environment. There are melatonin receptors on the SCN cells. Exogenous melatonin can produce phase-shifting effects, but the *required timing* of administration for a given direction of shift is opposite to bright light. A few hours before the traditional dark period, ingestion of melatonin induces phase advance whereas bright light phase delays. Melatonin's phase-shifting effects are not as potent as light and may require several days of medication. Experiments in animals and humans show that there is a limitation to how much the internal cycle can be phase-shifted at any one time (1–2 hours maximum). Thus, acclimization to a new time zone requires several days.

A number of maneuvers have been tried to minimize the difficulties of jet lag. Short-acting hypnotics, such as triazolam, improve the continuity of sleep but do not shift the circadian clock. Therefore, awakening and resuming full alertness is still a problem because the internal circadian clock is not truly shifted. Bright light exposure in the morning in the advanced time zone may assist in phase advancing the internal circadian clock, but this is not always practical. Melatonin has been reported to both consolidate sleep and shift the circadian clock. For example, taken in the evening it can help phase advance an eastward traveler. *However, the effectiveness and safety of melatonin is not well-documented.* Traditional stimulants, such as caffeine, are widely used to assist in maintaining alertness. Another approach is to prepare for the eastward trip by going to bed progressively earlier and arising earlier for 1 week before the trip. This slowly shifts the circadian clock prior to travel. Despite these maneuvers, most individuals still do not feel truly alert in the morning for several days. Scheduling meetings in the afternoon in the East Coast time zone or arriving several days prior to an important meeting are helpful approaches.

The present patient tried phase advancing himself before his eastward trips by getting bright light exposure in the morning, avoiding light in the evenings, and going to bed earlier for 1 week prior to his trips. When possible, he attempted to arrive a day or two earlier than his scheduled meetings. While on the East Coast, he tried to get as much early-morning, bright light exposure as possible. These procedures improved but did not eliminate his symptoms.

# Clinical Pearls

1. The jet lag syndrome can be treated with behavioral and scheduling changes, timed daylight exposure, short-acting hypnotics, and, possibly, melatonin.
2. The jet lag syndrome worsens with increasing age.

## REFERENCES

1. Moline ML, Pollack CP, Monk TH, et al: Age-related differences in recovery from simulated jet lag. Sleep 1991; 14:42–48.
2. Graeber RC: Jet lag and sleep disruption. *In* Kryger MH, Roth T, Dement WC (eds): Principles and Practice of Sleep Medicine. Philadelphia, W. B. Saunders, 1994, pp 463–470.
3. Arendt J, Deacon S: Treatment of circadian rhythm disorders—melatonin. Chronobiol Internat 1997; 14:185–204.

# PATIENT 96

## A 40-year-old woman with fibromyalgia

A 40-year-old woman was referred for complaints of nonrestorative sleep. She had a history of generalized pain and chronic fatigue of 1-year duration. She retired every night at 10 PM and usually took about 1 hour to fall asleep. During the night, she was awakened by discomfort three to four times. She had taken medications, including narcotics, that relieved the pain, but she often felt groggy the next day. There was no history of the restless leg syndrome. The patient's bedpartner had not noted snoring or leg kicks.

*Physical Examination:* Blood pressure 120/76, pulse 80, temperature normal. Chest: clear to auscultation and percussion. Extremities: pressure on several points over the shoulders and back caused excruciating pain. Neurologic: normal.

*Laboratory Findings:* Complete blood cell count, thyroid studies: normal.

*Figure:* Below is a tracing obtained during a sleep study.

*Question:* What is your diagnosis?

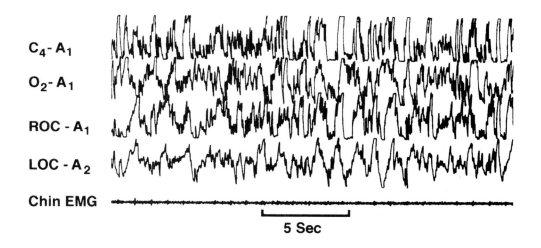

*Diagnosis:*   Fibromyalgia manifested as alpha-delta sleep.

*Discussion:*   Intrusion of alpha waves into slow wave sleep (alpha-delta sleep) was originally described in psychiatric patients, but the most well-known association is with fibrositis. Alpha-delta sleep is a **nonspecific polysomnographic finding.** It has been associated with rheumatoid arthritis, the posttraumatic stress syndrome, the chronic fatigue syndrome, and chronic pain syndromes. Other medical illnesses that disturb sleep can cause alpha-delta sleep, as well. Patients with alpha-delta sleep typically complain of **nonrestorative sleep** and **fatigue,** although frank, excessive daytime sleepiness usually is not prominent. The amount of alpha-delta sleep can vary considerably, and the amount of slow wave sleep often is decreased. Generally, no evidence of respiratory-related arousals or changes in the chin EMG is noted. Widespread alpha intrusion has been reported in some patients taking sedative-hypnotics. Therefore, diagnosis of alpha-delta sleep requires that the use of these medications be excluded.

**Fibromyalgia** is a syndrome usually affecting women that is associated with generalized musculoskeletal pain, chronic fatigue (without another explanation), widespread but localized tender points, and complaints of nonrestorative sleep. Despite these complaints, few objective findings are noted except for the tender points. Patients with fibromyalgia commonly show reductions in slow wave and REM sleep. However, in one study only 30% showed alpha-delta sleep. The usual treatment for sleep disturbance associated with fibromyalgia is **amitriptyline** (Elavil) 25–50 mg qhs. Amitriptyline may improve daytime symptoms as well as patient assessment of sleep quality, although alpha-delta sleep may persist. Complaints related to alpha-delta sleep and associated with other diseases, such as rheumatoid arthritis, also have been treated successfully with this medication. A recent study found that **fluoxetine** 20 mg qam or a combination of amitriptyline and fluoxetine was effective in treating patients with fibromyalgia.

In the present patient, monitoring showed alpha intrusion into slow wave sleep (see figure) consistent with alpha-delta sleep. This was not surprising given the history and physical findings. Treatment was begun with amitriptyline 25 mg qhs. The patient reported an improvement in perceived sleep quality and reduced musculoskeletal pain and fatigue.

## Clinical Pearls

1. Alpha-delta sleep is a polysomnographic finding that can be associated with psychiatric disease, fibromyalgia, rheumatoid arthritis, and chronic pain syndromes.

2. Alpha-delta sleep may be associated with complaints of nonrestorative sleep.

3. In fibromyalgia and other conditions associated with chronic pain, low doses of amitriptyline at bedtime or fluoxetine in the morning may improve sleep and daytime symptoms of pain.

REFERENCES
1. Hauri P, Hawkins DR: Alpha-delta sleep. Electroencephalogr Clin Neurophysiol 1973; 34:233–237.
2. Whittig RM, Zorick FJ, Blumer D, et al: Disturbed sleep in patients complaining of chronic pain. J Nerv Ment Dis 1982; 170:429–431.
3. Moldosky H, Lue FA, Smythe HA: Alpha EEG sleep and morning symptoms in rheumatoid arthritis. J Rheumatol 1983; 10:373–379.
4. Goldenberg D, Mayskiy M, Mossey C, et al: A randomized, double-blind trial of fluoxetine and amitriptyline in the treatment of fibromyalgia. Arthritis Rheum 1996; 39:1852–1859.

# PATIENT 97

## A 40-year-old woman with fatigue and disturbed sleep

A 40-year-old woman was evaluated for fatigue and disturbed sleep of 6-month duration. The patient went to bed at 11 PM and fell asleep in about 15 minutes. She reported about three awakenings nightly and an earlier-than-normal waketime (5:00 AM). During the day she felt very fatigued. There was no of history of cataplexy or sleep paralysis. The patient's husband reported that she frequently snored, but never kicked or moved her legs during sleep. She denied feeling depressed, but did admit to being under a lot of stress after a recent promotion and worrying that she was not spending enough time with her husband. There was no history of prior treatment for depression or episodes of mania.

*Physical Examination:*  Unremarkable.

*Sleep Study*  (Lights out 11:00 PM, Lights on 7:00 AM, Final awakening 5:10 AM)

| | | Sleep Stages | % SPT |
|---|---|---|---|
| Time in bed | 420 min (419–464) | | |
| Total sleep time | 302 min (402–449) | Stage Wage | 15 (0–11) |
| Sleep period time (SPT) | 355 min (408–456) | Stage 1 | 13 (3–7) |
| Sleep efficiency | .72 (.94–.98) | Stage 2 | 49 (51–64) |
| Sleep latency | 15 min (2–14) | Stages 3 and 4 | 2 (5–17) |
| REM latency | 40 min (65–99) | Stage REM | 21 (19–25) |
| Arousal index | 10/hr | | |
| | | AHI | 5/hr (<5) |
| | | PLM index | 0/hr |

*Question:*  What is causing the fatigue and sleep disturbance?

*Diagnosis:*   Major affective disorder—depression.

*Discussion:* Approximately 90% of patients with major depression complain of sleep disturbance. If the patient reports feelings of sadness and despair, the diagnosis is obvious. However, a patient may emphasize loss of energy and decreased appetite. Therefore, depression should be considered in anyone complaining of sleep disturbance and fatigue. A medical evaluation is essential to rule out anemia, hypothyroidism, and other causes of fatigue. Fifty percent of sleep studies performed in patients suffering from depression show objective abnormalities. Common findings include a **reduced REM latency**, **normal or increased amounts of REM sleep**, and **decreased stages 3 and 4 NREM sleep**. The REM latency typically is 40–60 minutes, but occasionally is in the range suggestive of narcolepsy (10–20 min). Additionally, the first REM episode is longer (20–25 minutes instead of the usual 10–15 minutes) and has a higher REM density than normal. These alterations in REM sleep may persist even after successful treatment of depression or between depressive episodes.

In patients with unipolar depression, insomnia with early-morning awakening usually is the major sleep complaint. Sleep complaints tend to be more pronounced in older patients. Typical sleep study findings are: increased sleep latency, decreased sleep efficiency, increased stage Wake and stage 1, reduced total sleep, and early-morning awakening. In the depressive phase of bipolar disorder, seasonal affective disorder, and atypical depression, hypersomnia typically is the major complaint, with a prolonged total sleep time and daytime sleepiness.

If the diagnosis of depression is obvious, a sleep study is not indicated unless another sleep disorder is suspected. The finding of a short REM latency by itself is not specific for depression, but in the absence of other pathology, it is suggestive. Sometimes it is difficult to determine if the major patient complaint is fatigue or daytime sleepiness. In addition, as stated above, some patients with depression complain of hypersomnia rather than sleep disturbance. Thus, the major utility of a sleep study is to rule out other sleep disorders. Psychological questionnaires also may help uncover suspected depression.

In the present case, a sleep study was ordered because of the history of snoring to rule out obstructive sleep apnea and the upper airway resistance syndrome. The study revealed a modestly shortened nocturnal REM latency, early-morning awakening, and an absence of evidence for sleep apnea and periodic leg movement. The upper airway resistance syndrome remained a possibility, but the arousal index was not very high. Interestingly, the first REM period was quite long (25 minutes) and the REM density (number of eye movements / time) was unusually high during this initial episode of REM. These findings suggested the presence of depression. Subsequently, symptoms of depression were explored in more detail when the sleep study results were discussed with the patient. At that time, she admitted that she felt torn between her responsibilities to her employer and to her husband and was overwhelmed at times. The patient was referred to a psychiatrist with whom she could explore these issues. Treatment with counseling and fluoxetine 20 mg qd resulted in improvement in symptoms and early-morning awakening.

# Clinical Pearls

1. A moderately short REM latency and a prolonged initial REM period with an increase in REM density is characteristic of depression. These findings may persist after successful treatment or be present between depressive episodes.

2. Depression can present with complaints of disturbed sleep and early-morning awakening (unipolar depression) or hypersomnia (bipolar depression).

3. Depression always should be considered when evaluating insomnia or excessive daytime sleepiness.

## REFERENCES

1. Rush AJ, Erman MK, Giles DE, et al: Polysomnographic findings in recently drug-free and clinically remitted depressed patients. Arch Gen Psychiatry 1986; 43:878–884.
2. Benca RM, Obermeyer WH, Thisted RA, et al: Sleep and psychiatric disorders: A meta-analysis. Arch Gen Psychiatry 1992; 49:651–668.

# PATIENT 98

**A 45-year-old man with persistent insomnia while on treatment for depression**

A 45-year-old man was referred by his psychiatrist for evaluation and treatment of insomnia. The patient had a long history of major depressive episodes, which generally responded to treatment with tricyclic antidepressants. However, he had difficulty with the side effects of the medication. The current episode was under treatment with fluoxetine 60 mg daily, and although the patient's energy level and feelings of sadness were much improved, he continued to have difficulty initiating and maintaining sleep. Frequent awakenings during the night were a major problem. The patient felt tired in the morning. There was no history of snoring, and the patient's wife reported an absence of leg kicks and apnea.

***Physical Examination:*** Height 6 feet, weight 200 pounds. Vital signs: normal. Neck: 16-inch circumference. Chest: clear. Cardiac: normal. Extremities: no edema.

***Question:*** What evaluation and treatment do you recommend?

*Diagnosis:*  Insomnia secondary to antidepressant therapy.

*Discussion:*  Insomnia is a common complaint of patients with depression. In patients with known depression, a sleep study adds little to the evaluation unless periodic limb movement in sleep is suspected. Today, most patients with mild-to-moderate depression are started on **selective serotonin reuptake inhibitors** (SSRIs), such as fluoxetine, paroxetine, sertaline, and luvoxetine. These agents have fewer **side effects** than the traditional tricyclic antidepressants. Unfortunately, insomnia is a common side effect of these medications.

Behavior techniques and improved sleep hygiene should be the first treatments of SSRI-induced insomnia. However, many patients may not respond. In these situations, low doses of **trazodone** (50–100 mg) at bedtime can be a useful adjunct to SSRI treatment. This medication also is sedating but has fewer anticholinergic side effects than tricyclic antidepressants. Men must be counseled about the side effect of priapism (persistent and painful erections). If a priapism occurs, surgery may be needed, as permanent impotence can result. Trazodone also can cause severe postural hypotension.

An alternative is the addition of a **benzodiazepine hypnotic** or the **nonbenzodiazepine hypnotic, zolpidem.**

A third option is to switch to a different type of antidepressant. **Nefazodone** is a mildly sedating antidepressant that is a useful treatment alternative in depressed patients with prominent insomnia. In one study comparing nefazodone and fluoxetine, both were effective antidepressants, but only nefazodone improved objective sleep quality. Interestingly, the fluoxetine group also reported subjective improvements in sleep quality. Thus, the traditional SSRIs may actually improve a patient's *perception* of sleep by improving *mood*. Nefazodone is a direct antagonist to postsynaptic serotonin receptors; it also inhibits the reuptake of serotonin and norepinephrine. It must be administered twice daily, and the most common side effect is dizziness. Nefazodone inhibits the cytochrome P450 system and has important potential drug interactions (cisapride should not be coadministered). Unlike most other antidepressants, it increases the amount of REM sleep and does not increase the REM latency. Bupropion is the only other available antidepressant that does not decrease REM sleep.

In the current case, since the patient's depression had responded so well to fluoxetine, trazadone 50 mg at bedtime was added to the regimen. On this combination of medications he reported improved sleep quality and felt rested on awakening in the morning.

## Clinical Pearls

1. Insomnia in depressed patients may be exacerbated by treatment with SSRIs.
2. The addition of a low dose of trazodone (50–100 mg) at bedtime may improve sleep in patients having persistent/worsened sleep difficulty on SSRI treatment.
3. Switching from an SSRI to nefazadone may improve sleep quality in patients with depression and persistent insomnia.

## REFERENCES
1. Nierenberg AA, Adler LA, Peselow E, et al: Trazodone for antidepressant-associated insomnia. Am J Psychiatry 1994; 151:1069.
2. Neylan TC: Treatment of sleep disturbance in depressed patients. J Clin Psychiatry 1995; 56(suppl 2):56–61.
3. Gillin JC, Rapaport M, Erman MK, et al: A comparison of nefazodone and fluoxetine on mood and on objective, subject, and clinician-rated measures of sleep in depressed patients. J Clin Psychiatry 1997; 58:186–192.

# PATIENT 99

## A 45-year-old man with hyperphagia and hypersomnia

A 45-year-old man was evaluated for a 6-month history of daytime sleepiness. During this time he had developed a tremendous appetite and had gained 20 pounds. He also had increased difficulty dealing with the stresses of his job. His wife reported that he was hypersensitive to criticism and that he seemed to believe she did not love him anymore. The patient usually retired at 10 PM and slept until the alarm clock awakened him at 6:30 AM. He had tremendous difficulty getting out of bed and was late to work on several occasions. On the weekends he sometimes slept from 11 PM until 10–11 AM. The patient was reported to snore, but his wife had not noticed any pauses in breathing.

***Physical Examination:*** Height 5 feet 11 inches, weight 210 pounds. Neck: 16 inch-circumference. HEENT: slightly edematous uvula. Chest: clear. Cardiac: normal. Extremities: no edema.

***Sleep Study*** (Lights out 10:30 PM, Lights on 6:00 AM)

| | | Sleep Stages | % SPT |
|---|---|---|---|
| Time in bed | 450 min (390–468) | | |
| Total sleep time | 391.5 min (343–436) | Stage Wake | 10 (1–12) |
| Sleep period time (SPT) | 435 min (378–452) | Stage 1 | 6 (5–11) |
| WASO | 43.5 min | Stage 2 | 60 (44–66) |
| Sleep efficiency | .87 (.85–.97) | Stages 3 and 4 | 4 (2–15) |
| Sleep latency | 15 min (2–18) | Stage REM | 20 (19–27) |
| REM latency | 40 min (55–78) | | |
| Arousal index | 15/hr | AHI | 5/hr |
| | | PLM index | 0/hr |

( ) = normal values for age, AHI = apnea + hypopnea index, PLM = periodic limb movement

***Question:*** What is causing this patient's hypersomnia?

*Diagnosis:*  Atypical depression.

*Discussion:*  A majority of patients with major depression present with complaints of disturbed sleep. In most cases, insomnia and fatigue are the major complaints, rather than daytime sleepiness. However, hypersomnia is commonly noted in patients experiencing the depressive phase of bipolar disorder, seasonal affective disorder (winter depression), or atypical depression. Atypical depression is characterized by **weight gain** (hyperphagia), **rejection hypersensitivity, hypersomnia,** and **leaden paralysis** (heavy feeling in the extremities). Treatment of depressed patients with hypersomnia typically involves selective serotonin reuptake inhibitors (fluoxetine, in particular) because these drugs are not sedating. Patients not responding to SSRIs have been treated with MAO inhibitors, but these drugs have the potential for serious drug and food interactions. In bipolar patients, adjunctive treatment with mood stabilizers is indicated to avoid inducing a manic episode. Seasonal affective disorder often responds to light therapy.

The differential diagnosis of hypersomnia with depression includes recurrent hypersomnia, sleep apnea, and PLM. Recurrent hypersomnia (Kleine-Levin syndrome) is characterized by episodes (at least once or twice yearly) lasting 3–21 days and featuring voracious eating, hypersexuality, and disinhibited behavior (e.g., irritability, aggression). Monosymptomatic forms (hypersomnolence only) also exist. This disorder typically affects males and starts in adolescence. Onset in adulthood and occurrence in women have been described. During intervals between periods of somnolence, individuals appear normal.

In the present case, the history of snoring and weight gain prompted a sleep study to rule out obstructive sleep apnea. The study showed minimal amounts of apnea. The upper airway resistance syndrome also was considered, but the arousal index was low. While personality change can be noted with obstructive sleep apnea, the rapidity of onset made this seem less likely. The REM latency was moderately short—a characteristic of a variety of disorders, including sleep apnea, narcolepsy, and depression. However, there was no history consistent with narcolepsy. Onset of recurrent hypersomnia is unlikely at age 45. Given the weight gain, hypersomnia, and recent onset of problems dealing with criticism and rejection, the diagnosis of atypical depression was considered a likely possibility, and the patient was referred to a psychiatrist for evaluation. Treatment with fluoxetine produced considerable improvement within 4 weeks, and the patient lost about 10 pounds. The symptoms of daytime sleepiness resolved.

# Clinical Pearls

1. The depressive phase of bipolar disorder, atypical depression, and seasonal affective disorder (winter depression) can present with symptoms of hypersomnia.

2. Patients with atypical depression may gain weight (hyperphagia) and thus may trigger a suspicion of sleep apnea.

## REFERENCES
1. Billard M, Dolenc L, Aldaz C, et al: Hypersomnia associated with mood disorders: A new perspective. J Psychosom Res 1994; 38(suppl 1):41–47.
2. Benca RM: Sleep in psychiatric disorders. Neurol Clin 1996; 14:740–748.
3. Pande AC, Birkett M, Fechner-Bates S, et al: Fluoxetine versus phenelzine in atypical depression. Biol Psychiatry 1996; 40:1017–1020.

# PATIENT 100

## A 50-year-old veteran of the Vietnam War with upsetting dreams

A 50-year-old man was evaluated for recurrent awakenings with frightening dreams at night. These awakenings had been a frequent problem since his service in the Vietnam War. The dreams often were related to memories of combat, and when they occurred he could not go back to sleep. The patient reported difficulty falling asleep on some nights, and he generally felt unrefreshed in the morning. His wife reported that he frequently thrashed about during the night while asleep. There was no history of snoring. Previous treatment with benzodiazepines had not improved his symptoms.

***Physical Examination:*** Unremarkable.

***Sleep Study***

| | | | |
|---|---|---|---|
| Time in bed | 470 min (378–468) | Sleep Stages | % SPT |
| Total sleep time | 365.5 min (340–439) | Stage Wake | 15 (2–7) |
| Sleep period time (SPT) | 430 min (361–453) | Stage 1 | 14 (4–12) |
| WASO | 64.5 min | Stage 2 | 51 (51–72) |
| Sleep efficiency | .78 (.88–.96) | Stages 3 and 4 | 0 (0–13) |
| Sleep latency | 30 min (1–22) | Stage REM | 20 (17–25) |
| REM latency | 70 min (65–104) | | |
| Arousal index | 30/hr | AHI | 4/hr |
| | | PLM index | 5/hr |

( ) = normal values for age, AHI = apnea + hypopnea index, PLM = periodic limb movement

***Question:*** What is causing the patient's sleep disturbance?

*Diagnosis:* Post-traumatic stress disorder.

*Discussion:* The post-traumatic stress disorder (PTSD) occurs in individuals who have experienced a traumatic event in their life, such as combat, physical attack, natural disaster, or traumatic injury. The disorder is characterized by reexperiencing the events in **flashbacks**, **intrusive recollections**, or **recurrent dreams**. While it once was thought that complex dreaming is confined to REM sleep, recent studies suggest dreams may occur in both REM and NREM sleep. Symptoms of PTSD can begin immediately after the event or have a delayed onset (up to years later). Patients with PTSD also report a heightened startle response. Given a common exposure to a traumatic event, PTSD appears to occur more frequently in women than men. Patients with PTSD also may have depression and may abuse ethanol or other substances.

The differential of awakening with anxiety includes sleep panic disorder, REM behavior disorder, and night terrors. Unlike patients with panic attacks during sleep, patients with PTSD can recount a dream of a specific traumatic event. In contrast to night terrors, patients become alert quickly after awakening. Sleep studies in patients with PTSD have produced conflicting results. The duration of REM latency and the amount of REM sleep have varied among studies. This may be a reflection of the fact that some patients with PTSD also are suffering from depression. Several studies have found in increase in REM density in patients with PTSD (as in depression), an increase in body movements during sleep, and the presence of periodic limb movements (PLM) in sleep.

The treatment of PTSD includes counseling and medication. Although many patients with PTSD have anxiety, benzodiazepines have not been effective, and withdrawal of these medications may produce a flair of symptoms. Any REM-suppressing medication might decrease the incidence of nightmares. However, medications without REM suppression also have been effective. Treatment with tricyclic antidepressants, MAO inhibitors, and selective serotonin reuptake inhibitors such as fluoxetine have been shown to be effective in selected patient groups. Open-label studies have found nefazadone and low doses of anticonvulsant medications (e.g., carbmazepine, valproate) to be helpful in some patients. Anticonvulsants do not decrease the amount of REM sleep. Patients with PTSD are a heterogeneous group, and if one medication does not work, others should be tried. For example, fluoxetine is activating and may increase anxiety or sleep disturbance. Nefazadone is mildly sedating, may cause less sexual dysfunction, and may be better tolerated in anxious patients. The main side effect of this medication is dizziness, and severe drug interactions can occur as nefazadone inhibits the cytochrome P450 system (cisapride and terfenadine are contraindicated). Clonidine and propanolol also have been used for severe anxiety symptoms. Abrupt withdrawal of any of the aforementioned medications can induce a rebound in symptom severity. When starting a new medication, it is wise to start with a low dose and titrate upward slowly.

In the present patient, a sleep study was ordered to rule out PLM (history of thrashing around in bed). However, no significant amount of PLM was noted. The sleep study shows a reduced sleep efficiency with increased waketime during the night, and stages 3 and 4 are absent. The patient was started on low-dose amitriptyline (50 mg qhs), resulting in improved sleep and fewer nightmares; however, he felt groggy the next day. This symptom usually resolves after 2 weeks of treatment, but it did not resolve in this patient. Medication was switched to fluoxetine, and nightmares were reduced. However, the patient reported continued frequent awakenings on this medication and increased anxiety during the day. Nefazadone was started at 100 mg po bid, and the patient reported improved sleep and a decrease in nightmares. His wife also noted less thrashing around in bed.

## Clinical Pearls

1. Sleep disturbance and awakenings with frightening dreams are common manifestations of PTSD.

2. Patients with PTSD have increased REM density but variable amounts of REM sleep.

3. Increased body movements and PLM during sleep also have been reported in PTSD.

4. A wide variety of medications are successful in different patient groups. Treatment must be individualized.

# REFERENCES

1. Ross RJ, Ball WA, Dinges DR, et al: Rapid eye movement sleep disturbance in posttraumatic stress disorder. Biol Psychiatry 1994; 35:195–202.
2. Brown TM, Boudewyns PA: Periodic limb movements of sleep in combat veterans with posttraumatic stress disorder. J Trauma Stress 1996; 9:129–136.
3. Davidson JR: Biological therapies for posttraumatic stress disorder: An overview. J Clin Psychiatry 1997; 58(Suppl 9):29–32.
4. Mellman TA, Nolan B, Hedding J, et al: A polysomnographic comparison of veterans with combat-related PTSD, depressed men, and non-ill controls. Sleep 1997; 20:46–51.

# PATIENT 101

## A 40-year-old woman with terrifying awakenings

A 40-year-old woman was evaluated for episodes of awakening from sleep with intense anxiety and fear. These awakenings were first noted at age 38. Similar attacks sometimes occurred during wakefulness, but they did not seem as intense. The patient experienced shortness of breath, palpitations, diaphoresis, and chest pain during these episodes, which usually occurred within 1–2 hours of bedtime. During one of the episodes she had been admitted to a hospital to rule out myocardial infarction. A subsequent evaluation for cardiac disease was negative. The patient denied having frightening dreams preceding the attacks and was able to remember the episodes the following morning. Previously, the patient was under the care of a psychiatrist for phobias related to elevators.

*Physical Examination:* Unremarkable.

*Question:* What treatment do you recommend?

***Diagnosis:*** Sleep panic attack.

***Discussion:*** Panic attacks are repeated occurrences of extreme anxiety accompanied by at least four of the associated symptoms: shortness of breath, choking, palpitations, chest pain, sweating, dizziness, nausea, paresthesia, fear of dying, flushing, and chills. Although panic attacks usually take place while the patient is awake, up to one-third of patients report nocturnal panic attacks as well. The attacks occur from NREM sleep, commonly at the transition from stage 2 to stages 3 and 4 sleep.

The differential of panic attacks includes night terrors, nightmares, post-traumatic stress disorder, and REM behavior disorder. Night terrors usually begin in childhood, and the effected individual is not well aware of his or her surroundings and does not remember the episodes in the morning. In nightmares, the patient usually is aware of a frightening dream. In contrast, patients with panic attacks remember the episode, but typically do not report a terrifying dream.

The treatment of panic attacks includes behavioral psychotherapy or relaxation techniques and pharmacotherapy. Although benzodiazepines (e.g., alprazolam, clonazepam) were the classic treatments for panic disorder, many psychiatrists prefer a trial of selective serotonin reuptake inhibitors (SSRIs) or tricyclic antidepressants. Both SSRIs (e.g., paroxetine, sertaline) and tricyclic antidepressants (e.g., imipramine) must be started at very low doses or panic attacks initially may be exacerbated. For example, paroxetine is started at 10 mg daily or imipramine at 10–25 mg daily. The doses are slowly increased to 20–40 mg for paroxetine or 100–200 mg for imipramine, as tolerated. As improvements may take 4–6 weeks or longer, some physicians add benzodiazepines during the early course of therapy.

In the present case, the patient was referred for psychiatric treatment. She was started on clonazepam 1 mg and imipramine 10 mg at bedtime. Over the next 2 months, the imipramine was slowly increased to 100 mg daily, and clonazepam was discontinued. The patient noted almost complete resolution of the nocturnal attacks.

# Clinical Pearls

1. Patients with sleep panic attacks usually have similar episodes when awake.
2. Treatment with benzodiazepines or tricyclic antidepressants usually is effective.

## REFERENCES

1. Mellman TA, Ude TW: Patients with frequent sleep panic: Clinical findings and response to medication treatment. J Clin Psychiatry 1990; 51:513–516.
2. Benca RM: Sleep in psychiatric disorders. Neurol Clin 1996; 14:750–751.
3. Hahn RK, Albers LJ, Reist C: Psychiatry—Current Clinical Strategies. Laguna Hills, CA, Current Clinical Strategies Publishing, 1997, pp 46–48.

## Sleep Disorders Classification

Sleep disorders comprise a diverse set of syndromes. The Diagnostic Classification of Sleep and Arousal Disorders (published in 1979) divided sleep disorders on the basis of the presenting complaint. The major categories included: disorders of initiating and maintaining sleep (DIMS), disorders of excessive sleepiness (DOES), parasomnias, and disorders of the sleep-wake schedule. Some disorders appeared in more than one category. Subsequently, the International Classification of Sleep Disorders (ICSD; published in 1990) used a different approach. Sleep disorders directly affecting sleep (dyssomnias) were classified on the basis of whether they developed from internal, external, or circadian rhythm causes. The 1997 revised classification outline appears below. The reader is referred to the valuable text by the American Sleep Disorders Association from which it comes.*

1. DYSSOMNIAS
   A. Intrinsic Sleep Disorders
      1. Psychophysiologic Insomnia
      2. Sleep State Misperception
      3. Idiopathic Insomnia
      4. Narcolepsy
      5. Recurrent Hypersomnia
      6. Idiopathic Hypersomnia
      7. Post-traumatic Hypersomnia
      8. Obstructive Sleep Apnea Syndrome
      9. Central Sleep Apnea Syndrome
      10. Central Alveolar Hypoventilation Syndrome
      11. Periodic Limb Movement Disorder
      12. Restless Legs Syndrome
      13. Intrinsic Sleep Disorder Not Otherwise Specified (NOS)
   B. Extrinsic Sleep Disorders
      1. Inadequate Sleep Hygiene
      2. Environmental Sleep Disorder
      3. Altitude Insomnia
      4. Adjustment Sleep Disorder
      5. Insufficient Sleep Syndrome
      6. Limit-setting Sleep Disorder
      7. Sleep-onset Association Disorder
      8. Food Allergy Insomnia
      9. Nocturnal Eating (Drinking) Syndrome
      10. Hypnotic-Dependent Sleep Disorder
      11. Stimulant-Dependent Sleep Disorder
      12. Alcohol-Dependent Sleep Disorder
      13. Toxin-Induced Sleep Disorder
      14. Extrinsic Sleep Disorder NOS
   C. Circadian-Rhythm Sleep Disorders
      1. Time Zone Change (Jet Lag) Syndrome
      2. Shift Work Sleep Disorder
      3. Irregular Sleep-Wake Pattern
      4. Delayed Sleep-Phase Syndrome
      5. Advanced Sleep-Phase Syndrome
      6. Non-24-Hour Sleep-Wake Disorder
      7. Circadian Rhythm Sleep Disorder NOS

2. PARASOMNIAS
   A. Arousal Disorders

        1. Confusional Arousals
        2. Sleepwalking
        3. Sleep Terrors
    B. Sleep-Wake Transition Disorders
        1. Rhythmic Movement Disorder
        2. Sleep Starts
        3. Sleep Talking
        4. Nocturnal Leg Cramps
    C. Parasomnias Usually Associated with REM Sleep
        1. Nightmares
        2. Sleep Paralysis
        3. Impaired Sleep-Related Penile Erections
        4. Sleep-Related Painful Erections
        5. REM Sleep-Related Sinus Arrest
        6. REM Sleep Behavior Disorder
    D. Other Parasomnias
        1. Sleep Bruxism
        2. Sleep Enuresis
        3. Sleep-Related Abnormal Swallowing Syndrome
        4. Nocturnal Paroxysmal Dystonia
        5. Sudden Unexplained Nocturnal Death Syndrome
        6. Primary Snoring
        7. Infant Sleep Apnea
        8. Congenital Central Hypoventilation Syndrome
        9. Sudden Infant Death Syndrome
        10. Benign Neonatal Sleep Myoclonus
        11. Other Parasomnia NOS

3. SLEEP DISORDERS ASSOCIATED WITH MENTAL, NEUROLOGIC, OR OTHER MEDICAL DISORDERS
    A. Associated with Mental Disorders
        1. Psychoses
        2. Mood Disorders
        3. Anxiety Disorders
        4. Panic Disorders
        5. Alcoholism
    B. Associated with Neurologic Disorders
        1. Cerebral Degenerative Disorders
        2. Dementia
        3. Parkinsonism
        4. Fatal Familial Insomnia
        5. Sleep-Related Epilepsy
        6. Electrical Status Epilepticus of Sleep
        7. Sleep-Related Headaches
    C. Associated with Other Medical Disorders
        1. Sleeping Sickness
        2. Nocturnal Cardiac Ischemia
        3. Chronic Obstructive Pulmonary Disease
        4. Sleep-Related Asthma
        5. Sleep-Related Gastroesophageal Reflux
        6. Peptic Ulcer Disease
        7. Fibromyalgia

4. PROPOSED SLEEP DISORDERS
    1. Short Sleeper
    2. Long Sleeper
    3. Subwakefulness Syndrome
    4. Fragmentary Myoclonus
    5. Sleep Hyperhidrosis
    6. Menstrual-Associated Sleep Disorder
    7. Pregnancy-Associated Sleep Disorder
    8. Terrifying Hypnagogic Hallucinations
    9. Sleep-Related Neurogenic Tachypnea
    10. Sleep-Related Laryngospasm
    11. Sleep Choking Syndrome

*Reprinted from American Sleep Disorders Association: International Classification of Sleep Disorders. Rochester, Minnesota, ASDA, 1997; with permission.

## Sleep Stage Characteristics

| Stage | Characteristics | | |
|---|---|---|---|
| | EEG | EOG | EMG |
| Wake (eyes open) | Low voltage, high frequency<br>Attenuated alpha activity | Eye blinks, REMs | Relatively high |
| Wake (eyes closed) | Low voltage, high frequency<br>> 50% alpha activity | Slow rolling eye movements | Relatively high |
| Stage 1 | Low amplitude, mixed frequency<br>**< 50% alpha activity**<br>**No spindles, K complexes**<br>Sharp waves near transition to stage 2 | Slow rolling eye movements | May be lower than in stage Wake |
| Stage 2 | **At least one sleep spindle or K complex**<br>**< 20% slow wave activity** | | May be lower than in stage Wake |
| Stage 3 | **20–50% slow wave activity** | | Usually low |
| Stage 4 | **> 50% slow wave activity** | | Usually low |
| Stage REM | **Low voltage, mixed frequency**<br>Saw tooth waves may be present | **Episodic REMs** | **Relatively reduced**<br>(equal or lower than the lowest in NREM) |

Notes:  Required characteristics for the determination of each stage are in boldface.  Slow wave activity has a frequency < 2 Hz and a peak to peak amplitude > 75 microvolts.

EEG = electroencephalogram, EOG = electro-oculogram, EMG = electromyogram, REM = rapid eye movements, NREM = non-rapid eye movements.

### Disorders Causing Excessive Daytime Sleepiness

Sleep apnea syndromes
Upper airway resistance syndrome
Narcolepsy
Depression
Periodic leg (limb) movements in sleep
Idiopathic hypersomnia
Withdrawal from stimulants
Inadequate sleep
Sedatives/medications
Post-traumatic hypersomnia

### Common Causes of Insomnia

| Primary Insomnia | Secondary* Insomnia |
|---|---|
| Psychophysiological | Other sleep disorders (sleep apnea, PLM) |
|   Acute (adjustment sleep disorder) | Psychiatric disorders (depression, panic attacks) |
|   Chronic | Drugs (nicotine, ethanol, caffeine) |
| Idiopathic | Medical conditions/medications |
| Sleep state misperception |   Fibromyalgia and chronic pain syndromes |
| |   COPD and other respiratory disorders |
| |   Medications for illness (theophylline, beta blockers) |
| | Circadian disorders |
| |   Delayed sleep-phase syndrome |
| |   Advanced sleep-phase syndrome |
| |   Shift work or jet lag syndrome |
| | Inadequate sleep hygiene |
| | Environmental sleep disorder |

*Secondary means another disorder can be diagnosed.
PLM = periodic leg movement, COPD = chronic obstructive pulmonary disease

**Advanced sleep-phase syndrome (ASPS)**—characterized by early sleep onset and final waketime relative to societal (clock) norms in the external world.

**Alpha activity**—EEG activity at 8–13 Hz

**Alpha-delta sleep**—prominent alpha activity occurring during slow wave sleep.

**Amplitude**—the magnitude of deflection in a signal; units depend on calibration. For slow wave activity, refers to peak-to-peak deflection.

**Apnea**—absence of airflow at the nose and mouth for 10 seconds or longer.

**Apnea + hypopnea index (AHI)**—the number of apneas and hypopneas per hour of sleep, expressed as total number/total sleep time in hours. Also called the respiratory disturbance index (RDI).

**Arousal**—abrupt awakening from sleep which may be brief. In NREM sleep, an abrupt shift in EEG frequency longer than 3 seconds; in REM sleep, the EMG also must show augmentation to qualify as an arousal (ASDA definition).

**ASDA**—American Sleep Disorders Association.

**Beta activity**—EEG activity > 13 Hz.

**Biocalibration**—the initial recording of maneuvers during wakefulness to determine if the corresponding deflections in EEG, EOG, chin EMG, leg EMG, and airflow channels are satisfactory and to adjust amplifier gains, if necessary.

**Bilevel pressure**—method of ventilation allowing separate pressure levels in inspiration (inspiratory positive airway pressure) and expiration (expiratory positive airway pressure).

**$C_4(C_3)$**—central EEG electrode on the right (left) side of the head.

**Calibration**—adjustment of amplifier baseline and gain. In polysomnography, the settings of EEG, EOG, and EMG amplifiers are adjusted so that a known reference square wave input voltage elicits the desired pen deflections (or output voltage deflections). The low and high filter settings at the time of calibration are documented, as these affect the amplitude and shape of the deflections for a given calibration voltage.

**Cataplexy**—sudden loss of muscle tone (especially antigravity muscles) at moments of high emotion (e.g., surprise, laughter, fear); characteristic of narcolepsy.

**Central apnea**—apnea associated with an absence of respiratory effort.

**Cheyne-Stokes breathing**—crescendo-decrescendo pattern of breathing with central apneas or hypopneas at the nadir.

**Chronic obstructive pulmonary disease (COPD)**—chronic bronchitis, emphysema, or a mixture.

**Continuous positive airway pressure (CPAP)**—maintenance of positive airway pressure during inspiration and expiration.

**Delayed sleep-phase syndrome (DSPS)**—characterized by delayed sleep onset and final waketime relative to societal (clock) norms in the external world.

**Delta activity**—EEG activity at < 4 Hz.

**Derivation**—the choice of two electrodes providing input to a differential amplifier (e.g., $C_4$-$A_1$).

**Desaturation**—fall in arterial oxygen saturation ≥ 4% from baseline.

**Diurnal**—pertaining to daytime.

**Early-morning awakening**—final awakening earlier than expected; characteristic of depression.

**Electroencephalogram (EEG)**—recording of brain electrical activity.

**Electromyogram (EMG)**—recording of the electrical activity of a muscle. In routine sleep monitoring, surface electrodes monitor EMG activity in the chin area.

**Electro-oculogram (EOG)**—recording of the electrical activity generated during eye movements.

**Epoch**—a period of time usually corresponding to 30 seconds (one page of recording at a paper speed of 10 mm/sec).

**Forced expiratory volume (FEV)**—$FEV_1$ is the volume of air in liters exhaled in the first 1 second of a maximal forced vital capacity maneuver. In this text, normal is assumed to be 80–120% of predicted.

**Forced vital capacity (FVC)**—volume of air in liters exhaled from maximal inhalation (total lung capacity) to residual volume (maximal exhalation) during a forced maneuver. In this text, normal is assumed to be 80–120% of predicted.

**Hypnagogic**—an event occurring on transition from wake to sleep.

**Hypnagogic hallucination**—vivid imagery at sleep onset; a feature of narcolepsy in which REM periods occur at sleep onset.

**Hypnopompic**—an event occurring on transition from sleep to wakefulness.

**Hypopnea**—reduction in airflow (usually by 30–50% of baseline) for 10 seconds or longer. Many clinicians also require either an associated arousal or an arterial oxygen desaturation of 2–4%.

**K complex**—large-amplitude biphasic deflection of 0.5-second or longer duration; a negative (up) sharp wave followed by a positive (down) slow wave.

**Left outer canthus (LOC)**—electrode placed lateral to the outer corner of the left eye.

**Maintenance of wakefulness test (MWT)**—test to determine the ability to stay awake.

**Mean sleep latency**—the mean of sleep latencies recorded during naps of the MSLT.

**Mixed apnea**—apnea composed of an initial central part followed by an obstructive component.

**Montage**—the particular arrangement of electrodes by which a number of derivations are displayed simultaneously in a polysomnogram.

**Multiple sleep latency test (MSLT)**—test to determine the mean sleep latency during daytime naps as an objective measure of daytime sleepiness. The presence/absence of REM sleep during the naps also is determined.

**Non-REM (NREM) sleep**—sleep stages 1, 2, 3, and 4.

**$O_2(O_1)$**—occipital EEG electrode on the right (left) side of the head.

**Obesity-hypoventilation syndrome (OHS)**—daytime hypoventilation (hypercapnia) not secondary to lung disease in an obese patient, usually accompanied by severe obstructive sleep apnea.

**Obstructive apnea**—apnea with persistent respiratory effort.

**Obstructive sleep apnea (OSA)**—syndrome characterized by obstructive and mixed apnea and hypopneas, as well as excessive daytime sleepiness.

**Overlap syndrome**—OSA + COPD.

**Parasomnia**—a condition associated with or occurring from sleep. Disorders of arousal or partial arousal. Examples include sleep walking, night terrors, and REM behavior disorder.

**Periodic leg (limb) movement (PLM)**—leg (arm) movements, such as foot flexion, big toe extension, and partial flexion at hip and knee, of about 1-second duration that occur every 20–60 seconds during sleep.

**Periodic leg movement index (PLM index)**—number of movements per hour of sleep.

**Periodic leg movement–arousal index (PLM-arousal index)**—number of periodic leg movements associated with arousal per hour of sleep.

**Phasic REM sleep**—REM sleep in which rapid eye movements are present.

**Popping artifact**—high-voltage artifact caused by temporary disconnection of electrodes from the skin.

**Rapid eye movement (REM)**—a sharp (short duration) eye movement.

**Rapid eye movement behavior disorder (RBD)**—a parasomnia occurring from REM sleep associated with body movement and violent behavior.

**Rapid eye movement density**—number of eye movements per time in REM sleep. Normally highest during the last REM periods of the night.

**Rapid eye movement sleep**—a sleep stage characterized by a low-voltage, mixed-frequency EEG; episodic rapid eye movements; and a relatively low-amplitude EMG.

**Recording time; time in bed (TIB)**—total time of sleep monitoring from lights out to lights on.

**REM latency**—time from sleep onset to the start of stage REM.

**Respiratory disturbance index (RDI)**—equivalent to the apnea + hypopnea index.

**Restless leg syndrome (RLS)**—syndrome marked by creeping sensation in the legs that can be temporarily relieved by movement.

**Right outer canthus (ROC)**—electrode placed lateral to the outer corner of the right eye.

**Saw tooth waves**—form of theta rhythm (jagged up and down) seen in stage REM.

**Sharp wave** (vertex sharp wave)—high-voltage, brief, negative (up) wave present in stage 1 near transition to stage 2.

**Sleep architecture**—the relative amounts of the different sleep stages composing sleep and timing of sleep cycles (also see Fundamentals of Sleep Medicine 7).

**Sleep efficiency**—usually defined as total sleep time * 100 / time in bed.

**Sleep hygiene**—conditions and practices that promote continuous and effective sleep.

**Sleep latency**—time from lights out (start of monitoring period) to the first epoch of any stage of sleep.

**Sleep maintenance insomnia**—difficulty maintaining sleep; frequent awakenings.

**Sleep onset insomnia**—difficulty falling asleep.

**Sleep paralysis**—inability to move while still awake at sleep onset (hypnagogic) or at the end of a sleep period (hypnopompic).

**Sleep period time (SPT)**—time from sleep onset until the final awakening; total sleep time (TST) plus wake after sleep onset (WASO).

**Sleep spindle**—EEG activity of 12–14 Hz occurring in bursts of 0.5-second or longer duration; characteristic of stage 2 sleep but can be seen in stages 3 and 4.

**Sleep stages**—(also see Appendix II)

**Stage 1**—sleep characterized by a low-voltage, mixed-frequency EEG; an absence of sleep spindles and K complexes; and an epoch with < 50% alpha activity.

**Stage 2**—sleep characterized by an EEG showing at least one sleep spindle or K complex and an epoch with < 20% slow wave activity (see three-minute rule).

**Stage 3**—sleep with an EEG showing slow wave activity meeting the voltage criteria for 20–50% of the epoch.

**Stage 4**—sleep with an EEG showing slow wave activity meeting the voltage criteria for > 50% of the epoch.

**Sleep terrors**—a parasomnia characterized by sudden awakening from NREM sleep (usually stages 3 and 4) with a cry or scream, confusion, and autonomic hyperactivity.

**Sleep walking (somnambulism)**—characterized by a partial awakening from NREM sleep (classically from stages 3 and 4) with complex movements including walking.

**Slow rolling eye movement**—smooth, undulating eye movements occurring during drowsy wakefulness and stage 1 sleep.

**Slow wave activity**—by convention, oscillations slower than 2 Hz ( > 0.5 seconds in duration) with a minimal peak-to-peak amplitude of 75 microvolts.

**Slow waves (delta waves)**—EEG waves with a frequency of 1–4 Hz.

**Stage REM**—*see* Rapid eye movement sleep.

**Sweat artifact**—slow undulations in EEG and EOG tracings secondary to sweat.

**Ten-twenty system**—an international standard for the placement of EEG electrodes in which spacing of electrodes is 10% or 20% of the distance between landmarks on the head.

**Theta activity**—EEG activity at 4–7 Hz.

**Three-minute rule**—epochs of sleep between two spindles or K complexes that otherwise would be scored as stage 2 sleep are scored as stage 1 if the time between the spindles/K complexes is ≥ 3 minutes and as stage 2 if the time is < 3 minutes.

**Time in bed (TIB); recording time**—total monitoring time, from lights out to lights on.

**Tonic REM sleep**—REM sleep in which rapid eye movements are absent.

**Total sleep time (TST)**—total minutes of stages 1, 2, 3, and 4, and REM.

**Upper airway resistance syndrome (UARS)**—syndrome characterized by daytime sleepiness secondary to frequent arousals related to increased respiratory effort during periods of high upper airway resistance (narrowing) without a high amount of frank apnea or hypopnea.

**Uvulopalatopharyngoplasty (UPPP)**—an upper airway surgery for sleep apnea and snoring; the uvula, a portion of the soft palate, and excess pharyngeal tissues are removed.

**Wake after sleep onset (WASO)**—wake after sleep onset but before the final awakening.

# INDEX

Abdominal movement
  during hypopnea, 81
  during obstructive sleep apnea, 72, 75, 79
Acetazolamide, as idiopathic central sleep apnea treatment, 176
Acromegaly, obstructive sleep apnea associated with, 76
Adenoid-tonsillar hypertrophy, 155–156
Adjustment sleep disorder, 228, 232–234
Advanced sleep-phase syndrome, 238–239
  definition of, 263
Airflow, diurnal variation in, 170
Airflow monitoring
  for apnea evaluation, 71–73
  nasal, 49
  oral, 49
  polysomnographic, 49, 50, 51
  temperature-sensitive devices for, 73
Airflow profile, of upper airway resistance syndrome, 136
Airway function, circadian rhythm of, 170
Airway obstruction, as obstructive and mixed apneas cause, 79
Alcohol use
  avoidance of, as snoring treatment, 13
  as insomnia cause, 230
  as obstructive sleep apnea cause, 94–95
  as snoring cause, 13, 95, 130, 131
  sleep architecture effects of, 46
Alertness
  relationship to maintenance of wakefulness test latency, 125
  requirements for, 86
Alpha activity
  definition of, 263
  during sleep onset, 22
  during sleep stage 1, 24
  during wakefulness, 5–6
Alpha-delta sleep
  definition of, 263
  fibromyalgia manifested as, 243–244
American Sleep Disorders Association, 257, 263
American Thoracic Society, 127
Amitriptyline, as fibromyalgia treatment, 244
Amnesia, night terrors-related, 221
Amplitude, definition of, 263
Anemia, iron-deficiency, as restless leg syndrome cause, 190
Antidepressants, as insomnia cause, 247–248
Apnea
  central, 69
    Cheyne-Stokes breathing associated with, 178, 179–180, 182
    congestive heart failure associated with, 76

Apnea (*Cont.*)
    definition of, 263
    idiopathic, 172–174, 175–176
    oxygen therapy-related decrease of, 154
  definition of, 69, 263
  as excessive daytime sleepiness cause, 76, 261
  exhaled carbon dioxide fluctuations during, 71–73
  mixed, 69, 78–79
    Cheyne-Stokes breathing associated with, 177–178, 181–182
    definition of, 264
    oxygen therapy-related decrease of, 154
  obstructive. *See* Obstructive sleep apnea
Apnea-hypopnea index
  in children, 156
  definition of, 69–70, 263
  in obstructive hypopnea, 81
  in obstructive sleep apnea, 86, 93, 95
    effect of weight loss on, 97
  in positional sleep apnea, 120
  in severe sleep apnea, 88
  uvolopalatopharyngoplasty-related reduction of, 111, 112
Apnea index, definition of, 69
Arousal
  central sleep apnea-related, 173
  definition of, 1, 263
  electrocortical, 34
  hypopnea-related, 81
  implication for sleep staging, 41, 42
  inspiratory effort-related, 136
  night terrors-related, 221
  periodic limb movements-related, 186, 187–188
  in REM sleep, 34
  respiratory effort-related, 85, 90
  somnambulism-related, 221
  upper airway resistance syndrome-related, 85
Arousal index
  in excessive daytime sleepines, 34
  in severe sleep apnea, 88
  in upper airway resistance syndrome, 85, 95
Arrhythmias, obstructive sleep apnea-related, 143–145
Arterial oxygen desaturation ($SaO_2$), 70
  alcohol use-related exacerbation of, 95
  chronic obstructive pulmonary disease-related, 157–159, 160–161, 166, 167
    low-flow oxygen therapy for, 162–163
    with obstructive sleep apnea, 166–168
  as heart failure cause, 86
  hypopnea-related, 81
  obstructive sleep apnea-related, 154
  in post-polio syndrome patients, 184
  premature ventricular contractions-related, 144, 145

Arterial oxygen desaturation (SaO$_2$) (*Cont.*)
  as pulmonary hypertension risk factor, 86
  saw-tooth pattern of, 88, 158, 166, 167
Artifacts
  EKG, 52–53
  electrode popping, 58–59
  sixty-cycle EMG, 55–56
  sweat or respiratory, 56–57
Artificial eyes, implication for biocalibration, 60–61
Asthma, nocturnal, 169–171
Auditory monitoring, 49
Automobile accidents, by obstructive sleep apnea patients, 126–127
Awakening
  early-morning, 263
    advanced sleep-phase syndrome-related, 238–239
  terrifying, 254–255

Bed partners
  of excessive daytime sleepiness patients, 76, 77
  of obstructive sleep apnea patients, 82, 83
Bedtime, delayed, as REM latency decrease cause, 209
Benzodiazepines
  as adjustment sleep disorder treatment, 233, 234
  adverse effects of, 233, 234
  hypoventilation as contraindication to, 194
  as night terrors treatment, 221
  obtructive sleep apnea-exacerbaring effects of, 194
  as panic attack treatment, 255
  as restless leg syndrome treatment, 192
  sleep architecture effects of, 45–46
  sleep spindle activity effects of, 3–4
  as somnambulism treatment, 218
Bereavement, as depression cause, 232–233
Bereavement counseling, 233
Beta-agonists, as asthma therapy, 170
Bilevel pressure, 101, 102, 106
  definition of, 263
  as obesity hypoventilation syndrome treatment, 151
  use in post-polio syndrome patients, 184
Biocalibrations
  definition of, 263
  EEG during, 22
  in patient with artificial eye, 60–61
  procedures for, 50–51
Biofeedback treatment, for insomnia, 230
Bipolar disorder, 245, 246, 249–250
"Blue bloater" variant, of chronic obstructive pulmonary disease, 166–168
Bright light therapy
  for delayed sleep-phase syndrome, 236, 237
  for jet lag, 241
Bronchodilator therapy, for chronic obstructive pulmonary disease, 161, 165
Bruxism, differentiated from nocturnal seizures, 223

Caffeine
  as insomnia cause, 230
  as restless leg syndrome cause, 190
Carbamazepine, as cataplexy treatment, 203

Carbidopa. *See* Levodopa/carbidopa
Carbon dioxide
  exhaled, apnea-related fluctuations in, 71–73
  partial pressure, in obesity hypoventilation syndrome, 148–149
Carbon dioxide retention, unexplained, obesity hypoventilation syndrome-related, 148–149
Cataplexy, 77, 195–196
  definition of, 263
  drug therapy for, 202–203
  narcolepsy-associated, 198, 199–200, 205
    delayed appearance of, 207
Catheters, esophageal, 90
Cerebrovascular accidents, Cheyne-Stokes breathing associated with, 180
Chest movements
  during hypopnea, 81
  during obstructive sleep apnea, 72, 75, 79
Cheyne-Stokes breathing, 173, 177–178
  central apnea associated with, 178, 179–180, 182
  congestive heart failure-associated, 177–180, 182
  definition of, 263
  mixed apnea associated with, 177–178, 181–182
  obstructive sleep apnea-associated, 177–178
Children
  airflow monitoring in, 72
  apnea-hypopnea index in, 156
  night terrors in, 221
  obstructive sleep apnea in, 155–156
Chronic obstructive pulmonary disease (COPD)
  arterial oxygen desaturation associated with, 157=159, 160–161
    low-flow nocturnal oxygen therapy for, 162–163
    with obstructive sleep apnea, 166–168
  "blue bloater" variant of, 166–168
  definition of, 263
  obstructive sleep apnea associated with (overlap syndrome), 88, 151, 154, 163, 166–168, 264
    arterial oxygen desaturation in, 157–159
    as hypnotics contraindication, 165
  oxygen therapy for, 161, 162–163
    with continuous positive airway pressure, 167
  pedal edema associated with, 162–163, 166–168
  "pink puffer" variant of, 164–165
  poor sleep quality associated with, 164–165
  REM-associated nocturnal desaturation in, 157–159
Chronopharmacology, 170
Chronotherapy, for delayed sleep-phase syndrome, 236, 237
Circadian rhythm
  of airway function, 170
  internal pacemaker for, 241
  of REM latency, 68, 209
Circadian rhythm sleep disorders, 236
Clonazepam
  as periodic limb movement treatment, 188
  as REM sleep behavior disorder treatment, 215, 216
  as somnambulism treatment, 218
Clonidine, withdrawal of, as shortened REM latency cause, 208–209
Congestive heart failure
  central sleep apnea associated with, 76, 174

Congestive heart failure (*Cont.*)
  Cheyne-Stokes breathing associated with, 177–181, 182
  sleep apnea associated with, 77
Continous positive airway pressure (CPAP), 56, 79, 83, 85
  effect of alcohol use on, 95
  alternatives to, 122–124
    oral appliances, 111
    tracheostomy, 121–123
    uvulopalatopharyngoplasty, 110–112
    weight loss, 111, 112, 122
  auto-titration, 101
  for congestive heart failure-associated Cheyne-Stokes breathing, 180
  for congestive heart failure, 182
  definition of, 263
  expiratory positive airway pressure, 105, 106
  full face mask (oronasal), 103–104
  humidification use with, 99
  as idiopathic central sleep apnea treatment, 176
  initial use of, arterial oxygen desaturation during, 107–109
  inspiratory positive airway pressure, 105, 106
  lower-than-optimal pressure, 101
  nasal symptoms associated with, 98–99, 103–104
  as obesity hypoventilation syndrome treatment, 149, 151
  as obstructive sleep apnea treatment, 89–90
    discontinuation following weight loss, 96–97
  optimal pressure, 90
  use with oxygen therapy
    as obesity hypoventilation syndrome treatment, 151
    as overlap syndrome treatment, 167
  patient's intolerance of, 100–102, 103–104, 105–106, 113–114
  as periodic limb movement cause, 193–194
  persistent daytime sleepiness on, 206–207
  postural change mode of, 101
  ramp mode of, 101, 102
  relationship to automobile accident risk, 127
  as REM-specific sleep apnea treatment, 93
  repetitive central apnea appearance during, 181–182
  sleep rebound following, 194
  snoring during, 134
  as snoring treatment, 134
Continuous positive airway pressure titration, 90, 100
Cor pulmonale
  chronic obstructive pulmonary disease-related, 163
    with hypercapnia, 166–168
  neuromuscular disorders-related, 184
  obesity hypoventilation syndrome-related, 149
  obstructive sleep apnea-related, 154
Crescendo pattern, of respiratory efort, 85

Daytime somnolence. *See* Excessive daytime sleepiness
Definitions, respiratory, **69–75**
Deflections
  in-phase, 16
  K complexes as, 25–26
  voluntary eye movement-related, 61

Delayed sleep-phase syndrome, 235–237, 263
Delta sleep. *See* Slow wave sleep
Depression, 245–246
  advanced sleep-phase syndrome-related, 239
  bereavement-related, 232–233
  bipolar, 245, 246, 249–250
  chronic low-grade, differentiated from idiopathic hypersomnia, 212, 213
  as excessive daytime sleepiness cause, 77, 249–250, 261
  hypersomnia associated with, 246, 249–250
  insomnia associated with, 76, 232–234, 246
  REM latency in, 43
  sleep efficiency in, 48
  unipolar, 245
  as weight gain cause, 249–250
Dextroamphetamine, as narcolepsy treatment, 200, 201
Diagnostic Classification of Sleep and Arousal Disorders, 257
Dopamine agonists, as restless leg syndrome treatment, 192
Dreams. *See also* Nightmares; Night terrors
  recurrent, posttraumatic stress disorder-related, 251, 253
  violent, 214–216
Driving risk, posed by obstructive sleep apnea patients, 124–127
Driving simulators, 125, 127
Drugs. *See also* specific drugs
  as excessive daytime sleepiness cause, 76
  sleep architecture effects of, 45–46
Dyspnea, chronic obstructive pulmonary disease-related, 164–165
Dyssomnias, classification of, 257


Edema, pedal
  chronic obstructive pulmonary disease-related, 162–163, 166–168
  post-polio, 183
EKG artifacts, 52–53
Electrocardiography (EKG), 49, 50
Electrocortical arousals, 34
Electrode popping artifact, 58–59
Electroencephalography (EEG)
  alpha activity of
    definition of, 263
    during sleep onset, 22
    during sleep stage 1, 24
    during wakefulness, 5–6
  in benzodiazepines use, 3–4
  definition of, 263
  high-amplitude activity of, electro-oculoraphic detection of, 16
  lead placement in, **7–10**
  occipital lead recordings in, 5–6
  patterns of, **1–6**
  polysomnographic measurement of, 49, 50
  saw tooth patterns of, in REM sleep, 1–2
  in seizure activity, 223, 224
  of sleep stage 4-related epochs, 9–10
  during wakefulness, 5–6, 32

Electromyography (EMG)
    anterior tibialis, 49, 51
    chin (submental), 1, **17–34**
        for daytime sleepiness evaluation, 23–24, 29–30,
            31–32
        for insomnia evaluation, 26
        for parasomnia evaluation, 27–28
        polysomnographic applications of, 49, 50, 51
        during REM sleep, 29–30, 31–32
        sixty-cycle artifacts in, 54–55
        for sleep arousal evaluatio, 33–34
        during sleep onset, 22
        for sleep-onset insomnia evaluation, 22–23
        for snoring evaluation, 131
        during stage REM sleep, 40, 41
    definition of, 263
    leg, 186
Electro-oculography (EOG), **11–12**
    definition of, 263
    high-amplitude EEG activity detection by, 16
    lead placement in, 11–12
    patterns of, **13–16**
    polysomnographic calibration of, 50
    standard two-channel, 15–16
Environmental precautions
    for night terrors management, 221
    for REM behavior disorder management, 215, 216
    for somnambulism management, 218
Environmental sleep disorders, 228
Epilepsy. *See also* Seizures
    juvenile myoclonic, 223
Epochs, 9–10
    definition of, 1, 263
    phasic REM, 16
    70–75, scored as stage REM sleep, 40–42
    sleep stage transitions within, 16
    tonic REM, 16
Epworth Sleepiness Scale, 76
Esophageal catheters, 90
Esophageal pressure monitoring, 81
    of continuous positive airway pressure, 90
    of respiratory effort, 75
    of snoring, 131
    of upper airway resistance syndrome, 85, 136
Excessive daytime sleepiness, 23–24, **76–85**
    arousal index in, 34
    Cheyne-Stokes breathing associated with, 177–180
    common causes of, 261
    depression-related, 77, 261
    EKG artifacts associated with, 52–53
    fluoxetine-related, 47–48
    gasping associated with, 76
    history of, 76–77
    hypnotics abuse-related, 213
    hypothyroidism-related, 138–139
    idiopathic central sleep apnea-related, 172–174
    idiopathic hypersomnia-related, 212–213
    insufficient sleep syndrome-related, 210–211
    multiple sleep latency testing of, 67–68
    narcolepsy-related, 195–196, 197–198, 206–206
        drug therapy for, 199, 200
    obstructive hypopnea-related, 80–81
    obstructive sleep apnea-related, 204–205

Excessive daytime sleepiness (*Cont.*)
        in children, 156
        effect of alcohol use on, 94–95
    onset age of, 76–77
    periodic limb movements-related, 185–186
    post-uvolopalatopharyngoplasty, 115–116, 122
    REM eye movements associated with, 15–16
    REM-specific sleep apnea associated with, 93
    sedative abuse-related, 213
Expiratory reserve volume (ERV), 88
Eye movements. *See also* Electro-oculography
    in closed-eye wakefulness, 32
    conjugate, as out-of-phase deflection cause, 16
    in open-eye wakefulness, 32
    polysomnographic monitoring of, 51
    during sleep stage 1, 23, 24

Fatigue
    fluoxetine-related, 47–48
    upper airway resistance syndrome-related, 84, 85
Fibromyalgia, 243–244
First-night effect, 22, 234
    reverse, 228
Flashbacks, 252
Fluoxetine
    as cataplexy treatment, 203
    as fatigue cause, 47–48
    as fibromyalgia treatment, 244
    as obstructive sleep apnea treatment, 129

Gasping
    excessive daytime sleepiness-related, 76
    obstructive sleep apnea-related, 83, 131
Genioglossus advancement, with hyoid suspension,
        116
Glossary, 263–265
Glossectomy, laser midline, 122

Hallucinations, hyponagogic, 77, 196, 202, 203
    definition of, 264
    idiopathic hypersomnia-related, 213
Head trauma, as posttraumatic hypersomnia syndrome
        cause, 213
Health insurance coverage, for polysomnography, 228
Heart failure. *See also* Congestive heart failure
    arterial oxygen desaturation-related, 86
HLA haplotyping, for narcolepsy evaluation, 207
Homicide, somnambulism-related, 218
Hydrocephalus, 212, 213
Hyoid suspension, with geniogglossus advancement,
        116, 122, 123
Hypercapnia
    chronic obstructive pulmonary disease-related, with
        cor pulmonale, 166–168
    during intitial continuous positive airway pressure
        therapy, 108, 109
    obesity hypoventilation syndrome-related, 148–152,
        153, 154
Hyperphagia, depression-associated, 249–250
Hypersensitivity, rejection, 250

Hypersomnia
  depression-related, 246, 249–250
  idiopathic, 212–213
    as excessive daytime sleepiness cause, 212–213, 261
  posttraumatic, 213
Hypertension, 139
  obstructive sleep apnea associated with, 83, 140–142
  pulmonary, 86
  snoring associated with, 131
Hypertrophy, adenoid-tonsillar, 155–156
Hypnic jerks (sleep starts), 186
Hypnotics
  as adjustment sleep disorder treatment, 233, 234
  use in chronic obstructive pulmonary disease patients, 165
  guidelines for use of, 233
  as idiopathic central sleep apnea treatment, 176
  as jet lag treatment, 241, 242
  as selective serotonin reuptake inhibitors-induced insomnia treatment, 248
Hypopnea
  arterial oxygen desaturation in, 70
  chest and abdominal movements during, 75, 81
  chronic obstructive pulmonary disease-related, 158
  definition of, 69, 264
  effect of inspiratory positive airway pressure on, 106
  obstructive, 80–81
Hypothyroidism, obstructive sleep apnea associated with, 77, 138–139
Hypotonia
  loss of, idiopathic hypersomnia-related, 214–216
  REM-associated skeletal muscle, 30, 158
Hypoventilation
  central sleep apnea-related, 173
  as contraindication to benzodiazepines, 194
  hypopnea-related, 81
  nonapneic, initial nasal continuous positive airway pressure-related, 107–109
  post-polio, 183–184
Hypoxemia
  chronic obstructive pulmonary disease-related, 158
  during intitial continuous positive airway pressure therapy, 108, 109

Imipramine, 203
Insomnia, **225–255**
  alcohol use-related, 230
  antidepressants-related, 247–248
  biofeedback treatment for, 230
  central sleep apnea-related, 173, 174
  comon causes of, 261
  delayed sleep-phase syndrome-related, 235–237
  depression associated with, 76, 232–234, 246
  EEG during
    alpha activity associated with, 5–6
    of sleep stage 4-related epochs, 9–10
  good sleep hygiene therapy for, 230, 231
  periodic limb movements-related, 186
  psychophysiologic, 227–228
    transient, 228, 232–234
  relaxation therapy for, 230, 231

Insomnia (*Cont.*)
  sleep-maintenance, 43, 264
    sleep-onset, 21–22
    definition of, 264
    delayed sleep-phase syndrome as, 235–237
    sleep latency in, 43
  stimulus control therapy for, 230, 231
Inspiratory effort, arousal-inducing effect of, 136
Inspiratory positive airway pressure-expiratory positive airway pressure, in obesity hypoventilation syndrome, 151
Insufficient sleep syndrome, 210–211
International Classification of Sleep Disorder, 257
Ipratropium bromide, use in chronic obstructive pulmonary disease patients, 165

Jet lag, 240–242

K complexes, 25–26, 259
  definition of, 1, 264
  in stage 1 sleep, 39
  in stage 2 sleep, 39
Kleine-Levin syndrome, 250

Laser-assisted palatolasty, as snoring treatment, 111, 130–131, 134
Laser midline glossectomy, 122
Laser therapy, carbon dioxide, for nasopharyngeal stenosis, 118
Leg jerks. *See* Periodic limb movements
Levodopa/carbidopa
  as periodic limb movement treatment, 186, 188
  as restless leg syndrome treatment, 190, 191–192
    rebound effect in, 191–192
Lung disease. *See also* Chronic obstructive pulmonary disease (COPD)
  arterial oxygen desaturation in, 30
  obstructive, 88

Macroglossia, hypothyroidism-related, 139
Maintenance of wakefulness test, 124–125
  definition of, 264
  use with drivers, 124–127
Medroxyprogesterone, as obstructive sleep apnea treatment, 129
Melatonin
  as delayed sleep-phase syndrome treatment, 236
  as jet lag treatment, 241, 242
Methamphetamine, as narcolepsy treatment, 200, 201
Methylphenidate, as narcolepsy treatment, 199, 200, 201
Modafinil, as narcolepsy treatment, 200
Multiple sleep latency test, **65–68**
  comparison with maintenance of wakefulness test, 124–125
  definition of, 264
  lack of correlation with driving risk, 127
  mean nap sleep latency in, 65, 66

Multiple sleep latency test (*Cont.*)
  mean sleep latency in, 67–68
  for narcolepsy diagnosis, 65, 77, 196, 197–198
  with coexistent obstructive sleep apnea, 204–205, 207
  effect of nocturnal sleep duration on, 211
  for upper airway resistance syndrome diagnosis, 84, 85
Myoclonus, nocturnal. *See* Periodic limb movements

Nap monitoring, 65
Narcolepsy, 195–196. *See also* Cataplexy
  differentiated from idiopathic hypersomnia, 213
  excessive daytime sleepiness associated with, 206–207, 261
  multiple sleep latency test for, 65, 77, 197–198
    with coexistent obstructive sleep apnea, 204–205, 207
  onset age of, 77
  REM latency in, 43, 48
Nasal cannulas, for airfow evaluation, 136
  in apnea, 72, 73
  in obstructive sleep apnea, 90
Nasal congestion, continuous positive airway pressure-related, 98–99
Neck circumference, as obstructive sleep apnea risk factor, 83, 97, 131
Nefazadone, 248
Neurologic disorders
  as Cheyne-Stokes breathing cause, 180
  chronic obstructive pulmonary disease-related, 163
  sleep disorders associated with, 258
Nightmares, 30
  differentiated from night terrors, 221
  posttraumatic stress disorder-related, 251–253
Night terrors, 215, 218
  amnesia associated with, 221
  differentiated from nightmares, 221
  differentiated from nocturnal seizures, 223
  somnambulism (sleepwalkng) associated with, 218, 221
Nocturnal Oxygen Treatment Trial, 163
Nocturnal penile tumescence, 30
NREM (nonrapid eye movement) sleep
  arousals in, 34
  arterial oxygen desaturation in, 88
  depression-related decrease of, 246
  somnambulism during, 218, 219
  stages of, 27–28

Obesity, obstructive sleep apnea associated with, 74–75, 87–88
  position therapy for, 120
  weight loss therapy for, 111, 112, 116, 122
Obesity hypoventilation syndrome, 148–154
  definition of, 264
Obstructive sleep apnea, 69, **86**
  abdominal and chest movements during, 72, 75, 79
  alcohol use-related, 94–95
  apnea-hypopnea index in, 88
  arterial oxygen desaturation in, 70, 87–88

Obstructive sleep apnea (*Cont.*)
  benzodiazepines-related exacerbation of, 194
  "blue bloater" variant of, 166–168
  Cheyne-Stokes breathing asssociated with, 177–178
  in children, 156
  chronic obstructive pulmonary disease-related (overlap syndrome), 166–168, 264
    arterial oxygen desaturation associated with, 157–159
  as contraindication to driving, 126–127
  definition of, 264
  gasping associated with, 83, 131
  heart rate in, 144
  hypertension-related, 83, 140–142
  hypothyroidism associated with, 77, 138–139
  as life expectancy decrease cause, 141
  mild-to-moderate, treatment of, 110–112, 129–130
  with mixed apnea, 78–79
  narcolepsy-related, 204–205, 207
  nasal continuous positive airway pressure therapy for. *See* Continuous positive airway pressure (CPAP)
  obesity hypoventilation syndrome-related, 149
  oxygen therapy for, adverse effects of, 154
  personality changes associated with, 250
  positional, 119–120
  post-uvulopalatopharyngoplasty, 115–118
  during pregnancy, 147
  relationship to premature ventricular contractions, 143–145
  REM latency in, 43, 65, 204–205
  REM-related, 92–93
  respiratory effort detection during, 74–75
  severe, 87–88
  severity assessment of, 86
  sleep stages in, 43
  snoring associated with, 131, 132
  tracheostomy treatment for, 122–124
  treatment for, 86
  uvulopalatopharyngoplasty treatment for, 114–118, 120
    lack of efficacy of, 111, 112, 122
Oral appliances
  as continuous airway pressure alternative, 111
  as obstructive sleep apnea treatment, 113–114
  as persistent obstructive sleep apnea treatment, 116
  as simple snoring treatment, 134
Osteotomy, inferior sagittal mandibular, 116
  maxillomandibular, 122, 123
Overlap syndrome, 88, 151, 154, 163, 166–168
  as hypnotics contraindication, 165
  oxygen therapy for, 161, 162–163
    arterial oxygen desaturation in, 157–159
    with continuous positive airway pressure, 167
Oximetry, nocturnal, 160
Oxygen therapy
  for central apnea, 154
  for chronic obstructive pulmonary disease, 161, 162–163, 167
  for congestive heart failure-associated Cheyne-Stokes breathing, 180

Oxygen therapy (*Cont.*)
    controlled, as obesity hypoventilation syndrome
        treatment, 151
    for idiopathic central sleep apnea, 176
    low-flow nocturnal, for chronic obstructive pulmonary
        disease, 163
    for mixed apnea, 154
    for nasal continuous positive airway pressure-related
        hypoxemia and hypercapnia, 108, 109
    for obstructive sleep apnea, adverse effects of, 154

Palatoplasty, laser-assisted, as snoring treatment, 111,
    130–131, 134
Panic attacks, 254–255
Paralysis, leaden, 250
Parasomnias, 28
    classification of, 257–258
    definition of, 264
    video recording of, 49–50
Pavor nocturnus. *See* Night terrors
PCO$_2$ (partial pressure of carbon dioxide), in obesity
    hypoventilation syndrome, 148–149
Pemoline, as narcolepsy treatment, 201
Periodic limb movements, 76, 77, 185–186, 187–
    188
    arousal in, 186 187–188
    clonazepam treatment for, 188
    definition of, 264
    differentiated from nocturnal seizures, 223
    as excessive daytime sleepiness cause, 76, 261
    insomnia-related, 228
    posttraumatic stress disorder-related, 252
    relationship to narcolepsy, 196
    restless leg syndrome associated with, 186, 188, 190,
        192
    unmasked by continuous positive airway pressure,
        193–194
Pickwickian patients, 149
"Pink puffer" variant, of chronic obstructive pulmonary
    disease, 164–165
Plethysmography, respiratory
    impedance, 75
    inductance, 72, 73
Pneumotachography, 72, 73, 90, 136
Polysomnography, **49–64**, 65
    ambulatory, 83
    calibration procedures for, 50–51
    definition of, 49
    for idiopathic central sleep apnea diagnosis, 173
    lack of health insurance coverage for, 228
    for narcolepsy diagnosis, 196, 198
    for obstructive sleep apnea diagnosis, 83
    for psychophysiologic insomnia diagnosis, 228
    for REM sleep behavior disorder diagnosis, 215, 216
Popping artifacts, 58–59, 264
Position therapy
    for obstructive sleep apnea, 1191–20
    for simple snoring, 134
Post-polio syndrome, 182–183
Posttraumatic hypersomnia syndrome, 213
Posttraumatic seizure activity, 223
    differentiated from night terrors, 221

Posttraumatic seizure activity (*Cont.*)
    nightmares associated with, 215
Posture, during sleep. *See also* Position therapy
    monitoring of, 49
Pregnancy, snoring during, 196–197
Premature ventricular contractions, 143–145
Protriptyline
    as cataplexy treatment, 203
    as obstructive sleep apnea treatment, 129
    as simple snoring treatment, 134
Prozac. *See* Fluoxetine
Psychiatric disorders, sleep disorders associated with,
    258
    somnambulism as, 218
Pulse oximetry, 70

Rapid eye movements. *See* REM eye movements
Recollections, intrusive, 252
Relaxation therapy, for insomnia, 230, 231
REM behavior disorder, 30, 214–216
    definition of, 264
    differentiated from night terrors, 221
    differentiated from nocturnal seizures, 223
REM eye movements
    definition of, 264
    electro-oculographic patterns of, 13–14, 15–16
    in excessive daytime sleepiness, 15–16
    sleep onset, 48
REM latency, 43, 48
    age-related decrease of, 209
    alcohol use-related increase of, 95
    benzodiazepines-related increase of, 46
    circadian factors-related decrease of, 68, 209
    clonidine withdrawal-related decrease of, 208–209
    definition of, 48, 68, 264
    depression-related decrease of, 246
    diurnal variation in, 68, 209
    fluoxetine-related decrease of, 47–48
    multiple sleep latency test evaluation of, 65, 67–68
    obstructive sleep apnea-related decrease in, 204–205
    sleep-onset, 209
REM rebound, nonapneic, 108, 109
REM rule, 42, 43
REM sleep, 1
    alcohol use-related decrease of, 95
    arousals in, 34
    arterial oxygen desaturation in, 88, 158
    atypical, 249–250
    benzodiazepines-related decrease of, 46
    chin EMG during, 29–32
    in chronic obstructive pulmonary disease, 165
    definition of, 264
    in depression, 246
    determination of episodes of, 40–42
    EEG patterns in, 1–2
    epochs associated with, 16
    in obstructive sleep apnea, 92–93
    in patient with artificial eye, 60–61
    phasic, 16, 29–30
    in posttraumatic sleep disorder patients, 251, 252
    sleep-onset, 48
    somnambulism during, 218

REM sleep (*Cont.*)
  tonic, 16
  unequivocal, 13–14
REM sleep-suppressing drugs, withdrawal of, 43, 46,
    48, 65, 215
Renal failure, periodic limb movements associated with,
    76, 186
Respiratory disturbance index. *See* Apnea-hypopnea in-
    dex
Respiratory effort, 49
  arousal associated with, 85, 90
Respiratory failure
  obesity hypoventilation syndrome-related, 150–152,
    153–154
  post-polio, 183–184
Restless leg syndrome, 186, 189–192
  definition of, 264
Retrolingual procedures, 122

Salmeterol, use in chronic obstructive pulmonary dis-
    ease patients, 165
$SaO_2$. *See* Arterial oxygen desaturation
Seasonal affective disorder, 246, 250
Sedatives, as excessive daytime sleepiness cause, 213,
    261
Seizures
  daytime, 223
  nocturnal, 50, 218, 222–224
    differentiated from night terrors, 221
    differentiated from REM sleep behavior disorder,
      215, 216
    differentiated from somnambulism, 218
    NREM sleep-related, 215
Selective serotonin reuptake inhibitors, 46, 47–48
  as insomnia cause, 248
  as night terrors treatment, 221
  as obstructive sleep apnea treatment, 129
  as somnambulism treatment, 218
Sleep
  continuity of, 34
  duration of, 34
  restorative function of, 34
  standard variables in, 43–44
  sustained, 22
Sleep architecture, **43–48**
  definition of, 43
  effect of benzodiazepines on, 45–46
Sleep attacks, 196
Sleep diary
  for excessive daytime sleepiness evaluation, 211
  for multiple sleep latency evaluation, 65, 66
  for psychophysiologic insomnia evaluation, 228
Sleep disorders
  classification of, 257–259
  proposed, 258
Sleep efficiency, 43
  chronic obstructive pulmonary disease-related im-
    pairment of, 165
  definition of, 264
  depression-related impairment of, 48
Sleep latency, 21–22, 43. *See also* REM latency
  definition of, 22, 65, 68, 264

Sleep latency (*Cont.*)
  depression-related increase of, 246
  diurnal variation in, 68
  multiple sleep latency testing of, 67–68
  nap, 65
  in narcolepsy, 197, 198
  normal, 211
  in sleep-onset insomnia, 21–22
Sleep log. *See* Sleep diary
Sleep onset, chin EMG during, 22
Sleep paralysis, 77
  idiopathic hypersomnia-related, 213
  narcolepsy-related, 196
Sleep period time, 43
Sleep position treatment
  for obstructive sleep apnea, 119–120
  for simple snoring, 134
Sleep rebound
  following continuous positive airway pressure,
    194
  slow wave, as somnambulism cause, 219
Sleep restriction therapy, for insomnia, 230
Sleep spindles
  definition of, 1, 264
  in sleep stage 2, 39
Sleep stages, **1–6**
  characteristics of, 259
  determination of episodes of, 40–42
  stage 1, 1, 23–24
    definition of, 265
    K complexes of, 39
  stage 2
    benzodiazepines-related increase of, 45, 46
    definition of, 265
    K complexes of, 25–26, 39
  stage 3
    benzodiazepines-related decrease of, 45, 46
    definition of, 265
    during NREM sleep, 27–28
  stage 4
    benzodiazepines-related decrease of, 45, 46
    definition of, 265
    during NREM sleep, 27–28
  stage REM, 40–42
Sleep state misperception, 228
Sleep terrors. *See* Night terrors
Sleepwalking. *See* Somnambulism
Slow wave sleep, 43
  age-dependency of, 44
  benzodiazepines-related decrease of, 46
  chronic obstructive pulmonary disease-related de-
    crease of, 165
  definition of, 1, 265
  somnambulism during, 18, 219
  during stages 3 and 4, 16
Smoking cessation, by chronic obstructive pulmonary
    disease patients, 161
Snoring, 31–32, 38–39, 56–57
  age factors in, 131
  alcohol-related exacerbation of, 13, 95, 130, 131
  in children, 155–156
  definition of, 131
  excessive daytime sleepiness-related, 76

Snoring (*Cont.*)
    gender differences in, 131
    laser-assisted palatoplasty treatment for, 111,
        130–131, 134
    mixed apnea-related, 78–79
    obesity hypoventilation syndrome-related, 148–
        149
    obstructive sleep apnea-related, 83, 89–90, 92–93,
        119–120
    positional obstructive sleep apnea-related, 119–120
    post-uvolopalatopharyngoplasty, 117–118
    pregnancy-related, 196–197
    simple, 130–132
    somnoplasty treatment for, 111
Somnambulism, 27–28, 215, 217–219
    definition of, 265
    differentiated from nocturnal seizures, 223
    night terrors associated with, 218, 221
Somnoplasty, 111
Stage REM. *See* REM sleep
Stenosis, nasopharyngeal, 111, 117–118
Stimulants
    as narcolepsy treatment, 199, 200, 201
    withdrawal from, as excessive daytime sleepiness
        cause, 261
Stimulus control therapy, for insomnia, 230, 231
Stress, as adjustment sleep disorder cause, 233
Sweat artifacts, 56–57, 265
Sympathomimetics, indirect, as narcolepsy treatment,
    200, 201


Temporomandibular joint disorders, as oral appliances
    contraindication, 114
Theophylline
    as asthma treatment, 170
    use in chronic obstructive pulmonary disease pa-
        tients, 165
    as congestive heart failure-associated Cheyne-Stokes
        breathing treatment, 180
    as idiopathic central sleep apnea treatment, 176
Thermocouples
    in apnea evaluation, 71, 72
    limitations of, 136
Three-minute rule, 41, 42, 265
Thyroid replacement therapy, 139
Time in bed (TIB), 43, 265
Time zone change syndrome, 240–242
Tonsillectomy, with adenoidectomy, 155–156
Total sleep time (TST), 43
    definition of, 265
Tracheostomy
    as obesity hypoventilation syndrome treatment, 149,
        154, 154
    as obstructive sleep apnea treatment, 122–124
Transducers, pressure, 72, 90
Trazadone, 248
    as adjustment sleep disorder treatment, 233
    adverse effects of, 233
Triazolam
    as adjustment sleep disorder treatment, 234
    use in chronic obstructive pulmonary disease pa-
        tients, 165

Triazolam (*Cont.*)
    as idiopathic central sleep apnea treatment, 176
    as jet lag treatment, 241
Tricyclic antidepressants
    as insomnia treatment, 233
    as night terrors treatment, 221
    as panic attack treatment, 255
    as somnambulism treatment, 218


Upper airway, in obstructive sleep apnea, 97
Upper airway muscle tone, drug augmentation of,
    128–129
Upper airway resistance syndrome, 84–85, 90, 135–
    137
    arousal index in, 85, 95
    definition of, 265
    as excessive daytime sleepiness cause, 261
    laser-assisted palatoplasty treatment for, 111
    snoring associated with, 131, 132
Uremic neuropathy, as restless leg syndrome cause,
    190
Urine drug screens, 3, 4, 198
Uvolopalatopharyngoplasty, 110–112, 114–118
    definition of, 265
    efficacy of, 111, 112, 122
    excessive daytime sleepiness following, 115–116
    for positional sleep apnea, 120
    as snoring treatment, 134


Vascular insufficiency, as restless leg syndrome cause,
    190
Velopharyngeal insufficiency, post-uvulopalatopharyn-
    goplasty, 111
Ventilation
    during REM sleep, 30
    negative-pressure, use in post-polio patients, 184
    positive pressure volume-cycled
        as obesity hypoventilation syndrome treatment,
        151
        use in post-polio patients, 184
Ventilation-perfusion mismatch, chronic obstructive
    pulmonary disease-related, 158
Video recording
    of parasomnias, 49–50
    of seizure activity, 223, 224
Vietnam veterans, posttraumatic stress disorder in,
    251–253
Violent behavior
    during REM sleep, 30
    somnambulism-related, 218
Violent dreams, 214–216
Visual monitoring, 49–50. *See also* Video recording


Wake after sleep onset (WASO), 43, 265
Wakefulness, EEG during
    alpha activity of, 5–6
    eye-closed, 6
    eye-open, 6
        differentiated from stage REM sleep, 32
Waketime, early. *See* Awakening, early-morning

Weight gain, depression-related, 249–250
Weight loss
    effect on continuous positive airway pressure effi-
        cacy, 101, 102
    as obstructive sleep apnea treatment, 96–97, 111,
        112, 116, 122
    as persistent obstructive sleep apnea treatment,
        116

Weight loss (*Cont.*)
    as simple snoring treatment, 134


Zolpidem
    as adjustment sleep disorder treatment, 233, 234
    use in chronic obstructive pulmonary
    as insomnia treatment, 248 disease patients, 165